EPIDEMIOLOGY
A Research Manual for South Africa
2nd Edition

EDITED BY
GINA JOUBERT
RODNEY EHRLICH

CONTRIBUTING EDITORS
JUDY KATZENELLENBOGEN
SALIM ABDOOL KARIM

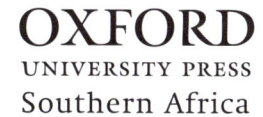

OXFORD
UNIVERSITY PRESS
Southern Africa

OXFORD
UNIVERSITY PRESS

Southern Africa

Oxford University Press Southern Africa (Pty) Ltd

Vasco Boulevard, Goodwood, Cape Town, Republic of South Africa
P O Box 12119, N1 City, 7463, Cape Town, Republic of South Africa

Oxford University Press Southern Africa (Pty) Ltd is a wholly-owned subsidiary of
Oxford University Press, Great Clarendon Street, Oxford OX2 6DP.

The Press, a department of the University of Oxford, furthers the University's objective of
excellence in research, scholarship, and education by publishing worldwide in

Oxford New York

Auckland Dar es Salaam Hong Kong Karachi
Kuala Lumpur Madrid Melbourne Mexico City Nairobi
New Delhi Shanghai Taipei Toronto

With offices in

Argentina Austria Brazil Chile Czech Republic France Greece
Guatemala Hungary Italy Japan Poland Portugal Singapore South Korea
Switzerland Turkey Ukraine Vietnam

Oxford is a registered trade mark of Oxford University Press
in the UK and in certain other countries

Published in South Africa
by Oxford University Press Southern Africa (Pty) Ltd, Cape Town

Epidemiology: A Research Manual for South Africa 2e
ISBN 978 0 19 576277 8

© Oxford University Press Southern Africa (Pty) Ltd 2007

The moral rights of the author have been asserted
Database right Oxford University Press Southern Africa (Pty) Ltd (maker)

First published 1997

All rights reserved. No part of this publication may be reproduced,
stored in a retrieval system, or transmitted, in any form or by any means,
without the prior permission in writing of Oxford University Press Southern Africa (Pty) Ltd,
or as expressly permitted by law, or under terms agreed with the appropriate
designated reprographics rights organization. Enquiries concerning reproduction
outside the scope of the above should be sent to the Rights Department,
Oxford University Press Southern Africa (Pty) Ltd, at the address above.

You must not circulate this book in any other binding or cover
and you must impose this same condition on any acquirer.

Publishing Manager: Alida Terblanche
Commissioning Editor: Zarina Adhikari
Project Manager: Lindy-Joy Dennis
Editor: Adrienne Pretorius
Designer: Ian Norris
Medical Proofreader: Tony Westwood
Indexer: Ethné Clarke
Permissions Researcher: Pat Rademeyer

Set in Plantin Std Regular 10 pt on 12 pt by Barbara Hirsch
Printed and bound by ABC Press, Cape Town
106367

Contents

List of contributors — viii
Foreword — xi
Preface — xii
Acknowledgements — xiii

SECTION A Contextualising epidemiology — 1

1 Why do epidemiological research? A South African perspective — 2
Scientific research — 3
Public health — 4
Public health research — 5
Epidemiology — 6
Epidemiology in South Africa — 7
Conclusion — 10

2 Key concepts in epidemiology — 12
Causation — 12
Levels of prevention — 16
Measures of the frequency of health events — 19
Demography — 24

3 Research ethics, human rights and community participation — 30
Ethics, advocacy and human rights — 30
Community participation — 37

SECTION B Epidemiological research methods and protocol development — 45

4 Planning a research project — 46
Introduction — 46
Assembling the research team — 46
The study protocol — 47
Bias in research — 52
Conclusion — 54

5	**Setting objectives for research**	55
	Introduction	55
	Steps to formulating research objectives	55
	Conclusion	63
6	**Literature review**	66
	Introduction	66
	Functions of literature reviews	66
	How to conduct a literature review	68
	Writing up the literature review	74
7	**Study design**	77
	Introduction	77
	Analytical study designs	78
	Experimental studies	88
	Conclusion	93
8	**Population and sampling**	94
	Study (target) population	94
	The sample	94
	Random sampling	95
	Non-random sampling	100
	Sampling bias	101
	Sample size	102
	Conclusion	104
9	**Data collection and measurement**	106
	Introduction	106
	Measurement instruments	106
	Review of records	106
	Questionnaires	107
	Steps in questionnaire development	107
	Quality of the data collected	116
	Other issues related to data collection	120
	Conclusion	122

SECTION C Data presentation, analysis and interpretation — 125

10	**Exploring, summarising and presenting data**	126
	Introduction	126
	Variables	127
	Data checking before analysis	127
	Exploratory data analysis	129
	Summarising the sample data	135
	Conclusion	138

11 Analysing and interpreting epidemiological data — 141
Introduction — 141
From the sample to the population — 142
Hypothesis (significance) testing — 145
Statistical versus clinical or public health significance — 146
Parametric versus non-parametric methods — 147
What to consider when choosing an appropriate analysis — 147
Analyses commonly used in epidemiology — 148
Conclusion — 154

12 Precision and validity in epidemiological studies: error, bias and confounding — 155
Introduction — 155
Factors that influence precision of study results: random error — 157
Factors that influence validity of study results: bias — 160
Conclusion — 168

SECTION D   Epidemiology applied to specific areas — 171

13 Routine health information systems and disease surveillance — 172
Introduction: what is a routine health information system? — 172
What are the main routine health information systems in South Africa? — 172
Disease surveillance as part of routine health information systems — 176
The epidemiology of disease surveillance — 179
Examples of other surveillance systems — 182
Health indicators — 184
Limitations of routine health information systems — 185

14 Community surveys — 188
What are community surveys? — 188
Conducting a community survey — 189

15 Burden of disease and mortality studies — 200
Introduction — 200
Mortality rates — 201
Cause of death statistics — 203

16 Social epidemiology — 210
Introduction — 210
The epidemiological study of poverty and health — 212
Measuring socioeconomic position — 213
Social networks and health — 214
Race as a variable in epidemiological studies — 216
Conclusion — 218

17 Infectious disease epidemiology	221
Introduction	221
Key concepts in infectious disease epidemiology	221
Measuring infectious disease occurrence and transmission	223
Study designs in infectious disease epidemiology	225
18 Outbreak investigation	229
Introduction	229
Steps in outbreak investigation	230
Conclusion	239
19 Epidemiology of HIV/Aids	242
Introduction	242
Studying transmission of HIV	243
Monitoring the evolving HIV epidemic	244
Identifying risk factors for HIV infection	245
Studying prevention	246
Conclusion	246
20 Environmental epidemiology	251
Introduction	251
Considerations in the planning and design of environmental epidemiology studies	252
Study designs in environmental epidemiology	254
Conclusion	259
21 Occupational epidemiology	260
Introduction	260
Uses of occupational epidemiology	261
The healthy worker effect	264
Exposure assessment	266
Typical outcomes and study designs in occupational epidemiology	267
Conclusion	268
22 Measuring disability in surveys	272
Introduction	272
Conceptualising disability	273
Methodological issues in surveys of disability prevalence	276
Current national and international data on disability prevalence	277
23 Psychiatric epidemiology	281
Introduction	281
Measurement challenges in psychiatric epidemiological research	282
Mental health services research	287

24 Nutritional surveys — 293
- Introduction — 293
- Dietary assessments in the evaluation of nutritional status — 293
- Anthropometric evaluation of nutritional status — 299

SECTION E Multidisciplinary approaches complementary to epidemiology — 305

25 Health services research — 306
- Introduction — 306
- Health services as systems — 306
- Evaluating health service quality — 308
- Different research methods used in health services research — 310
- Evaluation of programmes and projects — 311
- Epidemiological studies of health care — 311
- Conclusion — 315

26 Qualitative methodology: an introduction — 318
- Introduction — 318
- Philosophical approach — 319
- Methods of data collection — 319
- Methodological issues in qualitative research — 323

27 Economic evaluation — 328
- Introduction — 328
- Basic concepts in economic evaluation — 328
- Characteristics and types of economic evaluation — 329
- Scope of costs and outcomes — 331
- Decision-making 'rules' — 334
- Other issues in economic evaluation and potential limitations — 336

Appendices

I Standardisation (adjustment) of rates — 339

II Random number table — 343

III Writing a report — 344

IV Sample size calculation — 346

Index — 349

Contributors

Primary editors

Gina Joubert (Chapters 2, 4, 8, 9, 10, 11, 24, Appendix I)
BA, MSc

Associate Professor and Head, Department of Biostatistics, Faculty of Health Sciences, University of the Free State.

Rodney Ehrlich (Chapters 1, 2, 16, Appendix III)
BBusSc, MBChB, DOH, MFOM, FFCH (SA), PhD

Professor, School of Public Health and Family Medicine, University of Cape Town.

Contributing editors

Judy Katzenellenbogen (Chapters 1, 2, 4, 5, 8, 9)
BSc (Occ Ther), BSc (Hon) (Epidemiol), MSc

Doctoral candidate, School of Population Health, University of Western Australia.

Salim Abdool Karim (Chapter 12)
MBChB, MMed(CH), FFPHM (SA), MS, PhD

Pro Vice-Chancellor (Research), University of KwaZulu-Natal and Director, Centre for the Aids Programme of Research in South Africa (CAPRISA), Durban; Professor of Clinical Epidemiology, Columbia University.

Authors

Quarraisha Abdool Karim (Chapter 19)
PhD

Head, Women and Aids Programme, Centre for the Aids Programme of Research in South Africa (CAPRISA), Durban; Director, Columbia University-Southern African Fogarty Aids International Research and Training Program.

Max Bachmann (Chapter 25)
MBChB, DOH, MSc, PhD, MFPH (UK)

Professor of Health Care Interfaces, Medical School, University of East Anglia, United Kingdom.

David Bourne (Chapter 2)
BSc, BPhil (Environ Sci)

Chief Research Officer, School of Public Health and Family Medicine, University of Cape Town.

Debbie Bradshaw (Chapter 15)
MSc, DPhil

Director, Burden of Disease Research Unit, South African Medical Research Council; Honorary Associate Professor, School of Public Health and Family Medicine, University of Cape Town.

Marianela Castillo-Riquelme (Chapter 27)
BSc (Bus Admin), MSc (Health Mgt)

Research Officer, Health Economics Unit, School of Public Health and Family Medicine, University of Cape Town.

Susan Cleary (Chapter 27)
BA, BA (Hon), MA

Research Officer, Health Economics Unit, School of Public Health and Family Medicine, University of Cape Town.

David Coetzee (Chapters 17, 18)
BA, MBBCh, DTM&H, FFCH (SA), MS

Director, Infectious Diseases Epidemiology Group, School of Public Health and Family Medicine, University of Cape Town.

Nicol Coetzee (Chapter 18)
MBChB, FFPH

Consultant in Communicable Disease Control, Shropshire and Staffordshire Health Protection Unit, Health Protection Agency, Stafford, United Kingdom.

Aislinn Delany (Chapter 14)
BSoc Sci, MA (Research Psychology)

Senior Researcher, Community Agency for Social Enquiry, Johannesburg.

Alan Flisher (Chapter 23)
MSc (Clin Psych), MMed (Psychiatry), MPhil (Child and Adolescent Psychiatry), PhD, FCPsych (SA), DCH

Professor, Division of Child and Adolescent Psychiatry; Director, Adolescent Health Research Institute, University of Cape Town; Adjunct Professor, Research Centre for Health Promotion, University of Bergen, Norway.

John Gear (Chapter 1)
BSc, MBBCh, DPH, DTM&H, DPhil, FCP (SA), FAdEundem (CMSA)

Professor Assignatus, School of Public Health, University of the Witwatersrand.

Margaret Hoffmann (Chapter 2)
MBChB, BSc (Hon) (Epidemiol), DCM

Associate Professor, Women's Health Research Unit, School of Public Health and Family Medicine, University of Cape Town.

Ashraf Kagee (Chapter 3)
MPH, PhD

Professor, Department of Psychology, University of Stellenbosch.

Bongani Khumalo (Chapter 14)

Field Work Manager, Community Agency for Social Enquiry, Johannesburg.

Zaid Kimmie (Chapter 14)
BA, BSc (Hon), PhD, MPH

Research Director, Community Agency for Social Enquiry, Johannesburg.

Hassan Mahomed (Chapter 13)
MBChB, MMed (Public Health)

Epidemiologist, South African Tuberculosis Vaccine Initiative, University of Cape Town.

Angela Mathee (Chapter 20)
MSc, PhD

Director, World Health Organization Collaborating Centre for Urban Health; Director, Environment and Health Research Unit, South African Medical Research Council, Johannesburg.

Carol Metcalf (Chapter 18)
MBChB, MPH

Chief Research Specialist, Social Aspects of HIV/Aids and Health, Human Sciences Research Council, Cape Town; Honorary lecturer, London School of Hygiene and Tropical Medicine (Distance Learning Programme).

Chelsea Morroni (Chapter 7)
BA, MPH, MPhil, PhD

Senior Research Officer, Women's Health Research Unit, School of Public Health and Family Medicine, University of Cape Town.

Landon Myer (Chapters 7, 12, 16)
BA, MA, MPhil, PhD

Senior lecturer, Infectious Disease Epidemiology Group, School of Public Health and Family Medicine, University of Cape Town.

Rajen Naidoo (Chapter 21)
MBChB, DOH, MPH, PhD

Associate Professor and Deputy Director, Centre for Occupational and Environmental Health, School of Family and Public Health Medicine, University of KwaZulu-Natal.

Abdul-Rauf Sayed (Appendix IV)
BS, MSc

Senior Biostatistician, School of Public Health and Family Medicine, University of Cape Town.

Marguerite Schneider (Chapter 22)
BSc, MA

Chief Research Manager in Disability Studies within the Child, Youth, Family and Social Development Programme, Human Sciences Research Council, Pretoria.

Jerome Singh (Chapter 3)
PhD

Head: Bioethics and Health Law Programme, Centre for the Aids Programme of Research in South Africa (CAPRISA), Durban; Adjunct Professor, Department of Public Health Sciences and Joint Centre for Bioethics, Faculty of Medicine, University of Toronto.

Donald Skinner (Chapter 26)
MA (Clin Psych), PhD

Chief Research Specialist, Human Sciences Research Council, Cape Town.

Leslie Swartz (Chapter 3)
MSc, PhD

Professor and Chair, Department of Psychology, University of Stellenbosch; Honorary Research Associate, Human Sciences Research Council, Cape Town.

Stephen Tollman (Chapter 1)
MMed, MPH, MA

Head, Health and Population Division, School of Public Health, University of the Witwatersrand; Director MRC/University Unit in Rural Public Health and Health Transitions Research (Agincourt).

Jimmy Volmink (Chapter 6)
BSc, MBChB, DCH, MPH, DPhil

Professor and Deputy Dean (Research), Faculty of Health Sciences, University of Stellenbosch.

Corinna Walsh (Chapter 24)
RD (SA), PhD

Senior lecturer, Department of Human Nutrition, Faculty of Health Sciences, University of the Free State.

Foreword

In the foreword to the first edition of this multi-authored text a decade ago, one recognised the early budding in South Africa of epidemiology as a discipline. This was in sharp contrast to the withered blooms of the preceding half-century of the apartheid era. During that unhappy time, by contrast, one might safely assert that at best students could have plucked some of those withered blooms from three or four lectures. There was small likelihood, for instance, that their attention would have been directed to the fate of masses of Black workers labouring in the depths of the gold mines thousands of metres underground, threatened by rock falls, by silica dust from crushed rock, by scurvy from diets free of Vitamin C, and by the sexually transmitted diseases rampant among men living disrupted family lives far from their rural homes for nine months of every year. For Blacks, although not for Whites, the resulting inability to work meant dismissal without recompense, and a return to their rural homes to endure chronic disability.

Clinical medicine governed medical education, and by contrast, maintained excellent standards. Epidemiology was taught, if at all, only in the medical schools. At that time, only a few exceptional teachers extended their vision beyond the perspective of the individual patient (among them at Wits, one may recall EH Cluver, James and Harry Gear, and Sidney Kark in particular). Today epidemiology is clearly alive and well and reaches out beyond the confines of medical schools. Other health professionals as well as statisticians, sociologists, anthropologists and social psychologists have been enlisted to broaden the bounds of the discipline. The second edition of this book continues the mode of the first, being self-contained, systematic and, wherever possible, South Africa-based. The chapters on methods, both theoretical and practical, have all been updated, with the welcome addition of new and younger authors. Contributors drawn from universities and research institutions across the country illustrate widespread growth and development of the discipline, and can be taken also as a sign of scientific collaboration among them.

Three new chapters have been added and will serve readers well. One deals with social disparities, surely relevant to the restitution of social justice in a country once ridden by apartheid laws and by racial segregation seemingly cast in iron. The chapter provides the focus on methods for population studies ultimately necessary to effect greater good for greater numbers. Another much needed chapter deals with infectious diseases. The newly rampant HIV epidemic rightly has a chapter to itself. These chapters too reflect growth and new research directions in the country. The book will undoubtedly serve as a useful primer for the study of epidemiology and public health.

Mervyn Susser
Sergievsky Professor of Epidemiology Emeritus
Columbia University, City of New York

Zena Stein
Professor of Epidemiology and Psychiatry Emerita
Columbia University, City of New York

Preface

The earliest version of this book had its origin in training workshops organised by the South African Medical Research Council during the late 1980s and early 1990s in tandem with conferences of the then Epidemiological Society of Southern Africa (ESSA). The demand for copies and reprints of the manuals and booklets produced for these workshops prompted the production of a manual which incorporated aspects of the earlier material, but with a broader epidemiological scope. A wide range of contributors provided the material for publication, with technical assistance from the Medical Research Council, and the manual was launched at the ESSA Conference in July 1991.

In 1997 a fresh version of the manual was published as the First Edition under the Oxford University Press imprint. In the past decade, this book has enjoyed wide use in introductory Epidemiology and Research Methods courses. Its combination of guidance on developing a research protocol, basic epidemiological techniques, applied epidemiology with numerous South African examples and ancillary methods, such as qualitative research and economic evaluation, served such courses with their diverse student populations well.

In 2005 the editors were approached by Oxford to edit a second edition, and with the addition of a new primary editor, undertook the task. A mix of previous and new contributors were approached in order to retain the core of the First Edition while at the same time bringing fresh perspectives into the project. We are immensely grateful to the contributors who, despite all being busy, put in the time and effort to update their chapters or write new chapters, and to make the required changes through the long editorial process. All royalties will go to developing the disciplines of epidemiology and biostatistics in South Africa or to other projects concerned with public health and welfare.

As in the First Edition, we have aimed to provide an introduction to both the concepts and the application of epidemiology with a specific South African emphasis. The manual is aimed at health researchers – whether in the health professions, including nursing, or any of the disciplines contributing to public health – who have little or no experience of epidemiology, and particularly those starting research careers or carrying out research as part of their training. It is designed to help them understand the concepts of epidemiological research methods and to assist them in developing their research proposals and in undertaking their research.

Although it includes chapters on analysis of data, there are a minimum of statistical formulae and the manual does not replace a good introductory biostatistics text. We have also sought to emphasise that epidemiology is primarily an applied science which makes use of both routine and specially collected data, and to this end we have included chapters on routine information and disease surveillance, as well as burden of disease and mortality statistics. The list of chapters devoted to specific disease categories or health problems cannot be comprehensive in a book of this size, but has been expanded to include new chapters on infectious disease and HIV/Aids epidemiology, while retaining important but neglected subject areas such as occupational health, mental health and disability.

In recognition of the multidisciplinary nature of public health, the book ends with chapters on health services research, qualitative research and economic evaluation, in the hope that readers will complement their epidemiological research with ideas and techniques drawn from these disciplines.

The first three sections of the book should be read by all readers new to epidemiological research method, preferably in order, to enable optimal use of the last two sections, in which epidemiological and survey approaches in selected areas of public health are described. The reader can focus on a specific subject of interest or gain exposure to a number of applications of epidemiology.

The First Edition appeared at a time when public health researchers in a newly democratic South Africa were seeking to achieve a full accounting of its health problems as a basis for building a health system serving the needs of all. A decade later, this task persists; hence the continuing emphasis in the book on survey research and measurement of burden of disease. However, there is also a need to move beyond descriptive research and to draw on the evolving techniques of epidemiology as a public health science to test causal hypotheses and the effectiveness of proposed solutions.

We have aimed for a homegrown product. All the authors are active researchers in South Africa, and we have included mainly South African studies to demonstrate the achievements and possibilities of local work. Much remains to be done, however. We hope that this book serves its purpose and inspires its readers to build good research practice into their efforts to improve public health in South Africa and elsewhere.

Gina Joubert
Rodney Ehrlich
Primary editors

Judy Katzenellenbogen
Salim Abdool Karim
Contributing editors

Acknowledgements

The authors and publisher gratefully acknowledge permission to reproduce copyright material in this book. Every effort has been made to trace copyright holders, but if any copyright infringements have been made, the publisher would be grateful for information that would enable any omissions or errors to be corrected in subsequent impressions.

For full details of publications, please see the references in each chapter.

Text, figures & tables: Ch 2: Figs. 2.1 & 2.2 from Rothman & Greenland. 2005. *American Journal of Public Health*, 95:S144-S150. Reprinted by permission of the American Public Health Association. p14; Fig. 2.6 (3 figures) from Statistics South

Africa. 2003. Pretoria: © Statistics South Africa, Statistics South Africa, [online] http://www.statssa.gov.za. pp25 & 26; **Ch 5:** Fig. 5.1 from Varkevisser *et al*. 2003. Amsterdam: KIT Publishers; Ottawa: International Development Research Centre. Reprinted by permission of IDRC. p58; **Ch 6:** Fig. 6.1 from PubMed® website: http://www.nlm.nih.gov, a service of the US National Library of Medicine (NLM®). p71; Fig. 6.2 from Egger *et al* (eds). 2001. London: BMJ Publishing Group. Reprinted by permission of BMJ Publishing Group. p73; **Ch 7:** Fig. 7.4 from Kawachi *et al*. 1997. *American Journal of Public Health*, 87(9):1491-8. Reprinted by permission of the American Public Health Association. p88; **Ch 8:** Fig. 8.1 from Pick *et al*. 1990. Cape Town: Department of Community Health, University of Cape Town. Reprinted by permission of WM Pick. p96; **Ch 9:** Fig. 9.3 from Botha & Yach. 1986. *South African Medical Journal*, 70:766-72. Reprinted by permission of *SAMJ*. p118; **Ch 10:** Fig. 10.8 from Mathews *et al*. 1990. *South African Medical Journal*, 78:511-6. Reprinted by permission of *SAMJ*. p136; **Ch 13:** Fig. 13.1 from National Institute for Communicable Diseases. 2004. Johannesburg: National Institute for Communicable Diseases, National Health Laboratory Service, [online] http://www.nicd.ac.za. Reprinted by permission of NICD. p180; Fig. 13.2 from South Africa: Department of Health. 2005. p181; **Ch 14:** Fig. 14.1 from City of Johannesburg: Corporate Geo-Informatics, [online] http://www.eservices.joburg.org.za/joburg/eservices. Reprinted by permission of Corporate Geo-Informatics, City of Johannesburg. p191; **Ch 15:** Fig. 15.1 from Bradshaw *et al*. 2003. *South African Medical Journal*, 93(9):682-8. Reprinted by permission of *SAMJ*. p201; Fig. 15.4 adapted from Norman *et al*. 2006. Cape Town: South African Medical Research Council. Reprinted by permission of MRC. p.208; **Ch 16:** Fig. 16.2 adapted from information in Norman *et al* in Bradshaw & Steyn (eds). 2001. Medical Research Council pp53–103. p213; Table 16.2. from Bradshaw & Steyn (eds). 2001. Cape Town: South African Medical Research Council. Reprinted by permission of MRC. p.215; Table 16.3. adapted from Kaufman *et al*. 2001. *American Journal of Epidemiology*, 154:291-8. Reprinted by permission of Oxford University Press. p218; **Ch 17:** Fig. 17.1 adapted from Webb *et al*. 2005. Cambridge: Cambridge University Press. p222; **Ch 18:** Fig.18.1 adapted from J Giesecke. 2002. London: Arnold. Reproduced by permission of Edward Arnold (Publishers) Ltd. p232; **Ch 19:** Figs.19.1 & 19.2 from Siegfried *et al*. 2003. *Cochrane Database of Systematic Reviews*, 2003, Issue 3. Art CD003362. DOI: 10.1002/14651858. US, Cochrane Collection. ©Cochrane Collaboration, reproduced with permission of John Wiley & Sons Ltd and the author, NL Siegfried. pp248 & 249; **Ch 20:** Excerpt adapted from an article in World Health Organization (WHO). 1983. Geneva: World Health Organization. p252; Table 20.2 from Sexton *et al*. 1995. *Journal of Exposure Analysis and Environmental Epidemiology*, 5(3):233-56. p253; Fig. 20.2 first published in *Environmental Research* by Mathee *et al*. 1990. Copyright © Elsevier 2002 pp181-4. p256; **Ch 21:** Fig. 21.3 adapted from Naidoo *et al*. 2002. *SIMHEALTH, 607*. Mine Health and Safety Council, Johannesburg. Reprinted by permission of MHSC. p269; **Ch 23:** Fig. 23.1 adapted from Thornicroft & Tansella. 1999. Cambridge: Cambridge University Press. p288; **Ch 24:** Table 24.5 from RS Gibson. 2005. © New York: Oxford University Press. p301. **Photographs:** Section B: Jonny Myers; Section D: Eric Miller (supplied by Dr Andrew Boulle, Infectious Disease Epidemiology Unit, UCT); Section E: Jenny Altschuler. **Original artwork:** Fig. 24.2: Craig Booth.

Section A

Contextualising epidemiology

1. Why do epidemiological research? A South African perspective
2. Key concepts in epidemiology
3. Research ethics, human rights and community participation

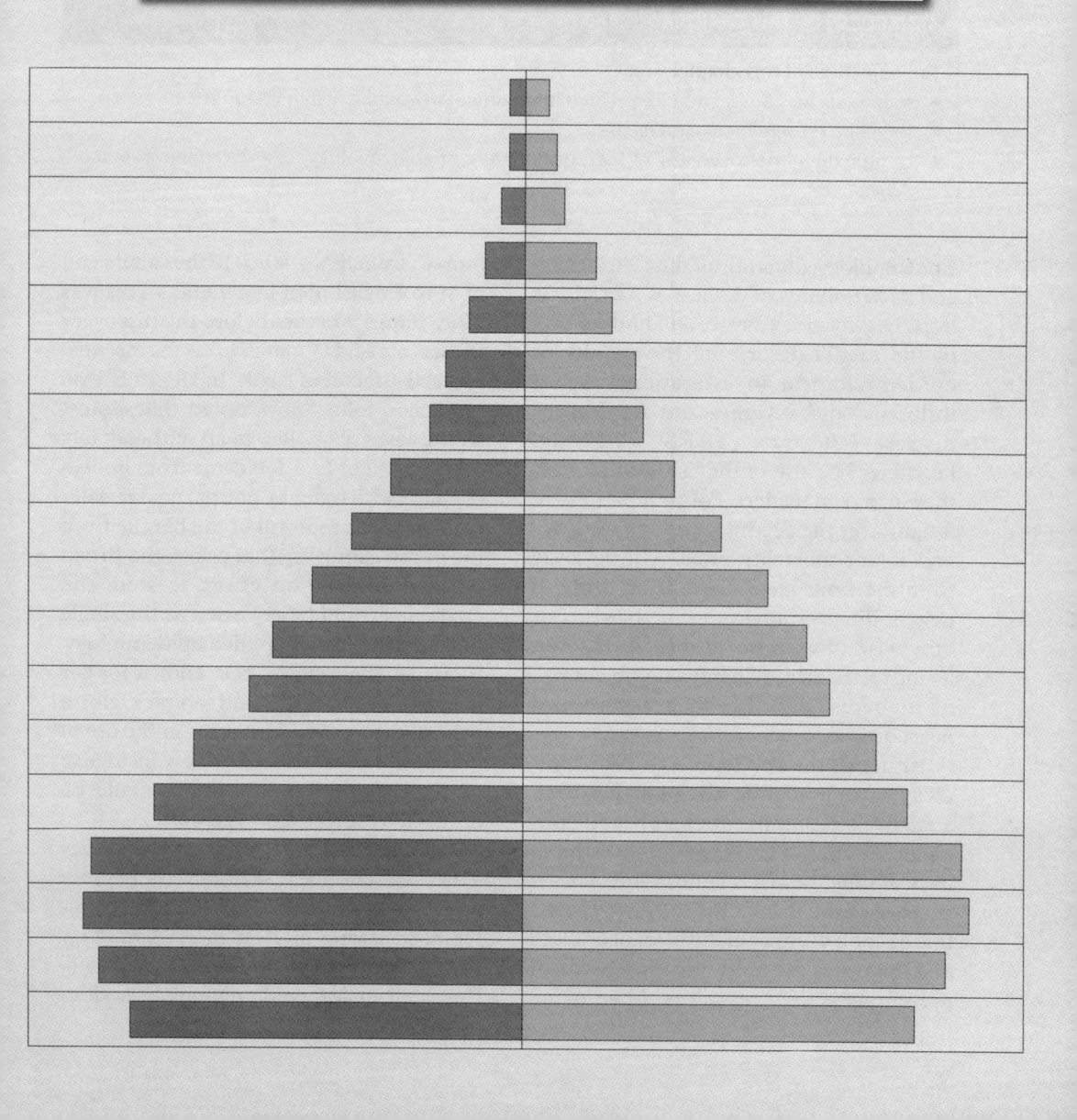

1

Why do epidemiological research? A South African perspective

Rodney Ehrlich Judy Katzenellenbogen Stephen Tollman John Gear

> **OBJECTIVES OF THIS CHAPTER**
>
> The objectives of this chapter are:
> - to provide an introduction to research and particularly public health research
> - to define epidemiology and its uses
> - to provide a brief overview of the development of epidemiology as a discipline in South Africa.

Epidemiology, the study of the distribution and determinants of disease, is part of our lives. On any given day we will find reports in the media describing the results of epidemiological investigations. Avian influenza and severe acute respiratory distress syndrome (SARS) catch the headlines because of the fear and interest they inspire in readers. Political battles are fought over the accuracy of Aids statistics and infant mortality rates. A little away from the front page, there is an array of new findings or advice on the benefits or otherwise of exercise, special diets, even loving relationships, in influencing our risk of diabetes, high blood pressure and heart attacks.

Although the development of epidemiology as an academic discipline has been a relatively recent phenomenon, epidemiological inquiries and experiments stretch back in time. In 1747, James Lind, a naval surgeon in the British Royal Navy, proved that a ration of citrus in the form of oranges and limes was the most effective means of preventing scurvy in sailors. (The name 'limey', from limes, stuck to the sailors and then to Englishmen in general.) This was more than 150 years before the discovery of ascorbic acid (Vitamin C) as the essential protective factor in citrus. In 1854 a British physician, John Snow, noted that almost all the cases of cholera in an outbreak in a certain area of London came from houses supplied with water by one particular water company. His removal of the handle from the pump supplying that water, the Broad Street pump, in an effort to stem the epidemic, could be regarded as the single most famous act in applied epidemiology. Florence Nightingale, best known for her innovations in nursing and sanitary reform in hospitals, was an innovator in the use of 'medical statistics' to show how incidence of disease in military hospitals could be reduced by improved hygiene.

Science, politics, detective work, advocacy – these all continue to feature in the practice and uses of epidemiology – and account for the growing interest in epidemiology as a method, field of inquiry and profession. But what makes epidemiology a modern science and how can it make a difference to people's health? To answer this question we need to consider briefly what research is and why it is done.

Scientific research

What is research?

Research is the systematic inquiry into nature and society leading to new knowledge. The methods of science are applied to observations about the world so as to arrive at valid generalisations. Every discipline has its own set of research tools which can be used to further knowledge in the field. Research methods and findings have to be open to scrutiny by others – therefore *peer review* is an essential aspect of the scientific research process.

Broadly speaking, there are two types of research: basic and applied research. While both types of research are aimed at the creation of new knowledge, basic research generates 'fundamental' knowledge that does not necessarily have immediate practical application. Although they may project possible uses for their research, basic scientists focus their energies on developing new techniques and on finding out how the world works, whether it is an enzyme in a cell, the human brain or the cosmos. Applied research, on the other hand, is usually directed at a problem already identified by society, whether by the researcher, industry, the public or the government. Epidemiology is therefore primarily an applied science.

The way that new knowledge is generated, and in particular how cause and effect come to be accepted, continues to challenge philosophers of science. Most scientists, including epidemiologists, do not usually engage in these debates but nevertheless, explicitly or implicitly, reflect some philosophical position in the way they practise their science.

Currently, there are two main schools of thought on how knowledge grows. One school, known as Verificationists, sees the growth of knowledge as proceeding via repeated observations of a particular association in nature or society. This association becomes new knowledge when, through repetition, the findings are 'sufficiently' verified. The findings may be linked together with others to form a theory which can then be expanded by other types of observation. This process of *induction* is probably closest to how most of us think and practise.

An opposing school, the Falsificationists, associated particularly with the work of the philosopher Karl Popper, rejects the idea that 'truth' can be ever by reached by accumulating observations. Rather, we start with hypotheses or conjectures and *deduce* predictions from these to test against the data. For this school, all theories or observed associations are tentative, and the role of scientific method is to seek observations or 'critical tests' that might refute these theories or conjectures. The validity of a theory is strengthened if it survives these tests. However, this knowledge always remains provisional and new techniques or theories may emerge in the future which enable critical tests that are not available today.

Beliefs about cause and effect underlie medical practice (e.g. disease treatment) and public health practice (e.g. government regulation or a campaign to change behaviour). Both medicine and public health are practical activities and action is needed today on the basis of 'good enough' evidence, whether such knowledge is derived through researchers using inductive or deductive methods or a combination of methods. However, the debate should alert researchers and practitioners to the tentative nature of observations, their dependence on some sort of prior theory held by the researcher, and the possibility that our most strongly held beliefs about cause and effect may be shown tomorrow to be false.

Public health

> **Defining public health**
>
> 'Public health' can be defined as
>
> *'one of the efforts organised by society to protect, promote and restore the health of the population. It is a combination of sciences, skills and beliefs that are directed to the maintenance and improvement of the health of the people through collective and social action. The programmes, services and institutions involved emphasise the prevention of disease and the health needs of the population as a whole. Public health activities change with changing technology and social values but the goals remain the same: to reduce the amount of disease, premature death, discomfort and disability in the population. Public health is thus a social institution, a discipline and a practice'.*
> (Last, 1988)

So in contrast to clinical medicine, which focuses largely on the medical care of ill individuals who present themselves for examination, diagnosis and treatment, public health focuses on the population or the community at large. The scope of public health is comprehensive, i.e. incorporating prevention as well as treatment, and considering the health system as a whole and the way the different levels of the system support each other.

Public health has its origins in attempts to control epidemics of infectious disease through the segregation and quarantine of affected individuals. With urbanisation and particularly the industrial revolution in Britain in the 19th century, appalling living conditions developed in the new factory cities with their slum housing, air pollution, child labour and long working hours. Life expectancy consequently initially declined with industrialisation (Szreter, 1999). A sanitary reform movement emerged, expressed through the work of national reformers and farsighted municipal leaders. Combined with wider political pressure as the vote was extended to include the working classes, the movement eventually led to improvements in housing, water supplies and working conditions in Britain.

The discovery of vaccination, of which smallpox had been the first, provided further impetus to mass public health improvement. At the beginning of the 20th century, high-risk groups such as children were targeted for health promotion activities, introducing an aspect of personal health to public health practice.

In Britain, the Medical Officer of Health (MOH) emerged to direct public health activities at municipal level, establishing a dominant role for medically trained people in this field. By contrast, in the United States, students and practitioners were from the outset drawn from a wide variety of disciplines, creating a stronger multidisciplinary tradition.

Worldwide, public health has been marginalised since the 1940s by an increasing curative focus on health. The doctrine of 'prevention is better than cure' has failed to win political and economic support, and public health programmes – which have the potential to improve the health of large groups – have had relatively low priority in national health budgets.

> **Public health professionals**
>
> Professionals from a variety of fields are centrally involved in public health practice, including doctors, nurses, environmental health officers (formerly known as health inspectors) and engineers, and increasingly those from a diversity of disciplinary backgrounds including economics, sociology and anthropology.

Public health programmes in fact require a variety of skills to ensure adequate planning, implementation and evaluation. The biological sciences are needed for the understanding and modification of the environment (for example, mosquito control) and for treatment of disease. The management sciences are needed for planning, staffing and financing health services and programmes. The social sciences are increasingly necessary for the understanding and modification of social and individual behaviour, for example, through economic incentives, health promotion and health education. Finally, the measurement sciences provide the tools for describing patterns and trends, finding causal linkages and evaluating effectiveness. As measurement sciences, epidemiology and biostatistics are therefore core disciplines of public health.

Public health research

People come to public health research in many ways. Professional training in the health professions requires demonstration of an ability to carry out a piece of research, even among those not contemplating research careers. This will include many readers of this book. Some will continue into academic careers in higher education in which they will be expected to do research in addition to teaching, and in fact to use their research to inform their teaching. There are an increasing number of public health research jobs in government-funded research agencies such as the South African Medical Research Council and the Human Sciences Research Council and in the many non-governmental organisations that have developed, for example, to support health systems improvements or to fight the HIV/Aids epidemic. Some researchers will have an international focus, whether dealing with the African continent and its sub-regions or through agencies associated with health and development – such as UNICEF or the World Health Organization.

The choice of *what* to research is often determined by funder or client specifications or health service requests. However, many researchers will choose their topic based on a prior or emerging interest or a need to answer questions arising out of their day to day work. The research results may be used to assist in making decisions, to change the way things are done, to argue for resources from funders and government agencies, to monitor progress or evaluate existing programmes. Research can also be used to empower the subjects of the research by providing them with the ability to gather information needed to demand changes in resource allocation.

The role of research in improving the health of populations, and promoting 'health equity' between groups, was set out in an important report by the Commission on Health Research for Development (1990). The Commission saw health research as serving two main purposes. First, country-specific research is essential to determine a society's health problems, analyse ways of dealing with them and help decide on actions to achieve health improvements with limited resources. Second, global health research aims at the development of new knowledge and technology to cope with the major unsolved problems worldwide.

This category of research requires global co-operation.

The Commission called these two enterprises – country-specific and global health research – 'essential national health research' (ENHR). Essential, because they address each country's priority health problems, and national, because of the importance of targeting research at local or national level problems while at the same time trying to build a 'transnational' scientific capability. The ENHR approach encourages a national strategy for setting priorities and managing and developing a country's resources for health research. It depends crucially on mutual understanding and active partnerships between researchers, health policy makers, managers and providers and communities. The idea is that priorities will not be set purely at national level or by the government, but rather that national priorities will emerge from a synthesis of local, regional and national concerns. By implication, research capacity and resources need to be available at all of these levels and should not merely be held centrally.

However, while research questions are undoubtedly shaped by funding flows and influenced by national co-ordinating efforts, advances in knowledge still require creative or dissenting thinkers to ask questions which may not have occurred to others to ask, or pose questions derived from a critical analysis of the status quo and of received wisdom.

Epidemiology

Defining epidemiology

'Epidemiology' can be defined as

the study of the distribution and determinants of health-related conditions and events in populations, and the application of this study to the control of health problems'. (Last, 1988)

Epidemiology is therefore an important research arm of public health, providing the scientific basis upon which public health policy decisions are made. *Descriptive* epidemiology describes the occurrence of disease and other health-related characteristics in human populations, classically with respect to person ('the who', such as age, sex, social class), place ('the where', such as region or altitude) and time (the 'when', such as season or year). *Analytical* epidemiology investigates the association between various factors and disease or health status to try to establish if those factors are causative or protective. *Experimental* epidemiology, in which the researchers introduce a treatment or intervention to determine its effectiveness, can be regarded as a third category. All of these approaches are discussed in detail in Chapter 7.

We need to make a distinction between the epidemiology of a specific disease and epidemiology, the discipline. The epidemiology of a disease is a description of what is known about the distribution and determinants of that disease. For example, the epidemiology of HIV infection reveals that young adults aged 16 to 30 years have the highest incidence rate of infection, that women have a threefold higher risk of HIV infection than men, and that in the absence of prophylaxis approximately 25% of children born to HIV positive women will be infected. In contrast, epidemiology, the discipline, is a methodology for gaining valid information about the distribution and causes of disease and about the

Epidemiology in South Africa

effectiveness of control methods. It is epidemiology the research methodology that forms the content of this book, although its value will be illustrated with reference to a number of important disease categories in South Africa.

As a result of industrialisation in the 20th century, the South African population was exposed to diseases of overcrowding and urbanisation. The mining industry, in particular, heralded an explosion in respiratory disease. Phthisis, a combination of what we today would call silicosis, tuberculosis and pneumonia, was a huge problem among goldminers at the beginning of the 20th century and a number of government commissions were established to try to describe and deal with these problems. The story of changing theories about the epidemiology and control of tuberculosis among miners and the community at large is particularly well told in Packard's book *White Plague, Black Labour* (Packard, 1989).

F Spencer Lister, one of the early directors of the South African Institute for Medical Research, studied the occurrence of pneumonia and the impact of a newly developed pneumococcal vaccine. The 1918 influenza epidemic led the health planners of the day to lay down strict national health measures to control and monitor the spread of infectious disease. Their rules were guided by emerging epidemiological principles. Siegfried Annecke helped to reduce malaria dramatically in South Africa through his surveillance of malaria and observation of the efficacy of DDT in mosquito control. However, it was in the realm of what we might today call 'primary health care epidemiology' that South Africa was a world leader by the mid-1940s.

Pholela and the roots of primary health care

Given South Africa's painful history, many people are surprised to learn that sixty years ago the country embarked on a series of primary health care experiments which gained the attention of practitioners and researchers worldwide.

This started in 1938 with a nutrition survey which documented, for the first time, the health status of South Africa's African majority. The study, initiated by Harry Gear (then Deputy Chief Medical Officer of the Union), Sidney Kark and Harding Le Riche, concluded that:

'[d]iet deficiency diseases, syphilis, malaria, bilharzia, tuberculosis, scabies and impetigo, and preventable crippling ... form no small array of factors contrary to the maintenance of good health ... No amount of juggling can succeed in separating the influence of one as opposed to the others ... The outstanding fact is that they are all preventable .... (Kark & Le Riche, 1994)

Faced with this reality, and without a ready-made solution, in 1940 the government initiated a rural health unit at Pholela in Natal (today Kwazulu-Natal) staffed by Sidney Kark, his colleague and wife Emily Kark, and Edward and Amelia Jali. Within five years, work at Pholela provided evidence for a revolutionary model of health care provision (Slome, 1962; Tollman, 1994). They introduced a number of innovations (Kark & Steuart, 1962), of which we single out three on the next page.

Today, although we take at least the third innovation for granted, we have yet to incorporate fully our understanding of these determinants in effective health promotion efforts, whether the problem is diarrhoea and the use of oral rehydration therapy, ischaemic heart disease and exercise programmes, or HIV infection and safe sex.

> **Innovations introduced by Kark's revolutionary model of health care provision**
>
> The following three innovations can be singled out:
> - An analysis of the health and health-related issues of groups or communities (community diagnosis) parallel with individual patient assessment.
> - Epidemiology as a tool for daily use, to monitor, evaluate and inform health actions.
> - Recognition that social, cultural and environmental factors are crucial determinants of community health status.

In the mid-1940s, Henry Gluckman, later Minister of Health, was appointed to chair a National Health Service Commission. In 1944, this commission recommended a countrywide network of health centres as the basis for fundamental health reform in South Africa. Their recommendation was based on the Pholela experience, the pilot study. Forty health centres were established. Eight centres in and around Durban formed practice-research sites for an Institute of Family and Community Health. Linked to the University of Natal, the Institute trained staff for health centre teams, including a new category – 'health recorders' – to maintain community, household and family records.

Although abruptly curtailed by the political events following the ascent of the National Government to power in 1948, such efforts caught the international imagination, by having demonstrated the links between community epidemiology, primary care and community health. Based on adaptations in many countries – the USA, Israel, Spain, Nicaragua, Britain – this approach became known as 'community orientated primary care'. As an important research base for the World Health Organization and UNICEF's 'Health for All' strategies, community-orientated primary care continues as one of several broad strands making up the fabric of contemporary primary health care.

South Africa, however, stagnated. 'Failure to build upon [such] early models cost the country dear, not only in financial terms but also, and more importantly, in terms of preventable death, disease and disability' (Yach & Tollman, 1993). Local models were tried, for example in Alexandra in Johannesburg, where Mervyn Susser and Zena Stein applied Kark's principles (Susser, 1957; Susser & Stein, 1959), and later in Mamre in the Western Cape and Gelukspan in what is now the province of North West. However, primary health care as national strategy had to await the establishment of democracy in the 1990s.

South African epidemiology in the 1950s through to the 1970s

From the 1950s to the mid-1970s, epidemiology did not feature prominently in South African health research. The pages of the *South African Medical Journal* from this period yield relatively little on the epidemiology of gastroenteritis, pneumonia, malnutrition, tuberculosis, cervical cancer and cardiovascular disease, all major killers. Information about the distribution, causation and control of many of these disorders was inadequate, with little useful baseline information to assess the effectiveness of any interventions. In the mid-1970s, priorities were still the exotic and the intellectually novel.

There are a few notable exceptions. In the area of nutrition, ARP Walker, Tom Bothwell and others documented the changing nutritional status of South African populations and linked these to current and future burden of disease. James Gear's work on the *Coxsackie* virus, poliomyelitis and rickettsial diseases such as tickbite fever had a strong epidemiological foundation.

Epidemiological information on rheumatic heart disease, a major cause of morbidity and mortality in urban blacks, was limited until Margie McLaren persuaded the cardiologists of Johannesburg to join her in a large survey of Soweto schoolchildren. This survey revealed many cases of advanced and previously undetected rheumatic heart disease (McLaren et al, 1979). The authors recognised the importance of socioeconomic improvement in preventing this disease as well as the need for public health measures in the form of primary prophylaxis (prevention of streptococcal throat infection leading to rheumatic fever) and secondary prophylaxis (treatment of children with rheumatic heart disease with antibiotics to prevent progression).

Epidemiology in the 1980s

Until the 1980s, much of South African epidemiology had been targeted at disease description, had been conventional in its focus on biomedical factors, and had with a few exceptions steered away from confronting the social disease of apartheid. There was little in the way of disciplinary development or training. This changed in the 1980s.

Within the Department of Health, a notable activity was the training of nurses in field epidemiology in its small Epidemiology Unit. This unit, with limited resources, analysed routinely collected national data and reported the findings monthly in the publication *Epidemiological Comments*. The first postgraduate epidemiology qualifications were introduced in Cape Town, while the South African Medical Research Council established the influential Centre for Epidemiological Research in Southern Africa (CERSA).

Epidemiological publications of this period reveal a new scope and thrust, with a strong social orientation in comparing health status by race ('population group') and social class. This has been described in detail by Myer et al (2004). (See also Chapter 16.) For example, in occupational health, researchers identified the role of occupational status and occupational hazards in contributing to common diseases such as hypertension and tuberculosis (Myers et al, 1982; White, 1982).

Other studies from this period focused on the unequal availability of health services as a critical pathway through which apartheid policies shaped the health of different population groups. Gross health resource inequalities were identified, e.g. in the number of health care personnel in relation to population in the 'homelands' compared to the 'rest of' South Africa (Botha et al, 1986). Immunisation rates in white municipalities were high; in black townships, abysmally low. Differences in health status between population groups were related explicitly to the apartheid system by researchers who were members of the anti-apartheid National Medical and Dental Association (Jinabhai et al, 1986). These writers argued that the World Health Organization objective of 'Health For All' in South Africa required the elimination of apartheid at the political level as well as socioeconomic advance. Many of these activists contributed to the 1990 Maputo Conference, recognised as a seminal event in the transition from oppositional critique to planning for a new public health system in South Africa (Critical Health and the Maputo Conference Co-ordinating Committee, 1990).

Coming of age

A feature of the 1990s was the emergence of Schools of Public Health at a number of universities. Epidemiology is now being widely taught in postgraduate courses dedicated to the subject together with complementary disciplines such as biostatistics and demography. Efforts to strengthen the explanatory force of these quantitative approaches has led to engagement with more qualitative research disciplines such as anthropology and sociology.

Specific areas of strength have emerged – at universities, the Medical Research Council, the new National Health Laboratory Service and elsewhere – in infectious disease epidemiology, demographic surveillance, occupational and environmental epidemiology, women's reproductive epidemiology and health systems research. Within the Medical Research Council, specialised units have emerged investigating burden of disease, health systems and policy, chronic diseases of lifestyle and health transitions.

The first comprehensive national health survey, the *South African Demographic and Health Survey*, was conducted in 1998, yielding a wealth of data (Department of Health et al, 2001). We have included many examples from the survey in this book. Aids epidemiologists have also been called upon to defend the accumulating body of research on this disease against denialists who have questioned (successively) the cause, extent and treatment of Aids, and continue to do so. Aids has also led to an increasingly critical citizenry who are interested in research findings and the implications of epidemiological debates. Aids vaccine trials are currently underway and raise huge ethical issues. More generally, there is increasing interest in research ethics with the expansion of internationally-funded research into the developing world. It has been argued that we need to widen the scope of research ethics to include an assessment of the benefits and effectiveness of research in respect of public health impact and not restrict this scope to informed consent and confidentiality.

The challenge remains to convert research evidence into health policy and practice at all levels of the health system. 'Evidence-based', a phrase originally applied to clinical medicine, is no less applicable to public health. Epidemiological findings need to be communicated in ways and in forums that influence policy, prevent wastage of resources and point to effective interventions.

Epidemiology in South Africa today

International recognition and collaboration, minimal in the pre-democracy years, are now abundant and epidemiology in South Africa has benefited. Organisations such as the World Health Organization and international donors are drawing on South African epidemiological expertise to strengthen their programmes in the region. These new relationships also create a responsibility among epidemiologists to ensure that local priorities are not lost amid agendas imposed, even with good intentions, by the developed world.

Conclusion

This overview has presented the chequered history of epidemiology in South Africa: original contributions in the 1940s and 1950s; considerable achievement followed by a dormant period in the 1960s and 1970s; and re-engagement during the 1980s and 1990s, accompanied by the laying of a strong – though still incomplete – foundation.

A host of challenges lies ahead in developing the discipline of epidemiology in South Africa:

- For the Schools of Public Health, Departments of Community Health and Nursing to build up expertise and ensure that essential epidemiological skills are acquired by a new generation of public health practitioners and researchers. It is hoped that this book will contribute to this goal.
- For policy-makers, managers and health care providers to understand the importance of measurement and evidence in decision making, as well as the criteria for good quality evidence, at the population as well as at the individual patient level.

- For epidemiologists to make use of the growth in sophistication of epidemiological theory and analytical techniques to hypothesise and investigate causal pathways in addition to undertaking descriptive studies.
- For us all to extend our working relationships, strengthen our ability to work across disciplines and share expertise with our neighbours in Southern Africa and beyond.

References used in this chapter

Botha, JL, Bradshaw, D & Gonin, R. 1986. Who dies from what? A study of the distribution of health needs and services in South Africa. In Zwi, AB & Saunders, LD (eds). *Towards health care for all: NAMDA Conference 1985.* Johannesburg: National Medical and Dental Association. 41–55.

Commission on Health Research for Development. 1990. *Health research: essential link to equity in development.* New York: Oxford University Press.

Critical Health and the Maputo Conference Co-ordinating Committee. 1990. Health and welfare in transition: a report on the Maputo Conference, April 1990. *Critical Health*, 31–32:2–58.

Department of Health, Medical Research Council & ORC Macro. 2001. *South African demographic and health survey, 1998.* Full report. Pretoria: Department of Health.

Jinabhai, C, Coovadia, H & Abdool Karim, S. 1986. Socio-medical indicators of health in South Africa. *International Journal of Health Services*, 16:163–76.

Kark, SL & Le Riche, H. 1994. A health study of South African Bantu school children. Report on a somatometric and clinical study conducted during 1938–39. *Manpower. Scientific Journal Devoted to Manpower Research in South Africa*, 3:2–141.

Kark, SL & Steuart, GW (eds). 1962. *A practice of social medicine.* Edinburgh: E & S Livingstone.

Last, JM. 1988. *A dictionary of epidemiology.* 2nd ed. New York: Oxford University Press.

McLaren, MJ, Hawkins, DM, Koornhof, HJ, Bloom, KR, Bramwell-Jones, DM, Cohen, E, Gale, GE, Kanarek, K, Lachman, AS, Lakier, JB, Pocock, WA & Barlow, JB. 1975. Epidemiology of rheumatic heart disease in black schoolchildren of Soweto, Johannesburg. *British Medical Journal*, 3:474–8.

Myer, L, Ehrlich, RI & Susser, E. 2004. Social epidemiology in South Africa. *Epidemiology*, 26:112–23.

Myers, J, White, N & Cornell, J. 1982. Prevalence of hypertension in semi-skilled manual workers. *South African Medical Journal*, 62:894–8.

Packard, RM. 1989. *White plague, black labour: tuberculosis and the political economy of health and disease in South Africa.* Los Angeles: University of California Press.

Slome, C. 1962. Community health in rural Pholela. In Kark, SL & Steuart, GW (eds). *A practice of social medicine.* Edinburgh: E & S Livingstone. 260–91.

Susser, M. 1957. African township: a socio-medical study. *Medical World*, 86:385–400.

Susser, M & Stein, Z. 1959. A study of obstetric results in an underdeveloped community: Part IV. The causes and prevention of maternal and obstetric deaths. *The Journal of Obstetrics and Gynaecology of the British Empire*, 66:68–74.

Szreter, S. 1999. Rapid economic growth and the four Ds of disruption, deprivation, disease and death: public health lessons from nineteenth-century Britain for twenty-first-century China. *Tropical Medicine & International Health*, 4:146–52.

Tollman, S. 1994. The Pholela Health Centre – the origins of community-orientated primary health care (COPC). *South African Medical Journal*, 84:653–8.

White, N. 1982. Tuberculosis as an occupational disease. Medical Students Conference: *Consumption in the land of plenty – TB in South Africa.* Cape Town: Medical Students Association. 68–90.

Yach, D & Tollman, S. 1993. Public health initiatives in South Africa in the 1940s and 1950s: lessons for a post-apartheid era. *Annals of the Journal of Public Health*, 83:1043–50.

2

Key concepts in epidemiology

Causation
Rodney Ehrlich

Levels of prevention
Judy Katzenellenbogen   Margaret Hoffman

Measures of the frequency of health events
Gina Joubert

Demography
David Bourne   Gina Joubert

OBJECTIVES OF THIS CHAPTER

The objectives of this chapter are:
- to describe the different ways in which 'cause' can be understood in epidemiology, and guidelines for judging whether an association is causal
- to describe a framework for interventions aimed at prevention of disease
- to outline ways in which the occurrence of health events can be quantified and compared
- to describe basic concepts and indicators used in demography – the study of populations – and their usefulness in public health.

Causation

Rodney Ehrlich

What is a cause?

A large part of epidemiology focuses on the search for *associations* between various factors and disease outcomes. Consistent associations can be useful for predicting the likelihood of disease from the presence of predictive factors. The term 'risk factor' is frequently used to describe these predictive factors, without specifying whether they are true causes or just 'markers' of risk (i.e. are correlated with the true causes and are merely proxies or substitutes for them).

In fact, despite our everyday use of the phrase 'A is the cause of B', there is disagreement among epidemiologists on the meaning of a 'cause' as applied to health outcomes. Sufficient agreement on what causes disease is, however, critical to public health action. For example, public health intervention (the equivalent of treatment in clinical medicine) may involve costly investment in health services or programmes, campaigns to change behaviour, or government regulation to restrict or even ban commercial products. In particular, we need to have evidence we can trust that removing or modifying the cause of a disease will result in fewer occurrences of that disease.

The notion of 'cause' in epidemiology

The prevailing concept of cause in epidemiology is linked to the *effect* produced when comparing one value of a risk factor or exposure to another. This may, for example, be the effect of smoking a pack of cigarettes a day for 20 years compared to the effect of never smoking. In more complicated cases it may be the relative effects of different levels of exposure, e.g. smoking different numbers of cigarettes per day versus smoking none. Epidemiology measures these effects by comparing groups or populations with different levels of exposure to the risk factor. Note that the comparison is always of one exposure (or level of risk factor) *relative* to an alternative exposure.

Necessary, sufficient and component causes

Most conditions require a number of causes working together before the condition occurs. Therefore, infection with *Mycobacterium tuberculosis* is a cause of the clinical condition of tuberculosis. Because the disease of tuberculosis is defined by reference to the mycobacterium, the mycobacterium is a *necessary cause* of tuberculosis, i.e. it must be present in all cases of the disease. This is typical of infectious disease epidemiology, where the disease is defined by the presence of the infectious agent. Historically, infectious disease epidemiology has involved the search for this necessary agent, with epidemiologists working with laboratory scientists able to isolate the infectious agent in tissue samples taken from affected people and to reproduce the disease in laboratory animals.

However, not everyone infected with tuberculosis will develop the active disease. Other factors are needed to operate in concert with the infection to produce active disease. Usually there are a number of different combinations of these factors which together with the necessary cause are capable of resulting in disease. The individual factors are called *component causes*. Any particular combination of factors working together to produce disease in at least some people is termed a *sufficient cause*.

This is illustrated in a hypothetical example for tuberculous disease in Figure 2.1. Each pie represents a proportion of the disease incidence in a population. Only three pies are shown, but there could be many more. The segments are the component causes contributing to that proportion of disease frequency. So, for example, the factors tuberculous infection (A), crowded living conditions (B) and smoking (C) combine to produce the proportion of disease represented by pie I. An extra segment (U) is added for poorly understood or 'unknown' factors, including individual genetic susceptibility. As knowledge grows, U will be disaggregated into specific known causes. In the case of pie II, tuberculous infection again appears, but with HIV as the complementary cause in this case.

Taking an extreme case, there may be only one component cause participating in disease causation – the factor will therefore of itself be a *sufficient cause*, i.e. its presence will inevitably lead to disease. However, it is rare for one factor alone to be both a necessary and sufficient cause of a disease. Specific genetic defects with 100 percent expression (i.e. if the defect is present, the specific disease will occur) are one example. Among the infectious diseases, infection with the rabies virus, e.g. through the bite of a rabid dog, will always lead to the disease rabies in a person who has not been immunised.

When it comes to non-communicable diseases, most causes are neither necessary nor sufficient. Obesity is therefore linked to many cases of adult onset diabetes, but diabetes may occur in thin people and most

Figure 2.1 Different combinations of component causes making up sufficient causes of tuberculous disease

Source: Adapted from Rothman & Greenland (2005)

I: circle divided into A, B, U, C
II: circle divided into D, U, A
III: circle divided into A, E, U, F

One causal mechanism (bracket under I)
Single component cause (arrow pointing to A in II)

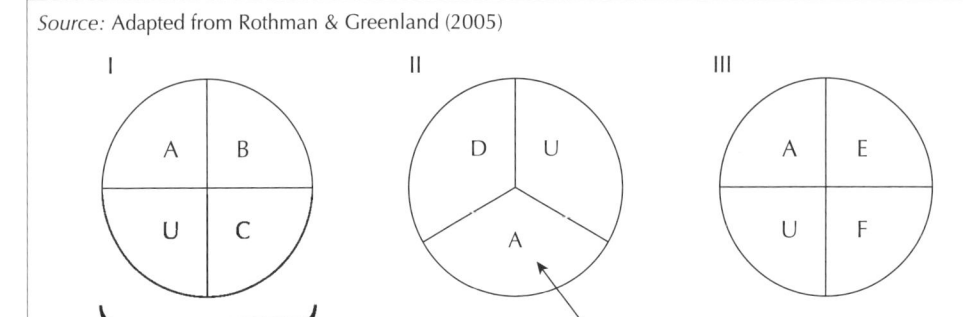

For example: A = infection with *Mycobacterium tuberculosis*; B = household crowding; C = smoking; D = HIV infection; E = under-nutrition; F = very young age; U = unknown factors including individual genetic susceptibility.

---

obese people do not get diabetes. Further, the disease is not usually defined with reference to a single necessary factor as with infectious diseases. Ischaemic heart disease (disease of the coronary arteries supplying the heart) is another example. This disease has a number of risk factors which, working together as component causes, make up a number of sufficient causes (Figure 2.2). Note that there is no factor that appears in every sufficient cause. (U does not necessarily represent the same set of factors in each case.) Similarly there is no sufficient cause made up of one factor alone.

Figure 2.2 Different combinations of component causes making up sufficient causes of coronary artery disease

Source: Adapted from Rothman & Greenland (2005)

I: circle divided into A, B, U, C
II: circle divided into D, U, E
III: circle divided into F, B, U

One causal mechanism (bracket under I)
Single component cause (arrow pointing to E in II)

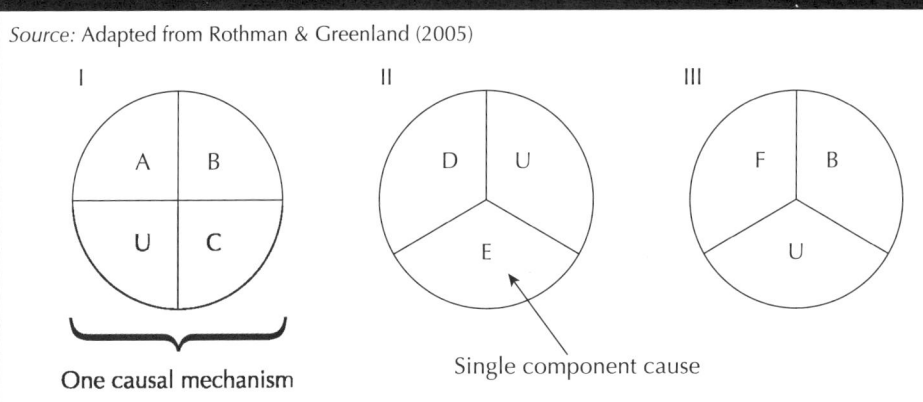

For example: A = high serum cholesterol; B = smoking; C = job strain; D = overweight; E = hypertension; F = lack of physical exercise; U = unknown factors including individual genetic susceptibility.

Levels of causation

There are many candidates for causal factors in epidemiology. These occur at different *levels*. For example, at the physiological level, genetic or biochemical markers may predict disease differences between populations or smaller groups as part of a biological model of disease. At the level of behaviour, we have become used to talking about infant feeding practices, smoking, diet, alcohol use and exercise as causes of disease. We also know that disease patterns may differ sharply by socially shaped characteristics such as gender, race/ethnicity and socioeconomic status. There is an increasing body of evidence showing that health status is influenced by purely *population level* characteristics such as degree of income inequality and social cohesion. It has proved difficult to incorporate all of these usages into a single agreed notion of 'cause'.

'Upstream' versus 'downstream' causes

We can make a distinction between 'distal' or 'upstream' causes and 'proximal' or 'downstream' causes. Upstream causes tend to be social and economic factors, e.g. lack of education, racial discrimination, and poor residential neighbourhoods, which have multiple related influences on people's life chances and behaviour and affect a wide range of health conditions. Downstream causes are those most closely associated with the individual, such as genetic predisposition or smoking behaviour. There may be a chain of causation leading from upstream to downstream factors, e.g. low socioeconomic status leading to poor diet leading to obesity leading to diabetes among those genetically susceptible. There is no point in trying to distinguish which is the 'real' cause, as they are all part of the same causal chain.

Guidelines for judging whether a relationship is causal

There are no rules or criteria that can be universally applied to decide whether an observed association is causal. As discussed in Chapter 1, it has been argued that no amount of observation can 'prove' cause and effect. Rather, the consistent observation of an association (in the absence of other explanations) can lead us to hold a causal view, but such a belief will always be provisional. In this view, science progresses by trying to refute causal hypotheses with new observations.

The most popular set of criteria for evaluating whether a relationship is causal in epidemiology is based on a list first proposed by Bradford Hill in relation to tobacco smoking and lung cancer (Bradford Hill, 1965). It should be emphasised that none of the criteria, except for temporality (see below), is *necessary* for causation. With this caution, the list provides a useful set of questions to ask about the relationship between the findings of a study, its design and other evidence that is available.

Temporality: The occurrence of the risk factor of interest precedes the outcome of interest. This criterion is sometimes difficult to apply when the exposures are ongoing and the disease is chronic with no detectable starting point. It therefore requires measurement procedures and a study design capable of making this temporal distinction.

Strength of the association: The occurrence of disease among those exposed to the risk factor is substantially greater than that among the unexposed.

Dose response: Where the risk factor of interest has a number of levels, e.g. low, medium and high (or is continuous), the risk of disease increases similarly from low to high.

Biological plausibility: The findings are supported by laboratory evidence or by a theory using biological reasoning.

Consistency: A similar association is obtained in different studies in different populations. For most causal associations a body of evidence is required based on a number of studies and careful evaluation of the study quality. This is discussed further in Chapter 6.

Other criteria suggested by Bradford Hill included:

- *specificity* (the disease has only one cause, and/or that cause is not associated with other diseases)
- *experimental evidence*
- *coherence* (the association does not contradict known facts about the natural history of the disease); and
- *analogy* (for example, exposures of the same general type have been shown to cause disease).

For an individual study to contribute causal evidence, it must itself be internally valid, i.e. free of bias. Methods to minimise bias will be discussed in detail in later chapters. Interpreting an effect in an individual study is also easier if the uncertainty due to random variation is minimised. However, statistical significance (having a large enough sample size to reduce the effect of random variation) should not be confused with validity or causality. This concept will also be explained in greater detail in Chapters 11 and 12.

Conclusion

Deciding on causal effects in epidemiology requires a thorough knowledge of the specific subject matter (e.g. the epidemiology and biology of a particular disease) and the ability to assess the quality of the evidence critically. As certainty is not achievable, trade-offs may be necessary between waiting (and paying for) more or stronger evidence and acting timeously in ways that may avert death, disease and disability.

Levels of prevention

Judy Katzenellenbogen
Margaret Hoffman

Dealing with the dangerous cliff

It was a dangerous cliff as they freely confessed,
Though the walk near its crest was so pleasant;
But over its terrible edge there had slipped
A duke and full many a peasant.
So people said something would have to be done,
But their projects did not tally;
Some said 'Put a fence around the edge of the cliff',
Some 'An ambulance in the valley'.

This anonymous poem describes one of the major dilemmas found in modern health care. Much time and money are spent providing ambulance and emergency services at the bottom of the proverbial cliff (Figure 2.3). Few resources are allocated to alternative strategies – be it building fences or putting up notices – that prevent the problem in the first place.

Figure 2.3 The dangerous cliff: what can be done?

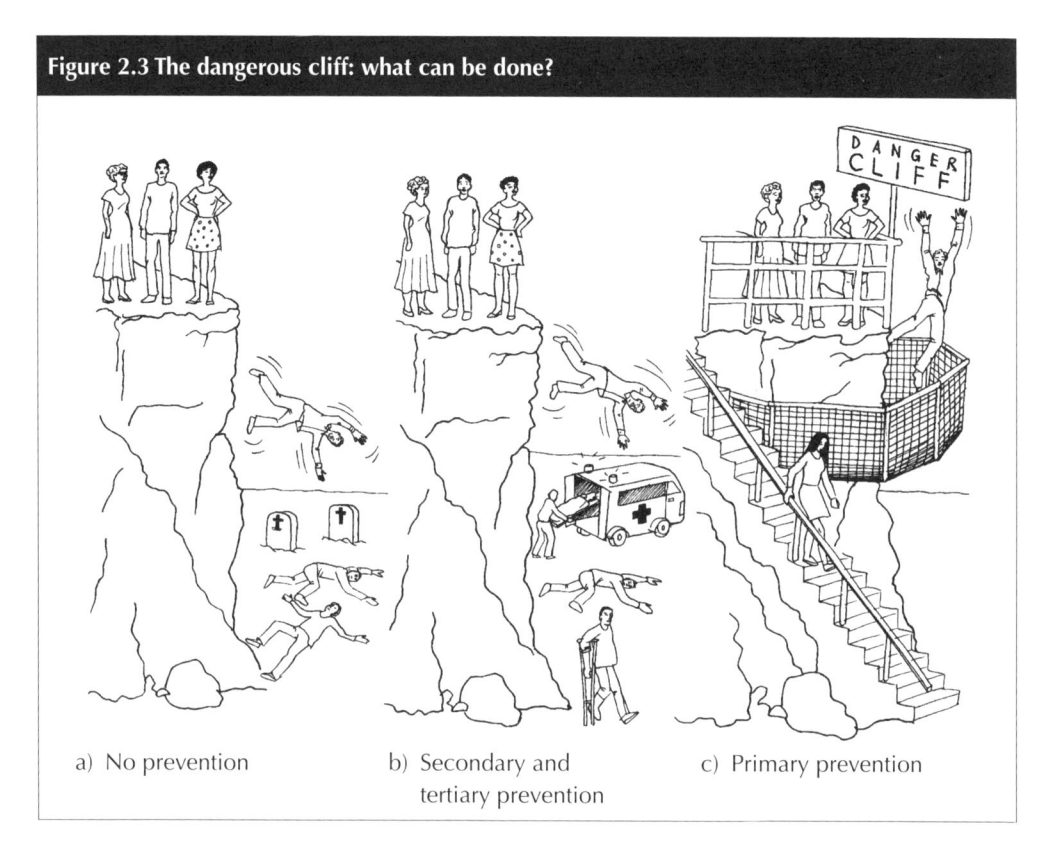

a) No prevention
b) Secondary and tertiary prevention
c) Primary prevention

While there seems to be agreement that prevention is better than cure, traditionally very little is done actively to promote prevention. The historical development of medicine has been dominated by efforts to treat the injured and the sick who present themselves to health services rather than to prevent these conditions. Only more recently has there been an appreciation that health responsibilities need to be more extensive.

In order to take fuller responsibility in the control and management of a disease, a thorough understanding is required not only of the multiple causes of the disease but also of its natural history.

Natural history of disease

The natural history of disease refers to the systematic description of the course of disease over time, unaffected by treatment. Several stages form part of the natural history.

- During the susceptibility phase, risk factors only are present.
- During the preclinical or pre-symptomatic phase, the biological process of the disease has started. There are some physical manifestations, but no obvious disease is present.
- In the clinical disease phase, signs and symptoms of disease are present.

The outcome of disease can include recovery, remission, disability or death.

Epidemiology, through the use of its different study designs, contributes substantially to the generation of knowledge concerning the natural history of diseases and therefore to prevention. This is done by identifying risk factors (stage of susceptibility), evaluating screening programmes (pre-symptomatic stage), and describing consequences of disease and treatment (stage of clinical disease and disability). On the basis of such information, interventions can be planned for the comprehensive management and control of particular diseases.

Intervention at different stages of disease

Interventions must be on as many levels as possible. Each level of action represents a level of prevention. There should therefore be an attempt to prevent the disease from occurring at all. Once the disease has occurred, it should be identified as early as possible and prevented from getting worse. If residual effects of the disease remain, these should be minimised, and disability prevented wherever possible.

A framework is needed for preventative endeavours. A common approach to prevention divides the process into four parts representing all potential levels of intervention.

Primordial prevention: This level aims to curb the development of unhealthy or injurious social, environmental or lifestyle patterns among groups/populations which have not yet developed them. The classical example of the need for primordial prevention is in the cardiovascular disease area, where communities which still have low levels of cardiovascular disease and the lifestyle associated with these should be targeted for prevention. In Southern Africa, communities undergoing urbanisation and cultural transition should be targeted for primordial prevention programmes that relate to both communicable and non-communicable diseases. Government and legislative support should protect the population from the promotion and sale of unhealthy products, while encouraging activities in all sectors of the community to promote health.

Primary prevention: At this level, interventions are aimed at healthy individuals or groups in order to reduce the development of new cases (incidence). Measures are taken to promote optimum health or provide specific protection of target groups against disease and injury. This can be done on a non-personal level, where the probability of the condition is reduced by engineering out the risk (for example, banning asbestos products), or on the personal level by providing vaccinations or promoting healthy lifestyles. Some primary prevention activities focus specifically on high risk individuals (for example, people with high blood pressure, to prevent stroke, or unborn babies of HIV-positive mothers, to prevent mother-infant transmission), while other activities promote the change of risk factors in the population as a whole (for example, change in diet, smoking or unprotected sex).

Secondary prevention: At this level, measures are aimed at people who have a disease. Secondary prevention measures include early diagnosis and prompt treatment to prevent the progression of clinical disease and complications from the disease, thereby reducing disease prevalence. For example, secondary prevention of tuberculosis can take place through screening in the workplace (for early diagnosis) and prompt treatment by means of medication. Similarly, screening for cervical cancer identifies the disease in its early phase, thereby improving prognosis.

Tertiary prevention: At this level, measures involve the treatment of the disease or condition in its later stages and rehabilitation to optimise function, thereby preventing or minimising impairment and disability. For example, a tuberculosis patient may be treated after going to a doctor with clinical symptoms. In most cases, the patient can be treated with medication and return to normal function (secondary prevention). In some cases, there may be residual respiratory problems and rehabilitation may be needed, including occupational training in a new type of job. Palliative care of terminal patients which prevents an undignified or painful death can also be considered tertiary prevention.

Figure 2.4 provides the outline of the framework for levels of prevention and gives examples of each type of activity.

Key concepts in epidemiology

Figure 2.4 Framework for levels of prevention

		ONSET OF DISEASE		DISEASE OUTCOME
Healthy state (pre-disease)	→	Pre-clinical disease → Clinical disease →		Recovery Chronic disease Disability Death

PRIMORDIAL PREVENTION	PRIMARY PREVENTION	SECONDARY PREVENTION	TERTIARY PREVENTION
Health promotion • prevent lifestyle factors with high disease risk • target groups where risks are not yet high	**Health promotion** • health education • nutrition • personal development • education • housing • recreation **Specific protection** • immunisation • personal hygiene • environmental controls • protection from occupational hazards and accidents	**Early diagnosis** • screening • case-finding **Prompt treatment** • arrest disease process	**Treatment** • prevention or limitation of disability **Rehabilitation** • retrain remaining capacities maximally • retrain maximal independence including employment

Conclusion

A comprehensive, multi-level approach is required to reduce the occurrence and impact of disease and injury on the population. Through epidemiological research, information is generated that is used to plan interventions at all levels of prevention of a disease. In doing so epidemiology forms one of the pillars of population health, which aims to improve the health of the population as a whole.

Measures of the frequency of health events

Gina Joubert

Most epidemiological studies focus on the occurrence or frequency of disease or risk factors. Disease frequency can be measured by incidence or prevalence.

Incident cases are the number of new cases reported during a specified period in a defined population (Figure 2.5). The number of new cases can be determined by making use of routine surveillance systems (such as notifications), although the quality of the surveillance system, for example, its completeness, has to be taken into account. Studies which follow individuals up for a specified time can also be conducted to determine the number of incident cases.

Prevalent cases are the number of people who have a particular disease at a specific time (Figure 2.5). Prevalence therefore focuses on existing cases at a specific time, regardless of when the disease onset was. It is also known as point prevalence, since it refers to the number of cases at a point in time. Period prevalence includes the number of cases which existed at any point during a specified period. Prevalent cases include new cases (incident cases) and cases which occurred any time previously as long as they still have the condition at the time of assessment. Cases who have died or recovered by the time of assessment are excluded.

Figure 2.5 Counting incident and prevalent cases

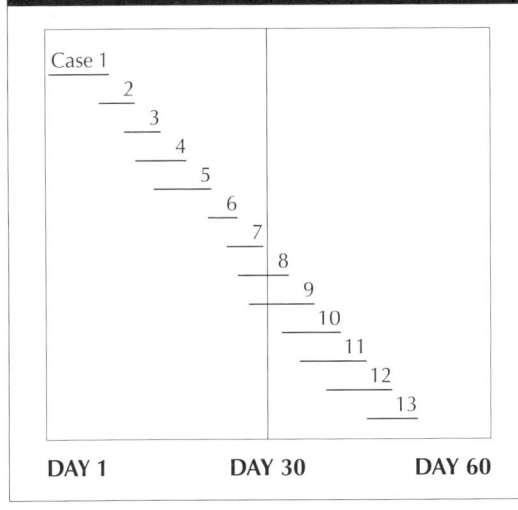

The day on which healthy individuals develop a disease is indicated by the point where the line under the case number starts. The duration of the disease is indicated by the length of the line. The number of incident cases in the period Day 1 to Day 30 is 9 cases (cases 1 to 9) and in the period Day 30 to Day 60 4 cases (cases 10 to 13). If a cross-sectional study is done on Day 30 to determine prevalence, the number of prevalent cases will be 2 (cases 8 and 9).

The longer the duration of a disease, the higher its number of prevalent cases. So if a disease is rapidly fatal, it may have a low number of prevalent cases in spite of a high number of incident cases. If treatment success improves so that more cases survive but with some residual disease, the number of prevalent cases would increase even if incidence remained unchanged.

Primary versus secondary prevention

Primary prevention strategies (see previous section) aim to reduce new cases of disease, that is, incident cases. Secondary prevention strategies aim to decrease prevalence by decreasing the severity and the duration of disease (thereby increasing the number of cases who are cured).

Rates, ratios and proportions

It is useful to know the absolute numbers of people with certain conditions to determine the case load on the health services. However, to be able to compare the frequency of disease in different groups or in a group over time, one has to calculate rates, since they relate the number of cases to the size of the population at risk in the specified group in the specified period. If it is determined that in Area A there are 50 cases of a disease and in Area B 500, it cannot be concluded that the disease is more common in Area B. What if there are only 100 people in Area A compared to 10 000 in Area B? For proper comparison, the size of the populations (and population structure with respect to age, for example) in the two areas has to be taken into account.

A *rate* is calculated by dividing the number of cases (numerator) by the population at risk and the period of

Key concepts in epidemiology

observation (denominator) (Table 2.1). Rates express the frequency of some characteristic per 1 000 (or 10 000 or 100 000) persons in the population per unit of time. Some key rates are listed in Table 2.2. For some rates the numerator is not actually part of the denominator, for example, in the case of the infant mortality rate (IMR), where the numerator is the number of deaths of children under the age of one in a given year, and the denominator is the number of live births in the same year. (A child of three months who dies in January will contribute to the numerator of that year's IMR despite having been born in the previous year and therefore not contributing to the denominator.) Strictly speaking such quantities are *ratios*, but the terminology 'rate' is firmly entrenched. A critical part of a rate is the period of observation/study expressed, for example, as 'per year' or 'per month'.

Table 2.1 Components of a rate: numerator and denominator

If there are two sick people in one year in a population of size 100,

$$\text{the disease rate} = \frac{2 \leftarrow \text{numerator}}{100 \times 1 \text{ year} \leftarrow \text{denominator}}$$

$$= 20 \text{ per } 1\,000 \text{ per year}$$
(or 200 per 10 000 or 2 000 per 100 000 per year)

In a rate, the numerator is a sub-part of the denominator. In the case of a *ratio*, however, the numerator is not necessarily part of the denominator. For example, if 20 boys and 25 girls are born, the ratio of boys to girls is 20:25 or 0.80.

Table 2.2 Key rates

Birth rate

$$\frac{\text{Number of live births during the year}}{\text{Total population}} \times 1\,000$$

Fertility rate

$$\frac{\text{Number or live births to women 15–49 years of age during the year}}{\text{Number of women 15–49 years of age in the population}} \times 1\,000$$

Mortality (death) rates

Crude mortality rate

$$\frac{\text{Total number of deaths during the year}}{\text{Total population}} \times 1\,000$$

Cause-specific mortality rate

$$\frac{\text{Number of deaths due to a specific cause during the year}}{\text{Total population}} \times 100\,000$$

Maternal mortality rate

$$\frac{\text{Number of deaths of women due to pregnancy or childbirth during the year}}{\text{Number of births (live and stillbirths) during the year}} \times 10\,000$$

Infant mortality rate (IMR)
$$\frac{\text{Number of deaths of children under 1 year of age during the year}}{\text{Number of live births during the year}} \times 1\,000$$

Neonatal mortality rate
$$\frac{\text{Number of deaths of children under 28 days of age during the year}}{\text{Number of live births during the year}} \times 1\,000$$

Perinatal mortality rate
$$\frac{\text{Number of foetal deaths (28+ weeks) and deaths of children under 7 days}}{\text{Number of foetal deaths (28+ weeks) and live births during the year}} \times 1\,000$$

To relate the number of incident cases to the population at risk, the cumulative incidence or the incidence rate can be calculated. The *cumulative incidence* is the *proportion* of the at-risk population who become diseased in a specified period. The at-risk population in this case consists only of individuals who are at risk of becoming new cases, that is, it excludes those who have the disease at the start of the time period. For example, to calculate the cumulative incidence of measles in the unvaccinated, the denominator excludes all existing cases at the start of the time period and those who have been vaccinated.

$$\text{Cumulative incidence} = \frac{\text{number of new cases in a specified time period}}{\text{number of people in at-risk population at the start of the time period}}$$

When cumulative incidences are calculated for large populations, for example, for a country as a whole, the denominator often consists of the total population, since excluding those who are already diseased will change the resulting cumulative incidence very little.

The cumulative incidence assumes that the entire population at risk at the beginning of the time period is followed up for the specified period (for example, one year). However, some individuals may be lost to follow-up and different members of the at-risk population may have differing lengths of follow-up.

The *incidence rate* (sometimes referred to as incidence density) takes into account the length of disease-free time each individual in the at-risk population remained under observation. The numerator is the number of new cases and the denominator is the sum of the individual time periods of observation until disease onset or loss to follow-up, in terms of person-time (person-days, person-months or person-years). For example, if person 1 is followed for the whole period of one year, without developing disease, this person contributes one year to the denominator, and nothing to the numerator. If person 2, on the other hand, is followed for 3 months, and then develops disease, this person contributes 0.25 years to the denominator and one disease case to the numerator. Person 3, who is followed for 6 months before being lost to follow-up, being healthy at that time, contributes 0.5 years to the denominator and nothing to the numerator.

$$\text{Incidence rate} = \frac{\text{number of new cases in a specified time period}}{\text{total disease free person-time of observation in the at-risk population}} \times 10\,000$$

The incidence rate is therefore expressed as the number of cases per person-time.

To relate the number of prevalent cases to the at risk population, the *prevalence* is calculated as follows. The numerator is the number of prevalent cases, i.e. all cases at a given time. The denominator is all at-risk people in the group investigated, i.e. all individuals at risk of being a case plus those who are already cases (Table 2.3). For example, to calculate uterine cancer prevalence, the denominator would be all adult women in the population of interest, excluding those who have had hysterectomies.

$$\text{Prevalence} = \frac{\text{number of existing cases at a specific point in time}}{\text{number of people in the at-risk population at that time}}$$

Prevalence is sometimes referred to as prevalence rate. This is incorrect, because it is not expressed per unit of time.

Table 2.3 summarises the differences between prevalence and incidence.

Table 2.3 Difference between incidence and prevalence

Incidence	Prevalence
Numerator = new cases	Numerator = all cases
Denominator = healthy population at risk at start of time period (cumulative incidence) OR Sum of disease-free person-time of observation (incidence rate)	Denominator = total population at risk of being a case
Measured over a specified time period	Measured at a point in time

Crude and specific rates

If the total number of cases in a population is divided by the size of the population at risk, a *crude (overall) rate* is calculated. For example, one can determine the crude mortality rate in a population. However, the epidemiologist is more interested in what the rates are for subgroups, for example, for the sexes or for different age groups. These are called *specific rates* and they enable the researcher to study the variation of the condition of interest between subgroups of a population. We could therefore have disease rates which are sex-, age-, and cause-specific, for example, heart disease mortality rates for men in the 55 to 64 year age group.

Comparison of rates

Epidemiologists often wish to compare disease or mortality rates between groups, for example, between countries, sexes or age groups, or in the same group over time. To be able to compare such rates meaningfully, we need to be sure that any observed differences in rates are real and not due to differences between the groups in the distribution of other factors. For example, what conclusions can we reach if the crude mortality rate in Group A is higher than that in Group B, but it is known that Group A has a larger proportion of elderly people than Group B? Because mortality rates increase rapidly with age, older populations will have higher crude mortality rates. If the mortality rate of a population has increased over the last century, is it due to a real change in mortality experience or to changes in the age structure of the population? If two populations are similar with respect to factors related to the disease, we could feel confident about comparing crude rates. If they differ, however, a comparison of crude rates may give misleading results.

Standardisation

Standardisation, also called *adjustment*, is a way of removing the effect of differences in the composition of various populations and so overcoming the problem of making erroneous comparisons based on crude rates. If age is related to the outcome of interest (for example, heart disease), and the two populations differ with respect to age distribution, we need to adjust the rates. Standardisation provides new summary rates which take into account the differences between the groups. (Details of direct and indirect standardisation are given in Appendix I.) It is, however, important always to examine the subgroup-specific rates (for example, age-specific rates) prior to standardisation. If the rates differ markedly between subgroups, standardisation will obscure these differences.

Demography

David Bourne
Gina Joubert

From the previous section on measuring health events, it is clear that knowledge of the size and characteristics of a population or community is necessary to be able to interpret health information meaningfully. The composition of the population also has implications for its pattern of health. To plan and deliver health services effectively it is necessary to know what the community looks like. For these reasons, there is a close relationship between public health, epidemiology and demography.

Defining demography

'Demography' is the scientific description of the characteristics of populations, and embraces all aspects of population structure and changes which can be measured numerically. This involves primarily the measurement of the size of a population (how many people there are), composition (what the characteristics, such as sex and age, of the people are), distribution (where the people in the region are), and changes in numbers of people. The main demographic processes which lead to changes in the number of people and composition of a population are fertility, mortality and migration.

Population-based rates are essential in epidemiology. While great care is often taken in establishing the numerator, less attention is given to obtaining an accurate estimate of the denominator – the population size. The primary source of demographic data is the national census, which aims to obtain data for the whole population. Censuses are usually conducted once every five or ten years. In using census data, it is important to realise that there is often an undercount, and it must be established whether the published census figures have been adjusted for this undercount or not. Census data are often supplemented by routine surveys, such as annual household surveys.

Key concepts in epidemiology | 2

Population composition

The composition of a population can be described in terms of factors such as age, sex, occupation, income, race or ethnicity, education and literacy. The population composition determines to a large extent the types of health problems experienced, and which health services have to be delivered.

Population pyramids

A population pyramid is a useful summary representation of certain aspects of population composition. It is a graphical display of the percentage composition of a population by age and sex. Age is usually grouped in five-year intervals. The percentages are represented by proportionately drawn horizontal bars. By convention, the percentages relating to the males are drawn on the left of the pyramid and the females on the right. The age groups are drawn from the youngest at the bottom of the pyramid to the oldest at the top.

The influence of births, deaths and migration on the population composition can be seen from the shape of the pyramid. A developing country with high birth rates and low life expectancy will have a high proportion of young people and therefore a population pyramid with a triangular shape and a broad base. On the other hand, a developed country with higher life expectancy will have a higher percentage of people in the older age groups and therefore a population pyramid with a narrower base and steeper sides. Events such as famines, wars, or mass migration in the recent past will be reflected by irregularities in the shape of the pyramid. Population pyramids of South Africa, Gauteng and the Eastern Cape are given in Figure 2.6. These provincial pyramids show the effects of migratory labour, particularly men from the Eastern Cape to Gauteng.

Figure 2.6 Percentage of the total South African, Gauteng and Eastern Cape population in each five-year age group by sex, October 2001

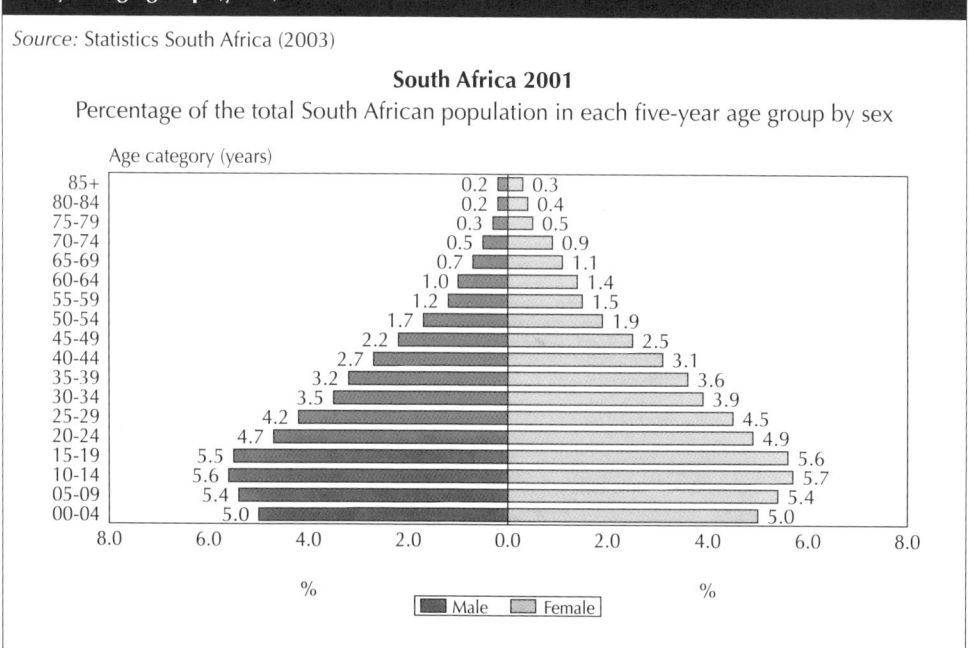

Source: Statistics South Africa (2003)

South Africa 2001
Percentage of the total South African population in each five-year age group by sex

Age category (years)	Male	Female
85+	0.2	0.3
80-84	0.2	0.4
75-79	0.3	0.5
70-74	0.5	0.9
65-69	0.7	1.1
60-64	1.0	1.4
55-59	1.2	1.5
50-54	1.7	1.9
45-49	2.2	2.5
40-44	2.7	3.1
35-39	3.2	3.6
30-34	3.5	3.9
25-29	4.2	4.5
20-24	4.7	4.9
15-19	5.5	5.6
10-14	5.6	5.7
05-09	5.4	5.4
00-04	5.0	5.0

A   Contextualising epidemiology

Source: Statistics South Africa (2003)

Gauteng 2001
Percentage of the Gauteng population in each five-year age group by sex

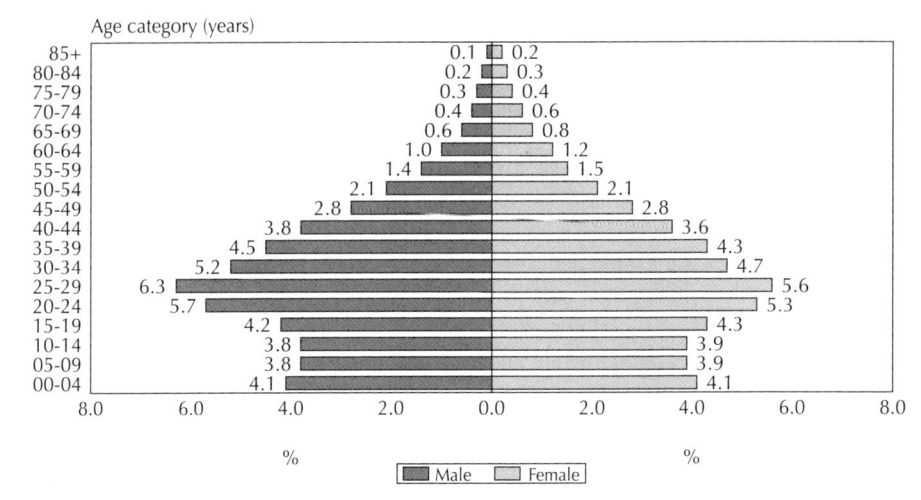

Age category (years)	Male	Female
85+	0.1	0.2
80-84	0.2	0.3
75-79	0.3	0.4
70-74	0.4	0.6
65-69	0.6	0.8
60-64	1.0	1.2
55-59	1.4	1.5
50-54	2.1	2.1
45-49	2.8	2.8
40-44	3.8	3.6
35-39	4.5	4.3
30-34	5.2	4.7
25-29	6.3	5.6
20-24	5.7	5.3
15-19	4.2	4.3
10-14	3.8	3.9
05-09	3.8	3.9
00-04	4.1	4.1

Source: Statistics South Africa (2003)

Eastern Cape 2001
Percentage of the Eastern Cape population in each five-year age group by sex

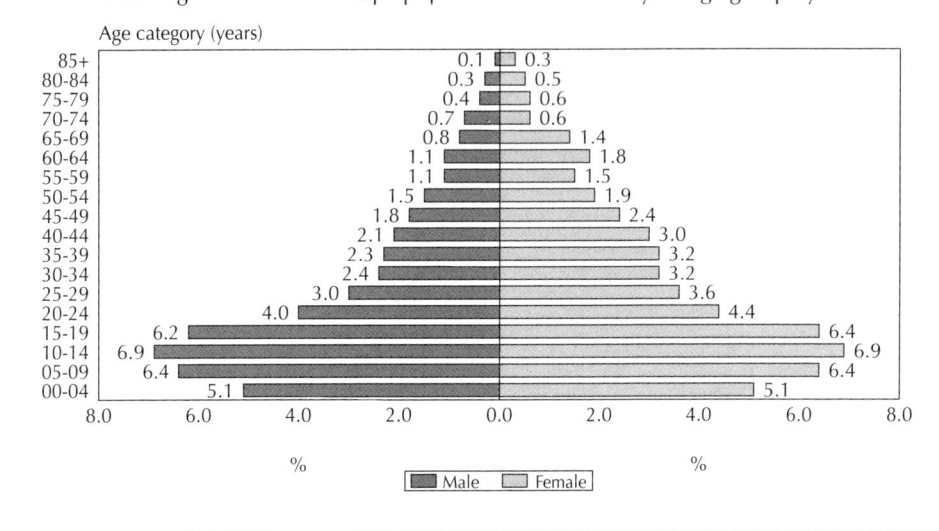

Age category (years)	Male	Female
85+	0.1	0.3
80-84	0.3	0.5
75-79	0.4	0.6
70-74	0.7	0.6
65-69	0.8	1.4
60-64	1.1	1.8
55-59	1.1	1.5
50-54	1.5	1.9
45-49	1.8	2.4
40-44	2.1	3.0
35-39	2.3	3.2
30-34	2.4	3.2
25-29	3.0	3.6
20-24	4.0	4.4
15-19	6.2	6.4
10-14	6.9	6.9
05-09	6.4	6.4
00-04	5.1	5.1

Key concepts in epidemiology

Demographic processes

Three processes determine the changing size of a population: fertility (births), mortality (deaths) and migration. The balance between these three determines whether a population increases, decreases or remains stable in size. The growth rate of a population is given by the following equation:

$$P_{t+1} = P_t + B_t - D_t + I_t - E_t$$

where P_t is the population in year t, P_{t+1} is the population in the following year, B_t are the births in year t, D_t are the deaths in year t, I_t is the immigration in and E_t is the emigration out in year t.

Fertility

The determinants of fertility are complex. We will restrict ourselves to some basic measures of fertility.

Crude birth rate

This is the number of live births per 1 000 persons in the population. This measure requires only total births and total population. It is a 'crude' measure in epidemiogical terminology because it does not take into account the age or sex structure of the population. It can be contrasted with an *adjusted* or *standardised* birth rate in which age and sex structure are taken into account.

General fertility rate

This refers to the number of births per 1 000 women aged 15 to 44 years. In this case, the denominator consists only of the females of child-bearing age in the population. Sometimes the age group used is 15 to 49 years. Note that for birth rates the denominator includes both sexes, whereas for fertility rates it includes women only.

Age-specific fertility rate

If the numbers of the female population and births are known by age of the mother, age-specific fertility rates can be calculated. These are obtained by dividing the total number of births to mothers in each age group (for example, 15 to 19 years) by the number of women in that age group.

Total fertility rate

The best single summary index of fertility (if the age-specific data are available) is the total fertility rate. It is calculated by adding the age-specific fertility rates together over the reproductive ages. This represents the average number of children who would be born to a group of women over the reproductive period as they experience current age-specific fertility rates. It incorporates the age structure of the reproductive female population, which the general fertility rate does not do.

Mortality

Mortality is of great importance in demography as well as epidemiology. In epidemiology it is often used as a substitute (although a biased one) for morbidity (disease), since mortality information is collected routinely and is more easily obtainable than morbidity information.

Crude death rate

The crude death rate expresses the number of deaths per 1 000 population. As pointed out in regard to fertility, other more specific death rates, for example by cause or age, may be more useful.

Infant mortality rate

The infant mortality rate is defined as the number of deaths under the age of one year divided by the number of live births in a given year. It is usually expressed as a rate per 1 000 live births. The infant mortality rate (IMR) is considered to be of great importance for public health. It is not only an indicator of health among the young, but the World Health Organization has also used the IMR as an indicator of the quality of the social, economic and physical environment of the whole community as well as of the effectiveness of health services. The current overall IMR for South Africa is about 60 per 1 000, with large disparities between social groupings, however.

Under-five mortality rate

The under-five mortality rate is defined as the number of deaths under five years of age divided by the number of live births in a given year. It is often expressed as a rate per 1 000 live births in a given year.

Note that the infant mortality rate and under-five mortality rate have the number of live births as their denominator, and not the population under one year or under five years. All other mortality rates use the population at risk as the denominator.

Life expectancy

A useful index of overall longevity is life expectancy. It is easily understood as it is expressed in years. Life expectancy *at birth* is, on average, the number of years a person just born can be expected to live. It is a theoretical concept which imagines a cohort of people just born experiencing the current age-specific mortality rates throughout their lives. Because of the differences in mortality rates of males and females, women have a longer expectation of life at birth than men. This index is often represented separately for males and females.

An increase in life expectancy at birth could be due either to people living longer or to fewer people dying in the young age groups. In most countries, increases in life expectancy have been brought about mainly by the reduction of infant mortality.

Life expectancies are usually calculated during census years, when reliable information on population size is available and reliable mortality rates can be calculated. As a result of the HIV/Aids epidemic, life expectancy at birth in South Africa has fallen from about 65 years in the 1980s to around 40 years in 2005.

Life expectancies can be calculated from any age, for example, life expectancy at 45 years. This takes into account only mortality rates in middle and old age, and is not influenced by mortality in childhood or young adulthood.

Estimates for South Africa of the above indicators are given in Table 2.4 for illustration. Note that considerable uncertainty surrounds these estimates and different sources give conflicting values.

Table 2.4 Table of main demographic indicators for South Africa 2005	
Total population	44 million
Infant mortality rate	59 per 1 000 live births
Under-5 mortality rate	95 per 1 000 live births
Total fertility rate	2.8
Life expectancy at birth	43 years

Migration and urbanisation

Migration refers to human movement in a geographical sense. Socioeconomic and political factors lead to the migration of people. Migration consists of immigration (people moving into a specific region) and emigration (people moving out of a specific region).

In recent decades, there has been rapid urbanisation in South Africa caused by migration to cities. The counting of the ever changing urban population for which services need to be provided is a public health priority. Urbanisation is also important to health in that it is associated with lifestyle or environmental changes which profoundly affect health. However, defining who is a migrant is difficult, as many people do not necessarily remain in the urban area they move to, but shift back and forth between rural and urban regions cyclically.

Demographic transition and epidemiological transition

Populations are not static. Over the last one to two hundred years, a number of societies experienced decreases in the birth and mortality rates. The drop in mortality occurred first, followed by a drop in fertility some time later. There was consequently a rise in the growth rate of the population in the intermediate period, with low or even negative rates of population growth occurring later. In many (usually poorer) countries the birth rate did not follow the fall in mortality rates, leading to rapid and continuing population growth.

These phenomena are known as the *demographic transition*. Historically, at the beginning of such a period of change, the majority of deaths were due to infectious diseases, whereas at the end the majority were due to the chronic diseases of later life. This change in disease pattern has been called the *epidemiological* (or health) *transition* (Omran, 1971).

Chronic diseases, previously referred to as 'conditions of affluence' (i.e. of developed countries and the upper socioeconomic strata in a society) now contribute substantially to the burden of disease in developing countries, especially among the poor. South Africa and other developing countries have in fact experienced a 'protracted transition' in which high rates of both chronic disease and infection are likely to co-exist for some time. In the last decade the emergence of HIV/Aids has led to a new phenomenon in sub-Saharan Africa, that of massive mortality among young adults. Violence and injury are other major sources of mortality in South Africa – making up the so-called 'quadruple burden' of disease (Bradshaw *et al*, 2003).

Conclusion

A knowledge of the structure of populations supplies considerable insight into the understanding of epidemiological problems and is fundamental to the accurate calculation of most rates.

Useful web sites

CIA World Factbook. [Online]. Available: http://www.cia.gov/cia/publications/factbook. [25 February 2007].

Health Systems Trust. [Online]. Available: http://www.hst.org.za. [25 February 2007].

References used in this chapter

Bradford Hill, A. 1965. The environment and disease: association or causation? *Proceedings of the Royal Society of Medicine*, 58:295–300.

Bradshaw, D, Groenewald, P, Laubscher, R, Nannan, N, Nojilana, B, Norman, R, Pieterse, D, Schneider, M, Bourne, DE, Timaeus, IM, Dorrington, R & Johnson, L. 2003. Initial burden of disease estimates for South Africa 2000. *South African Medical Journal*, 93:682–8.

Omran, AR. 1971. The epidemiologic transition. A theory of the epidemiology of population change. *Milbank Memorial Fund Quarterly*, 29:509–38.

Rothman, KJ & Greenland, S. 2005. Causation and causal inference in epidemiology. *American Journal of Public Health*, 95:S144–S150.

Statistics South Africa. *Census 2001: census in brief. Reports nos 03-02-03, 03-02-05 & 03-02-07 (2001)*. 2003. [Online]. Available: http://www.statssa.gov.za. [24 May 2007].

3

Research ethics, human rights and community participation

Ethics, advocacy and human rights
Jerome Amir Singh

Community participation
Ashraf Kagee   Leslie Swartz

OBJECTIVES OF THIS CHAPTER

The objectives of this chapter are:
- to define ethics, bioethics, and public health ethics
- to explore the applicability of the principles of biomedical ethics and public health ethics to epidemiology
- to outline specific ethical guidelines for epidemiological research
- to describe the processes of informed consent and maintaining confidentiality
- to examine the relationship between epidemiology, advocacy, and human rights
- to outline the rationale for community participation in health research
- to present an example of a South African model of community participation in epidemiological research.

Ethics, advocacy and human rights

Jerome Amir Singh

Ethics, bioethics, and public health ethics

Defining ethics

The *American Heritage Dictionary* (2000) defines 'ethics' variously as 'a theory or a system of moral values', 'the study of the general nature of morals and of the specific moral choices to be made by a person' and 'the rules or standards governing the conduct of a person or the members of a profession'.

The word 'bioethics' originated in the early 1970s, yet as an idea and guiding principle, it has been with us for thousands of years.

'Bioethics' has been defined as 'a branch of applied ethics that studies the value implications of practices and developments in the life sciences and medicine' (*Bioethics Thesaurus*, 1999). It helps health care professionals identify and respond to moral dilemmas in their work. It can also be described as a field of study concerned with the ethics and philosophical implications of certain biological and medical procedures, study methodologies, technologies, and treatments. Framed widely, bioethics encompasses the ethical considerations, implications, and impact of health research and clinical practice, including emerging technologies, on human or animal health, or the environment. Several guiding principles have emerged from the discipline of bioethics, the most prominent being the principles of biomedical ethics, which, like the practice of medicine, largely focus on the *individual*.

Public health can be distinguished from medicine in that it:
- identifies and measures threats to the health of *populations*
- develops governmental and community responses to these concerns
- seeks to ensure certain benefits.

Defining public health ethics

'Public health ethics' is increasingly being seen as a distinct branch of bioethics and has been described as

'[t]he principles and values that help guide actions among public health system actors, which are designed to promote health and prevent injury and disease in the population. The principal values of public health ethics include the salience of population health, safety, and welfare; fairness and equity in the distribution of services; and respect for the human rights of individuals and groups'. (Gostin, 2003)

The principles of biomedical ethics and public health ethics are explored below.

Making an ethical decision in the context of health research, like any other decision in health care, is not a precise art but a learned skill. *What* decision is ultimately made and *how* that decision is made have always been topics of intense debate. After the post-World War II trial of Nazi physicians in 1947, the *Nuremberg Code* outlined unacceptable research practices. In 1964 the *Declaration of Helsinki* followed and has been revised several times. Two major influences in the last half of the 20th century have shaped and defined the substance of modern day ethical principles in health research. These were the *Belmont Report* (National Commission for the Protection of Human Subjects of Biomedical and Behavioural Research, 1979) and the writers Beauchamp and Childress (1979) with their groundbreaking book *Principles of Biomedical Ethics*.

Principles of biomedical ethics

The *Belmont Report* summarises the basic ethical principles identified by the US National Commission for the Protection of Human Subjects of Biomedical and Behavioural Research. According to the *Belmont Report*, the expression 'basic ethical principles' refers to those general judgements that serve as a basic justification for the many particular ethical prescriptions and evaluations of human actions. The *Belmont Report* suggests that three basic principles, among those generally accepted in our cultural tradition, are particularly relevant to medical ethics involving human subjects:
- respect for persons
- beneficence
- justice.

Other writers such as Beauchamp and Childress have suggested that four basic principles are particularly relevant to health care ethics involving human subjects:
- autonomy
- beneficence
- non-maleficence
- justice.

The *Belmont Report* expounds just three principles since its first principle, 'respect for persons', includes and considers the principle of 'autonomy', while its second principle, 'beneficence', includes and considers the principle of 'non-maleficence'.

In the following part, we provide a brief summary of the principles of autonomy, beneficence, non-maleficence and justice.

Autonomy – respect for persons

Respect for persons incorporates at least two ethical convictions: first, that individuals should be treated as autonomous agents; and second, that persons with diminished autonomy are entitled to protection. The principle of respect for persons therefore divides into two separate moral requirements:
a) the requirement to acknowledge autonomy; and
b) the requirement to protect those with diminished autonomy.

An autonomous person is an individual capable of deliberation about personal goals, and of acting under the direction of such deliberation. To respect autonomy is to give weight to autonomous persons' considered opinions and choices, while refraining from obstructing their actions, unless these are clearly detrimental to others. To show lack of respect for an autonomous person is to repudiate that person's considered judgements, to deny an individual the freedom to act on those considered judgements, or to withhold information necessary to make a considered judgement, when there are no compelling reasons to do so.

Some persons are in need of extensive protection (for example, minors, comatose and unconscious individuals, and the mentally insane), even to the point of excluding them from activities which may harm them; other persons require little protection beyond making sure they undertake activities freely and with awareness of possible adverse consequences. The extent of protection afforded should depend upon the risk of harm, and the likelihood of benefit. The judgement that any individual lacks autonomy should be periodically re-evaluated, and will vary in different situations.

Even though patients, owing to their illness, may lose some measure of their independence, they still deserve to be treated with respect and remain in control of their lives. Health care professionals as well as health care students have specific professional responsibilities which help ensure that patients and research participants are treated with respect and that they are given an opportunity to retain control over their lives and their bodies. These include the responsibilities to respect the confidences of research participants or patients, to communicate with them honestly, and to obtain informed consent or refusal from them for treatment or research participation.

Beneficence and non-maleficence

Persons are to be treated in an ethical manner, not only by respecting their decisions and protecting them from harm, but also by making efforts to secure their well-being. Such treatment falls under the principle of beneficence. 'Beneficence' is often understood to cover acts of kindness or charity that go beyond strict obligation. Two general rules have been formulated as complementary expressions of beneficent actions in this sense:

a) do not harm; and
b) maximise possible benefits, and minimise possible harm.

It has been argued that beneficence captures the true moral essence of the professional responsibilities of health care professionals. The Hippocratic Oath requires physicians to benefit their patients 'according to their best judgement'. So the guiding principle of the health care professional's relationship with a patient may be characterised as attempting to move the patient from a state of health need to one of health benefit. Similarly, with a research participant, the guiding principle for investigators may be to conduct the research by minimising harm and maximising benefit. Examples of responsibilities which flow from the principle of beneficence are competency, professionalism, discernment and service.

The Hippocratic maxim 'do no harm' has long been a fundamental principle of medical ethics. However, avoiding harm requires learning what is harmful; and, in the process of obtaining this information, persons may be exposed to risk of harm. Nonetheless, the essence of the principle of 'non-maleficence' instructs us not to harm others deliberately.

Justice

The principle of justice asks, 'Who ought to receive the benefits and bear burdens?' This is a question of justice, in the sense of 'fairness in distribution' or 'what is deserved'. An injustice occurs when some benefit to which a person is entitled is denied without good reason, or when some burden is imposed unduly.

According to this principle, all patients or research participants should be treated alike or equitably. The notion of equity is important to consider in a research context. Whereas the notion of equality forbids the preferential consideration of one group over another, the notion of equity might suggest the opposite. For example, faced with selecting a research site in either an urban or a rural location, the notion of equity will require investigators to consider what is fair in the circumstances. This could equate to focusing on the vulnerable – for example women in the impoverished and disease-burdened rural location as opposed to their counterparts in the affluent urban location – because this is where the need for data may be most crucial or because such individuals could be at greater risk of falling prey to a particular pandemic. In these instances, the principle of justice might dictate that the notion of equity should assume precedence over the notion of equality.

Likewise, it is possible that the biomedical principles of ethics may occasionally conflict with one another. In these instances one principle may be judged as having priority over the other.

The appropriateness of applying the principles of biomedical ethics to epidemiology

The application of the biomedical principles of ethics to all research contexts is not always appropriate. Ethical issues arise throughout the conduct of epidemiological research: in the process of determining the study question, designing the protocol, and implementing the study. Moreover, the scope and methods of epidemiological research – particularly the collection, storage and use of data on individuals and communities – have raised concerns about the risks of abuse and led to calls for a consideration of the ethical issues implicit in such endeavours. Public health practitioners also use tools, in addition to epidemiology, to accomplish their work, focusing primarily on community-wide, typically prospective, approaches to improve health. Furthermore, some public health functions – such as surveillance, vital statistics, disease and injury reporting, and disease registries – relate to epidemiology and the collection of data. Strict adherence to the biomedical principle of autonomy in these instances would not be appropriate or practical. So while the founders of bioethics attempted to articulate ethics principles that were relevant to all contexts of health, public health ethicists are increasingly arguing that the guidelines and codes of health care ethics that have emerged through the years are an imperfect fit to the arena of public health and epidemiology. As a result, several frameworks of public health ethics have recently emerged. Key aspects of some of these frameworks will now be briefly explored.

Principles of public health ethics

Lawrence Gostin, Nancy Kass, Ross Upshur and James Childress, amongst others, have proposed various frameworks of public health ethics – analytical tools of sorts akin to the four principles of biomedical ethics – designed to help public health professionals such as epidemiologists consider the specific ethical implications of proposed public health interventions, policy proposals, research projects, and health programmes. The following seven-step framework (Table 3.1) is a brief attempt at synthesising their respective proposals. Students should consult this section's recommended readings list for more on these emerging principles.

Table 3.1 The principles of public health ethics

1. What are the public health goals of the proposed project? (the principle of harm prevention and necessity)
2. How effective is the project known to be in achieving its stated goals? (the principle of effectiveness)
3. What are the known or potential burdens of the project? (the principle of burden identification)
4. Can the burdens be minimised? Are there alternative approaches? (the principle of least infringement/restriction/coercion)
5. Is the project implemented fairly? (the principle of proportionality)
6. Can the benefits and burdens of the project be fairly balanced? (the principle of public justification and transparency)
7. Reciprocity (individuals who are affected by public health initiatives should be adequately supported or fairly compensated)

Epidemiology ethics guidelines

Ethical issues often arise as a result of conflict among competing sets of values. In the context of epidemiology, the conflict often occurs between the rights of individuals and the needs of communities. Research ethics guidelines, such as the *Belmont Report*, the *Declaration of Helsinki* (issued by the World Health Organization), the *International Ethical Guidelines for Biomedical Research Involving Human Subjects* (issued by CIOMS – the Council for International Organisations of Medical Sciences) focus strongly on biomedical ethics, and in particular, on the rights of the individual. Cognisant that these guidelines were not appropriate for epidemiological research, CIOMS published a dedicated set of ethics guidelines for epidemiology in 1991. Entitled *International Guidelines for Ethical Review of Epidemiological Studies* and currently under revision, the guidelines are intended for investigators, health policy-makers, members of ethical review committees, and others who have to deal with ethical issues that arise in epidemiology. The guidelines are also intended to assist in the establishment of standards for ethical review of epidemiological studies. The guidelines offer specific guidance on a wide range of issues including informed consent, confidentiality, conflicts of interests, scientific objectivity, randomisation, and advocacy. Because of space constraints only the notions of informed consent, confidentiality, and advocacy will be explored in the South African milieu. Advocacy will be explored in the context of human rights.

Informed consent

When individuals participate in epidemiological research their informed consent should always be sought and preferably recorded in writing. Where investigators believe that informed consent should not be solicited from research participants or recorded in writing they have an obligation to justify to the research ethics committee reviewing their research why the study will be ethical in its absence. Four elements characterise informed consent:

(1) Capacity: Research participants must be legally and mentally competent to participate in the proposed research. They must accordingly meet the age requirements stipulated in law (outlined in the National Health Act 61 of 2003) and be mentally competent to autonomously participate in a study (unless surrogate consent is given by an authorised caregiver).

(2) Disclosure: Investigators should disclose to research participants all relevant knowledge about the proposed study, including its purpose, potential risks, benefits, and social implications. In instances where this is not deemed feasible, (for example, if the disclosure of the study hypothesis to study participants could endanger the study's validity), investigators must seek guidance or approval from the research ethics committee for the non-disclosure.

(3) Understanding: In addition to providing participants with the relevant knowledge about the proposed study, investigators should ensure that the research participants understand the disclosure. Disclosure should accordingly be made in the language spoken by the participant and scientific concepts (such as coding and randomisation) should be explained in layman's terms.

(4) Voluntary nature: In addition to research participants possessing the legal and mental capacity to participate in research, and having disclosure about the nature of the study outlined to them in a manner that facilitates their understanding of the proposed endeavour, they must affirmatively volunteer to participate in the study. Factors that compromise the voluntary nature of consent include:
- duress (participants are pressured to participate in the study)
- undue inducement (participants are offered incentives to participate in a study over and above reasonable compensation, for example, for transport, or missed meals); and
- 'therapeutic misconception' (participants wrongly believe that their participation in the study will improve their health).

Confidentiality

Epidemiologists often make use of confidential data – such as medical records, tissue samples, and occupational records – in the course of their work. However, the purpose for the access is often not contemplated and/or consented to by patients or research participants at the time when such data are collected. As such, individuals or public representatives should normally be notified that certain types of data might be used in epidemiological research and how their confidentiality will be assured. In addition, where relevant, the permission of health authorities must also be sought for the data to be accessed. Ethically, investigators may be expected to either seek the consent of the individuals concerned, or to justify to a research ethics committee why they should enjoy such access without consent. South Africa's Medical Research Council (MRC) advises that access may be ethical on such grounds as minimal risk of harm to individuals, public benefit, and the stringent steps investigators will take to protect the confidentiality of research participants (such as anonymising the data or giving a firm undertaking not to identify participants in any published work that emanates from the study).

The regulation of health research in South Africa

Research ethics committees (RECs) in South Africa play a vital role in overseeing and regulating health research in the country. Most universities as well as the MRC and Human Sciences Research Council (HSRC) have ethics committees. If these are not accessible to a researcher, the researcher should contact the Department of Health. The National Health Act 61 of 2003 creates a formal national research ethics framework by codifying the mandatory regulation of research by RECs. The Act also addresses the accountability of RECs. In terms of the Act RECs would be accountable to the National Health Research Ethics Council (NHREC).

The Act stipulates that every institution, health agency and health establishment at which health research is conducted must establish or have access to a health research ethics committee which is registered with the NHREC.

Epidemiology, advocacy and human rights

'Advocacy' has been defined as 'the act of pleading or arguing in favor of something, such as a cause, idea, or policy' while 'human rights' have been defined as 'the basic rights and freedoms to which all humans are entitled' (*American Heritage Dictionary*, 2000). The right to health is widely recognised as a fundamental human right. Aside from its obvious link to health, epidemiology is linked to human rights and advocacy in at least four important ways.

1. Epidemiological research, with its focus on health at a population level, can potentially affect human rights at an individual level. The impact on an individual's right to privacy (a fundamental human right) when medical records are reviewed as part of epidemiological research is an example of such an effect.
2. Human right abuses are traditionally reported on a case-by-case basis and the cumulative morbidity or mortality impact of such practices have not traditionally been described. Recently, however, the value of population-based studies of the incidence of human rights violations caused by wars and political instability characterised by violations of human rights on a massive scale has been recognised. To address this emerging public health problem, a number of surveys have been conducted in recent years in troubled regions of the world in an attempt to establish methods of estimating the occurrence of human rights abuses in affected populations. Epidemiological methods have played an important role in such initiatives.
3. While conducting their research epidemiologists may encounter states of affairs that have health-related human rights implications. Such discoveries may entail their assuming an advocacy role and lobbying public health authorities to effect changes in policy.
4. Conversely, lobbying for changes in health policy using human rights instruments (such as a Bill of Rights) is made easier if the lobbying is underpinned by strong evidence. Epidemiology can play a central role in generating such evidence.

The latter two scenarios have emerged in the South African context and are discussed in Example 3.1.

Human rights advocates such as Bebe Loff and Jim Black have argued that when epidemiological research is undertaken, particularly among communities whose dignity is affronted or who suffer discrimination and are therefore not fully able to claim the benefits of societal membership, the research proposal should be assessed alongside relevant human rights criteria. According to them:

'The way a problem is characterised defines the solutions. There may well be a place for decontextualised epidemiological research, but we would argue that the greater endowment to human well-being will emerge from contextualised epidemiological research done in a framework cognisant of and with respect for human rights.'
(Loff & Black, 2003)

The CIOMS ethics guidelines on epidemiological research also address the issue of advocacy. It notes that investigators may discover health hazards that demand correction, and become advocates of means to protect and restore health. In this event, CIOMS advises that their advocacy must be seen to rely on objective, scientific data. Similarly, investigators must guard against subjective interpretation of their data, particularly in instances where they feel strong convictions about the result.

Conclusion

Ethics demands that research and practice ought to be carried out at the highest attainable level. Epidemiologists should subject their work to an ethics analysis to ensure the integrity of their proposals and to assure the public of their integrity. Practical issues regarding ethics which have to be considered in planning and conducting epidemiological research are outlined in Chapter 4.

Aside from having strong ethical dimensions, the discipline of epidemiology is also intimately linked to advocacy and human rights. Only by taking on an evidence-based advocacy role can epidemiologists balance the ends of science, human rights and ethics.

Community participation

Ashraf Kagee
Leslie Swartz

The assumption that informs epidemiological research is that findings should be relevant to people's lives, directly or indirectly. Directly relevant research findings usually take the form of policy or other recommendations aimed at enhancing the likelihood of positive health outcomes. Research of indirect relevance may take the form of detailed descriptions of phenomena or the elucidation of risk factors that may in turn inform further studies aimed at enhancing health outcomes. In either case, for research to be conducted that is viable and relevant to the needs and realities of the people for whom it is intended, the commitment of participants is required. Public health research, particularly, is frequently conducted in communities rather than in a laboratory setting.

What is community participation?

In its fullest scope, community participation is the active participation of people or their representatives in the conceptualisation, decision-making, and implementation of research projects.

It may be puzzling to health researchers why communities need to participate in matters that require specialised knowledge and training. Historically, in many parts of the world, including South Africa, it was not part of the culture of research to consult with the people being researched. Instead, a wide gap was maintained between the researcher and the researched, with scientists in possession of power and expertise. All that was expected from communities was that they comply with the expectations of the researchers and obey instructions. In

> ### What is a community?
>
> Traditionally, the term community refers to a group of people who inhabit a geographically circumscribed area that has identifiable physical boundaries, such as roads, railway lines, or rivers. This method of describing a community has been challenged by scholars who call attention to the fact that people who live in close proximity to one another do not necessarily constitute a community. Instead, it is argued that the defining feature of a community is the *common identity shared by people* (Campbell & Jovchelovitch, 2000). The term community may therefore refer to people defined by the work they do (e.g. teaching community); sexual orientation (e.g. gay community); or disability status (e.g. Deaf community). A community defined by a geographical catchment area is therefore not likely to be a homogenous entity but subject to competing interests among inhabitants that could limit a sense of homogeneity. So in any epidemiological research conducted among people living within a bounded geographical space, diversity and within-group differences are important to consider. For the purpose of this chapter we define community as a subset of the population that shares a common identity.

South Africa the gap between the researchers and the researched also coincided with racial divisions, so that power and authority were often located among white, usually male, scientists whose research subjects were people living under conditions of impoverishment and oppression. Such situations were often characterised by the absence of proper consultation and the potential for the abuse of power. Awareness on the part of researchers of their role in the community they are researching and the potential for the abuse of this role is therefore necessary to increase the likelihood of research being conducted within a framework of human rights and accepted ethical practice.

Community participation is an attempt to fairly distribute power inherent in science so that communities are able to assert greater control over what is researched, how it is researched, and what is done with research findings. Rather than top-down, expert-designed projects that are imposed on communities without their involvement other than as subjects, the principle of community participation places importance on collaboration between researchers and the communities where research takes place and on empowerment of communities. Empowerment refers to the understanding that people have of the way in which social conditions have created conditions of oppression, and the application of this understanding to collective action aimed at changing and improving their social circumstances.

There may be a tension between the scientific requirements of a research study and full community participation. For example, it may take a long time for a researcher to consult and win the trust of community organisations, or in some cases even facilitate the creation of community structures such as community advisory boards (CABs) where these are absent. It may be necessary for time and money to be invested in order to ensure that such bodies are indeed representative of the communities they purport to represent, and that they continue to do so over the time in which the research is carried out.

Considerable effort may also be required to ensure that each person living in a community is adequately informed about the research being conducted in their midst. As a result, in addition to the actual participants in research projects, persons in their vicinity may also need to be informed and consulted before research may proceed. An example of the need for wide consultation is research aimed at testing an Aids vaccine for efficacy. For an Aids vaccine to be tested in a community, many hundreds of HIV negative individuals at risk for contracting HIV will be needed to enrol in a trial. However, their enrolment may affect others in their lives, such as partners and family members. Trial participants, even though HIV negative, may also be discriminated against by others in their community because of the stigma attached to Aids. For an Aids vaccine trial to be successfully conducted in a community, the entire community would need to be consulted so that the likelihood of eligible persons participating is maximised and of participants dropping out or being discriminated against is minimised. Moreover, appropriate participation of communities in research will increase the likelihood of uptake of any empirically supported interventions or products when these become available.

Other epidemiological research may require lower levels of effort in securing community involvement. For example, household surveys in which data are based mainly on the self-report of respondents may require less active community involvement than studies that involve invasive procedures or products with a higher level of risk to participants. However, even studies in which participants are interviewed or asked to respond to paper and pencil questionnaires require researchers to enter a community respectfully and request participation from relevant organisations or committees. A particular example of community participation is in occupational epidemiology, where workers who are the subjects of research need to be consulted, for example, via their union.

A South African model of community participation in epidemiological research

The HIV Prevention Trials Network (HPTN) has developed a model for researchers that may be adopted more generally to ensure and assess community participation in epidemiological research. The model is described below.

1. Establishment of Community Advisory Boards

A Community Advisory Board (CAB) is a useful mechanism to facilitate community participation in a research project. Members of a CAB may include potential study participants, representatives of community organisations and NGOs, health workers, religious leaders and researchers. The CAB has many roles: to be a voice for the community and study participants; to ensure that study investigators consider the concerns of the community; to liaise between researchers and the community; to assist with community education; to disseminate study information to local communities; and to provide input in scientific decision making from a community perspective. A well-functioning CAB is generally in close contact with study investigators who in turn are responsive to its contributions. In the HPTN model, CABs are represented on the research study's various Science Working Groups and its Executive Committee.

2. Community assessment

CABs may play an important role in developing an accurate community profile that may guide resource allocation and scientific decision making. In respect of a needs assessment, CABs may help to answer questions communities have about the research study, identify optimal data collection strategies and convey to investigators basic community informational requirements. CABs may assist in providing important information on previous interventions that have been conducted in a community, their successes, failures, and lessons learned; on possible barriers to implementing research interventions; and on the availability of existing services that may be necessary to augment research efforts.

3. Community education and materials development

Educational efforts targeting the broader community, site and research staff and trial participants require the active involvement of CABs. For proper community participation to occur, it is necessary that communities understand the purpose of the research as thoroughly as possible. Therefore it is necessary to develop educational materials that are culturally and linguistically appropriate to the community in which the study is conducted. Materials may include fact sheets, brochures, informational packages, newsletters, and websites with incremental levels of detail for the various tiers of participant, from ordinary community members to prospective study participants. An adequate budget is therefore of importance to ensure appropriate materials development.

4. Protection of research participants

The protection of participants in a research study is paramount. Investigators therefore need to make clear efforts to build trust between themselves and the communities in which they conduct research. Study investigators in collaboration with CABs need to address issues related to informed consent, standards of care, management of adverse events and monitoring of incentives provided for research participation.

5. Media relations

The purpose of media relations is to communicate accurate information about research activities to the public and to ensure that misinformation about research activities is kept to a minimum. In addition, it is appropriate to have frequent opportunities for communication between research staff and study participants, advocates, and the community so that any confusion or misunderstanding can be resolved.

6. Evaluation

Evaluation processes provide feedback about the success of efforts to ensure community participation. The HPTN has identified several indicators that may be of use in evaluating community participation in research. These are listed in Table 3.2.

Table 3.2 Indicators of community participation in an HIV vaccine trial

1. Existence of a CAB recruitment and retention plan
2. Annual review of the recruitment and retention plan
3. Evidence of regular CAB meetings with proper quorum requirements being met
4. Evidence that CAB meetings include education activities related to scientific issues, e.g. study design, control groups, interventions
5. Evidence of a mechanism to ensure feedback from CABs on the content and quality of community participation
6. Participation of CAB members in scientific meetings
7. Summaries of community education activities
8. Evidence of regular feedback between CAB members and the community whom they represent and between CAB members and study staff and investigators

7. Capacity development

Another element of community participation is capacity building. In many formerly oppressed communities, the employability and skill level of residents are low owing to the effects of apartheid education. In an effort to contribute to community development, investigators may also build into their study procedures a skills development component that involves the training of community members in some aspect of the research.

> **EXAMPLE 3.1**

Epidemiology and advocacy: scaling up ARV treatment in South Africa

As noted earlier, advocacy is most effective when it is supported by compelling evidence. Epidemiological data can play a key role in this respect.

In 2001, at the height of government denial about the scale and severity of the HIV/Aids epidemic in South Africa, the Medical Research Council (MRC) published a landmark epidemiological study entitled *The impact of HIV/Aids on adult mortality in South Africa*. The study showed that approximately 40% of adult deaths in South Africa that occurred in the age group 15 to 49 years in 2000 were due to HIV/Aids. Moreover, that approximately 20% of all adult deaths in that year were due to Aids. When combined with the excess deaths in childhood, the study concluded that Aids accounted for 25% of all deaths in the year 2000 and had become the single biggest cause of death in South Africa. The investigators argued that if nothing was done to treat Aids, the number of Aids deaths could be expected to grow further to more than double the number of deaths due to all other causes, resulting in 5 to 7 million cumulative Aids deaths in South Africa by 2010. They concluded that the rapid change in the empirical death rates confirmed predictions of the profound impact of Aids on mortality and that these results needed to galvanise efforts to minimise the devastation of the epidemic.

This study was significant for at least three reasons. First, the authors' brave stance on the matter, despite considerable pressure from government to conclude otherwise (the South African government tried to delay, even prevent, the publication of the report (Mason 2001)), illustrates the important advocacy role epidemiologists can play in highlighting potential human rights abuses and lobbying for change in such instances. Second, it demonstrates the crucial role epidemiological research can play in highlighting emerging health threats to the country. The new monitoring system developed by the research team to estimate the extent of HIV/Aids mortality has since provided the most up-to-date information about the epidemic for planning purposes. Third, Aids treatment advocates hailed the study as the solid evidence they needed to spur government to act on the pandemic. Armed with the evidence highlighted in this report and the right to health care in South Africa's Constitution, Aids treatment advocates pressured government into eventually initiating the country's prevention of mother-to-child treatment programme and the antiretroviral rollout program. Although these programmes have been arguably slow to materialise and grow, they have already had a positive impact on the lives of thousands of South Africans.

References:
Anonymous. 2001. HIV/Aids: its impact on mortality. *MRC News*, 32(6), December. [Online]. Available: http://www.mrc.ac.za/mrcnews/dec2001/hivaids.htm. [19 March 2007].
Dorrington, RE, Bourne, D, Bradshaw, D, Laubscher, R & Timaeus, IM. 2001. *The impact of HIV/Aids on adult mortality in South Africa*. Cape Town: Medical Research Council.
Editorial. 2005. South Africa needs to face the truth about HIV mortality. *Lancet*, 365:546.
Mason, B. *South African report shows devastating impact of HIV/Aids (October 22, 2001)*.[Online] Available: http://www.wsws.org/articles/2001/oct2001/aids-022.shtml. [19 March 2007].

Useful readings

Beauchamp, TL & Childress, JF. 1979. *Principles of Biomedical Ethics*. 1st ed. New York: Oxford University Press.

Campbell, C & Jovchelovitch, S. 2000. Health, community and development: Towards a social psychology of participation. *Journal of Community and Applied Social Psychology*, 10:255–70.

Dickert, N & Sugarman, J. 1995. Ethical Goals of Community Consultation in Research. *American Journal of Public Health*, 95:1123–7.

Emanuel, EJ, Wendler, D, Killen, J & Grady, C. 2004. What makes clinical research in developing countries ethical? *Journal of Infectious Diseases*, 189:930–7.

Quinn, SC. 2004. Ethics in public health research. Protecting human subjects: the role of community advisory boards. *American Journal of Public Health*, 94:918–22.

Singh, JA & Ngwena, C. 2001 Bioethics. In: Dada, MA & Mcquoid-Mason, DJ (eds). *Introduction to medico-legal practice*. Durban: Butterworth Publishers. 33–52.

Useful web sites

Council for International Organisations of Medical Sciences. 2002. *International ethical guidelines for biomedical research involving human subjects (2002)*. [Online]. Available: http://www.cioms.ch/frame_guidelines_nov_2002.htm. [25 February 2007].

Department of Health and Human Services: Centers for Disease Control and Prevention. [Online]. Available: http://www.phppo.cdc.gov/dphsdr/FaithBase/PCE/part2.asp. [25 February 2007].

Medical Research Council, South Africa. 2002. *Guidelines on ethics in medical research. General principles (2002)*. [Online]. Available: http://www.mrc.ac.za/ethics/epidemiological.htm. [19 March 2007]

National Health Research Ethics Committee, South Africa. 2004. *Ethics in health research: principles, structures and processes*. [Online]. Available: http://www.doh.gov.za/docs/factsheets/guidelines/ethics/editors.pdf. [19 March 2007]

References used in this chapter

American Heritage Dictionary of the English Language. 2000. 4th ed. Boston: Houghton Mifflin.

Childress, JF, Faden, RR, Gaare, RD, Goshin, LO, Kahn, J, Bonnie, RJ, Kass, NE, Mastroianni, AC, Moreno, JD & Nieburg, P. 2002. Public Health Ethics: Mapping the Terrain. *Journal of Law, Medicine and Ethics*, 30:170–8.

Gostin, LO. 2003. Public health ethics: traditions, profession, and values. *Acta Bioethica*, 9(2):177–88.

HIV Prevention Trials Network. 2005. *Approach to ensuring community involvement in research: year one*. [Online]. Available: http://www.hptn.org/Web%20Documents/CommunityProgram. [25 February 2007].

Kass, N. 2001. An ethics framework for public health. *American Journal of Public Health*, 91(11):1776–82.

Kennedy Institute of Ethics. 1999. *Bioethics Thesaurus*. Washington, DC: Georgetown University. [Online]. Available: http://www.ruhr-uni-bochum.de/zme/Literatur/bioths99.htm. [25 February 2007].

Loff, B & Black, J. 2003. Principles for public health action on infectious diseases. *Issues of Medical Ethics*, 11(4):113–15.

National Commission for the Protection of Human Subjects of Biomedical and Behavioural Research. 1979. *The Belmont Report: ethical principles and guidelines for the protection of human subjects of research*. [Online]. Available: http://ohsr.od.nih.gov/guidelines/belmont.html. [25 February 2007].

South Africa. 2004. *National Health Act 61 of 2003*. Pretoria: Government Printer.

Uphsur, R. 2002. Principles for the justification of public health intervention. *Canadian Journal of Public Health*, 93:101–3.

Section B

Epidemiological research methods and protocol development

4   Planning a research project
5   Setting objectives for research
6   Literature review
7   Study design
8   Population and sampling
9   Data collection and measurement

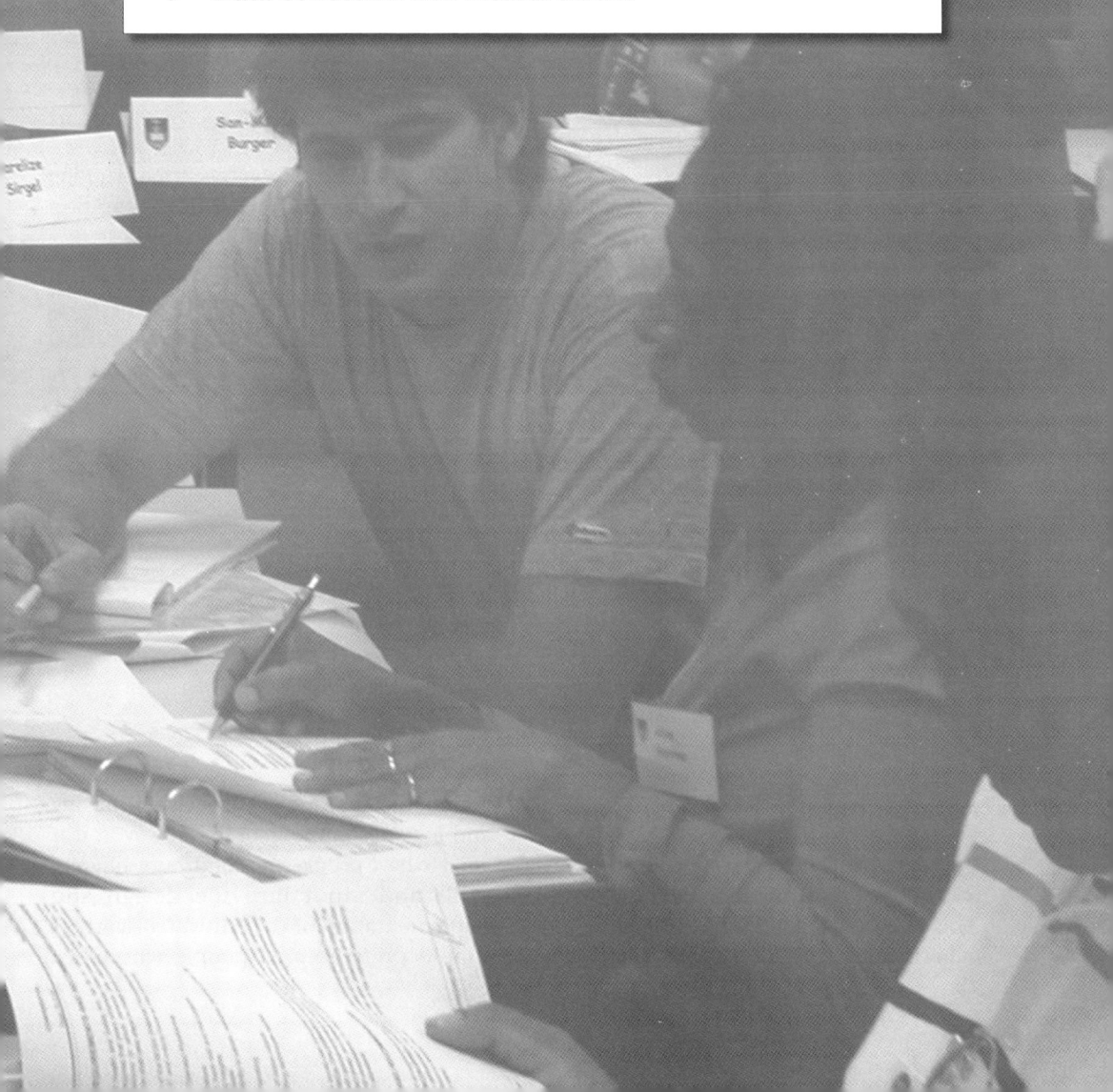

4

Planning a research project

Gina Joubert   Judy Katzenellenbogen

OBJECTIVES OF THIS CHAPTER

The objectives of this chapter are:
- to outline issues to consider in assembling a research team
- to explain the value of a well-planned research protocol
- to outline all the components of a research protocol
- to give a brief overview of bias in research.

Introduction

The research process includes planning, execution, analysis and reporting phases (Figure 4.1). This section covers the planning phase, which is the systematic preparation for a research study.

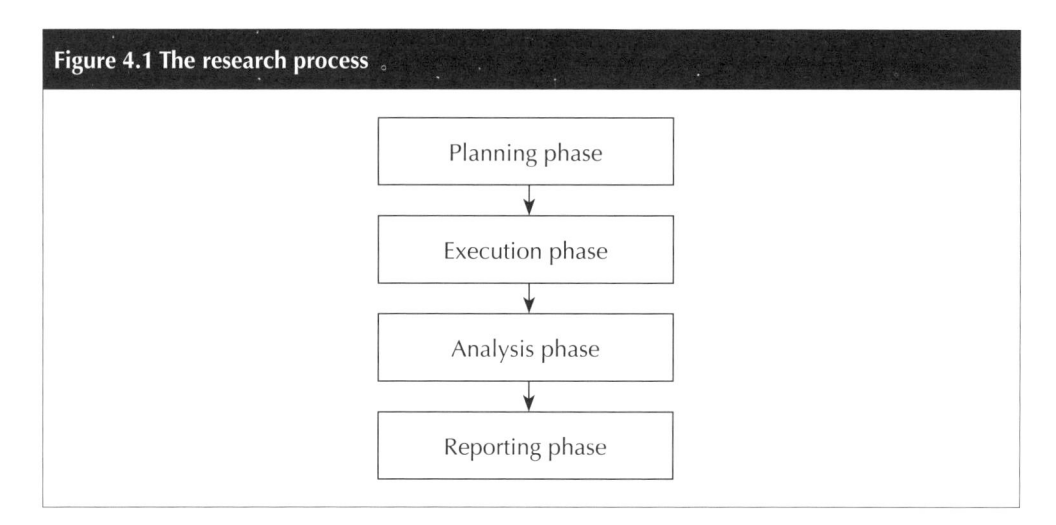

Figure 4.1 The research process

Planning phase → Execution phase → Analysis phase → Reporting phase

Assembling the research team

Epidemiological research is often done by research teams rather than by individuals. The research team should not have too many members, as this may hinder effective communication and make decision-making and logistics cumbersome. However, it is good to have people who contribute different skills and input into the design and implementation of the study. Co-workers should preferably be people whom the research leader knows will work well, are reliable, facilitate action and have good track records.

Potential users and beneficiaries (stakeholders) of the research information should be identified at the start of the project. These may include governmental and non-governmental service providers, and community-based organisations. It is important that the stakeholders closest to the unit of study should be involved; for example, village representatives and not only health department representatives, if the focus is on village level. Stakeholders should be involved in planning and where feasible could become members of the project team. (See Chapter 3, which deals with community participation.) The person who will be analysing the data should also be involved from the start since the proposed analysis of the data should form an integral part of the planning of the project.

The roles of the different team members must be spelt out to avoid duplication or omission of tasks. Researchers should be given clear areas of responsibility, for example data manager, fieldwork co-ordinator, questionnaire designer-in-chief, and sampling co-ordinator.

The team should hold regular meetings to keep everybody in touch with the study, to make joint decisions and to provide a forum for discussing concepts and understandings that are different among the different members. They will need to minute key decisions made at these meetings. They may need a memorandum of understanding or contract, particularly in a study involving more than one institution. Such a document would set out mutual responsibilities as well as the arrangements concerning rights to data, authorship, publication or presentation.

At the protocol development stage the team should discuss which team members will take responsibility for the writing up of publications resulting from the study. In this way, ambiguities and conflict about authorship can be avoided at a later stage. It should be made clear that there is no 'right' to authorship – it must be earned through intellectual contribution and work. (See http://www.publicationethics.org.uk/guidelines.)

The following two principles should be adhered to when assembling the research team:

- Try to avoid giving senior or high-profile people token co-investigator status on the project. Before the team can recognise any individual researcher as a co-investigator, that person must have a clear role and responsibilities.
- Avoid including overcommitted, uncommitted or even incompetent people who fail to do their tasks well and in time. It can be very frustrating for a group when they continually have to consider and compensate for one member's absence or failure to deliver.

The study protocol

The study protocol, sometimes called a research proposal, is a formal written document which is prepared prior to the study. It documents the background to and reasons for the study, the details of the methodology that will be used and important administrative aspects. In doing so, it gives a clear plan of exactly what will be done in the project.

The protocol is a dynamic document which keeps changing in the planning phase as the planning of the project progresses. A crude protocol might be presented in a session where colleagues review initial broad ideas and critically discuss their feasibility with the researcher. Based on input at these sessions, a more thorough and systematic protocol can be drawn up and discussed at later meetings. Changes and adaptations based on recommendations made by peers and consultants should be made so that the benefit of the peer review process is not lost. Key stakeholders in the

> **Purposes of the study protocol**
>
> The study protocol has many purposes:
> - It helps the researcher to focus on critical issues, clarify ideas and keep on track
> - It enables outsiders to understand what is planned so they can comment critically either on the written document itself, or at meetings where protocols are reviewed
> - A protocol is needed if funding is sought from funding agencies (for example the Medical Research Council)
> - A protocol needs to be submitted to an ethics committee for approval before the proposed research project can be started
> - Universities often require a protocol before confirming the registration of a student for postgraduate study
> - The protocol eventually helps in the writing up of the study since the motivation and methodology of the project are clearly described
> - A clearly written protocol enables other researchers to repeat the same design in another setting and allows for comparability of results

research should be involved in the protocol development:
- to ensure that there is agreement on the importance of the issues being studied
- to ensure that there is a commitment to act on the results; and
- to enhance participation.

Once the protocol has been accepted by an ethics committee, significant changes to the protocol, particularly those regarding subject recruitment, management or consent, have to be approved by the ethics committee.

The process of protocol development can be slow if the researcher is inexperienced, if there are few resources and consultants available, and if the area of research is a new one. However, a thorough protocol is essential for any project.

Contents of the protocol

The major headings to be used in a protocol are included in Table 4.1. A brief indication follows of what each heading covers. The main points are discussed in detail in the other chapters of this section. Various organisations have their own guidelines regarding the structure of a protocol. These structures, however, all cover the components outlined here. The protocol should describe only what is of relevance to the planned project. For example, certain studies may have many ethical issues that need to be described, while others have few. There must also be a clear theme throughout the protocol, sometimes called the 'golden thread', which links the title, the literature, the objectives and the methods to be used. Ultimately, the objectives are the hub around which the whole protocol and study revolve.

A protocol should start with a title and author's page. An informative (but not cumbersome) title which clearly describes the purpose of the study is important. This information is placed on many databases. Concise but not cryptic titles are desirable. The principal investigator's name, qualifications and institutional affiliation should then be stated. Some funding or reviewing institutions do not accept more than one principal investigator, while other institutions are more lenient. A list of co-investigators (either in order of importance to the study or in alphabetical order) with qualifications and institutional affiliations must also be included. Some ethics committees may require that the protocol should have the CVs of all investigators attached.

Table 4.1 Major headings in a protocol

Title, principal investigator, co-investigators, institutional affiliations, and qualifications

Summary/Abstract

1 Introduction
   1.1 Literature review
   1.2 Motivation for the study (problem)
   1.3 Purpose
   1.4 Specific objectives
   1.5 Implementation objectives
2 Methods
   2.1 Definition of terms
   2.2 Study design
   2.3 Study population and sampling
   2.4 Measurements
   2.5 Pilot studies
3 Logistics and time schedule
   3.1 Responsibilities of investigators
   3.2 Responsibilities of staff
   3.3 Time schedule
4 Data management and analysis
5 Resources
   5.1 Available resources
   5.2 Budget and budget motivation
6 Ethical and legal considerations
7 Reporting of results
8 References
9 Appendices

The title page is followed by a brief summary or abstract which gives the reader a general overview of the proposed study. A short statement of the purpose of the study, the major research questions to be asked or objectives pursued and the methods to be used, should be included.

Introduction: The introduction describes the problem to be studied and reviews relevant available information (referencing all sources consistently in the text, according to an accepted format). It provides the motivation for the research, and the specific research questions that are being asked. The overall purpose or aim, and specific objectives of the study should be clearly stated.

Methods: The methods section gives a comprehensive description of the methodology to be used.

- Include definition of terms which are used in a specific way in the study or which may be understood differently by different readers. Define all key terms referred to in the aim and objectives of the study. This ensures that all people reading the protocol have the same understanding. Definitions also help the researcher to clarify concepts for him- or herself.

- State which type of epidemiological study (study design) will be used to best meet the objectives.

- Identify the study population precisely with regard to sex, age, place, condition, or any other relevant factor. If sampling is to be used, describe the sampling strategy in detail. State the source of the sampling frame, and state the intended sample size (and reasons for this). (See Appendix IV for sample size calculation.)

- Specify the method of data collection (measurement), as well as the variables or characteristics to be measured. Describe measuring instruments, and provide an indication of their validity and reliability. Also indicate the desired characteristics of the people who will do the measurement and where it will be done.

- The protocol should state the intention to conduct a pilot study or briefly report on any such study which has already been carried out.

Logistics: Plan the practical logistics of the study carefully. These include clear task allocation, organisation of venues, shifts or duties, and transport. Attach a realistic approximate time schedule for carrying out

What is a pilot study?

A pilot study is a mini-study which tests part(s) of the study before the main study. Its objectives are to check the methods (for example, instruments or logistics), obtain data to assist in sample size estimation, and test the adequacy of field training. The protocol should indicate where and on how many people the pilot study will be done. Pilot data are not used in the main study.

various aspects of the study from planning to write up, and not only data collection. In particular, it is a common error to underestimate the time and effort required to recruit sufficient study subjects.

Data management and analysis: Give details of the steps in data management (such as data entry, data cleaning and ensuring data security) and data analysis (the methods of analysis, and any statistical support or advice received to date, or planned for the future). Useful additions to a protocol are 'dummy' or 'mock' tables which indicate how the final tables of results will look, i.e. with all the row and column headings in place but with no data in the table (see Table 4.2 for an example). Link the planned analyses clearly to the study objectives.

Table 4.2 Example of a dummy table describing participants' demographic characteristics

Demographic		Frequency	Percentage
Gender (n=):	Male		
	Female		
Age (n=):	15-24 years		
	25-34 years		
	35-44 years		
	45-54 years		
	55-64 years		
Highest school educational level completed (n=):	Less than Grade 8		
	Grade 8 or 9		
	Grade 10 or 11		
	Grade 12		

Resources: Record detailed estimates of personnel, equipment and financial resources (for salaries, travel costs, equipment, computing, telephone calls, stationery). An estimated budget is useful and often essential. Table 4.3 illustrates typical items in a budget. Depending on the project, we may list different items from those in the table. We must use whatever resources are available in the setting in which the research will take place. Service providers may second some health personnel to do fieldwork, and may provide some of the equipment needed. The researcher can submit a protocol to apply for research funds from the South African Medical Research Council, universities, private corporations or their social responsibility divisions and non-governmental organisations which focus on specific conditions (e.g. CANSA) or on strengthening health systems (e.g. Health Systems Trust). In recent years, there has been a large increase in international donor funding of local research. Proper timing of applications (well in advance of the desired starting date) and an understanding of the exact format required by each donor are essential.

Table 4.3 Budget for an Aids study – 1 March 2006 to 28 February 2007

A Recurrent expenses (Rand)

1. Personnel		270 000
1.1 Current employees		
Dr A (10% effort)	20 000	
Ms G (25% effort)	35 000	
Ms K (10% effort)	15 000	
1.2 To be employed		
Research officer	110 000	
Fieldworker (x 2)	80 000	
1.3 Consultants		
Dr Y (R 100 per hour)	10 000	
2. Supplies		15 500
2.1 Questionnaires (x 1 000)	2 000	
2.2 Blood collection kits (x 1 000)	12 000	
2.3 Stationery and photocopying	1 000	
2.4 Emergency first aid kit	500	
3. Travel		37 800
3.1 Lease of vehicle (x 12 months)	24 000	
3.2 Vehicle maintenance (40c per km x 18 000 km)	7 200	
3.3 Use of private vehicle (R1.10 per km x 6 000 km)	6 600	
4. Patient care costs		7 500
4.1 Hospital visits and in-patient stays	5 000	
4.2 Laboratory tests	1 500	
4.3 Drug treatments	1 000	
5. General		3 000
5.1 Cost of reprints	1 000	
5.2 Attending local conference	2 000	
Total recurrent expenses		333 800

B Capital expenses

1. Purchase of vehicle	120 000	
2. Equipment for laboratory tests	8 000	
Total capital expenses		128 000
Total direct costs		R461 800
C Administrative overhead (20%)		R92 560
TOTAL BUDGET		R554 360

Ethical and legal considerations: In the protocol, explain plans for safeguarding the rights and welfare of participants. You should specify steps which you will take to ensure ethical and legal access to communities, groups or records. In particular, describe the submission to an ethics committee and explain the method of obtaining informed consent. Other issues to be considered include permission for access, anonymity or confidentiality of data, the need for action on findings and procedures to adhere to when publishing results. Chapter 3 contains a full discussion of the ethical aspects of epidemiological research.

Reporting of the results: The protocol should state the specific format and manner in which results will be reported to the scientific community (for example conference presentations and peer-reviewed journal articles), the public in general, and particular individuals and groups. Identify target groups which can facilitate the implementation of recommendations based on the research findings. Give feedback to stakeholders directly, accessibly and promptly. For a research project to make a contribution to the solution of health problems, the researcher needs to be innovative, not only in generating new knowledge, but also in disseminating it to potential users (stakeholders), avoiding specialised terminology. Appendix III gives guidelines on how to write a report.

References: Include references, using an accepted format consistently. List only sources referred to in the protocol.

Appendices: Include in the appendices a copy of the questionnaire or data capture sheet, consent form, letter of permission and any other item needed by readers to assess quality and completeness of the intended research.

Appearance of the protocol

New researchers often have difficulty in conceiving what a protocol should look like. It should look similar to the Introduction and Methods sections of a journal article reporting on a research project. It differs from a journal article in that you must include details regarding logistics (a time schedule) and resources (a budget), as well as planned reporting of the results. In addition, you should attach examples of any relevant forms or letters.

Bias in research

Bias can enter the research process at any stage. Give special attention in the protocol to outlining how bias will be avoided at the various stages. In Chapters 7 and 12 ways of avoiding or controlling bias in specific study designs are discussed in more detail.

Defining bias

In ordinary language, bias means to favour one side against another, or prejudice. In research, bias takes on a more technical meaning, but remains true to the above definition in some ways. It is any process which produces results or conclusions that differ from the truth in a systematic (one-sided) way.

Bias can enter the research process at any stage:
- in the stage of reviewing the literature (for example, the researcher restricts articles to those that support a certain view or finding)
- in sample selection (for example, selection of non-comparable groups as cases and controls in a case-control study leads to wrong conclusions)
- in executing an intervention (for example, patients in the control group of a trial may unintentionally receive or be influenced by the intervention, thereby 'contaminating' the results)
- in measuring exposures and outcomes (for example, instruments can over- or under-score measurements taken, hiding real differences or showing differences where there are none)
- in data analysis (for example, deciding on categories into which variables are grouped after rather than before the analysis can lead to biased results)
- in interpreting the data (for example, there may be over-interpretation of results that are statistically significant but not of clinical or public health relevance)
- in publication of results (for example, the well-known tendency to publish only positive results gives a false impression of state of knowledge about the subject).

In this manual, we give attention to biases which can occur in the selection process (selection bias) or data collection process (measurement or information bias), and those which are due to confounding. We discuss these biases in detail in Chapter 12.

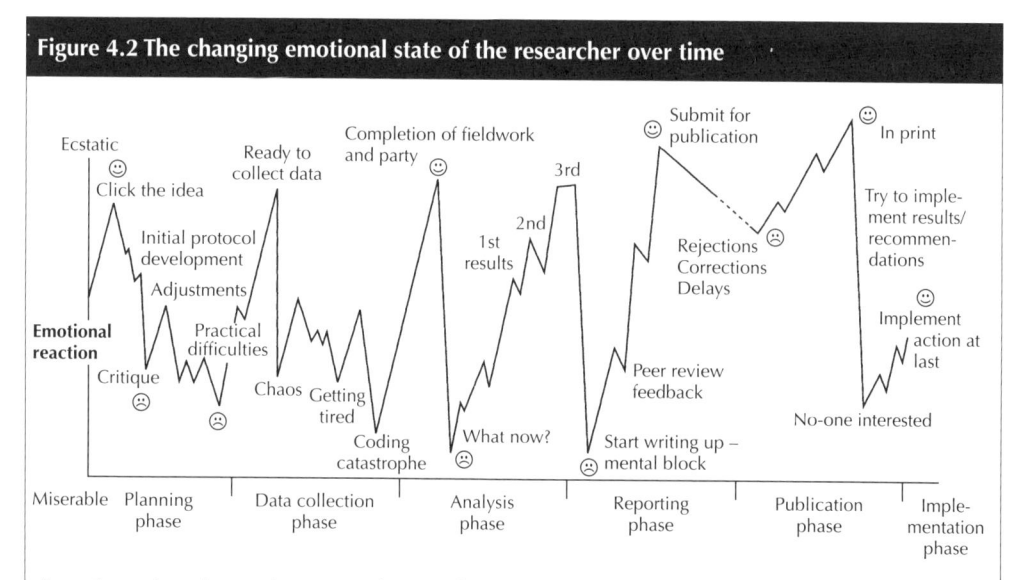

Figure 4.2 The changing emotional state of the researcher over time

Experience has shown that researchers undergo similar patterns of emotions while involved with any research project. Each stage of the research process tends to start on a positive note, but inevitably obstacles arise, with each stage having its own set of difficulties. Problem-solving abilities and persistence are tested to the utmost. Beginner researchers should note that once the fieldwork is completed, there is still a lot of work to be done.

The above graphic describes emotional reactions (Y axis) to typical events during the different phases of a study (X axis). It aims to help the researcher anticipate some of the emotional swings so that when (not if!) they occur, difficulties can be seen to fit into a common pattern.

Once present in the data, bias is difficult to deal with and it is well worth the effort to be cautious in the protocol design phase in order to avoid bias wherever possible.

Conclusion

However well a study is planned, difficulties do arise. Epidemiological research does not take place in an isolated, structured environment like a laboratory, and so the chances are high that something unforeseen will happen.

The development and completion of the protocol are merely the beginning of an often rather difficult emotional experience for the researcher. Figure 4.2 describes some of the ups and downs that researchers can anticipate during the different phases of research. The many ups experienced should compensate for the downs.

The other chapters in this section will describe the elements of the research process in detail. These include setting objectives for a study, literature review, study design, study population and sampling, and measurement.

Useful web site

Committee on Publication Ethics (COPE). *Guidelines on good publication practice.* [Online]. Available: http://www.publicationethics.org.uk/guidelines. [25 February 2007].

5

Setting objectives for research

Judy Katzenellenbogen

OBJECTIVES OF THIS CHAPTER

The objectives of this chapter are:
- to encourage a critical analysis of the health issue or problem being studied
- to assist potential researchers in narrowing the scope of their study
- to describe a step-wise process of formulating research objectives
- to highlight the link between study objectives and study design.

Introduction

Every research protocol must state what the intended study wants to achieve. The process of deciding on the research question might be lengthy, but is an extremely important one as it lays the foundation of the protocol before the methodological detail of the study is planned.

Steps to formulating research objectives

Most researchers use a similar step-wise approach to formulate research objectives, but they do not always call the steps by the same names. In particular, step 2 below may be referred to as setting the purpose, aim or general objective of the study. These all mean more or less the same thing in this context. It is therefore more important to understand the content of the steps than worry about the terminology. However, we should learn the convention used in our local context, e.g. in writing a dissertation or submitting a protocol for approval.

Step 1: Identification and analysis of the research problem

Just as necessity leads to invention, so a population health problem leads to population health research. However, prospective researchers often decide on a topic without thoroughly considering the original problem motivating the investigation or the most pressing information needs, and therefore skip an essential step in the process of identifying objectives.

Since a public health problem can be broad and complex, it is important for us to come to grips with all aspects of the problem before deciding on the focus and scope of our specific project. Exploring the problem thoroughly can help us to identify a suitable topic or research question.

B

> ### The value of critical thinking
>
> Any problem, whether it is a health system problem (for example, the clinic is crowded; why? what can be done about it?) or a problem relating to the relationship between exposure and outcome (for example, does smoking cause lung cancer?), should be broken down systematically into its major components so that the problem may be viewed critically.
>
> It is therefore important to develop skills in critical thinking. Such skills enable one to look at problems in such a way that preconceptions are put aside, and to consider issues beyond face value, from all angles, acknowledging complexities. This should lead to a better understanding and a clearer idea of which aspects of the problem would be most appropriate to tackle initially. Critical thinking is not a skill needed for research only – it is essential for any task requiring a good grasp of the problem and planning for effective action.

David Werner, community development theorist and health activist, has emphasised the need to develop a critical understanding of health issues. A much-used tool to facilitate critical thinking is the 'why' game (Werner & Bower, 1991). We use a South African example to illustrate the game and how it can help develop a critical understanding of health problems.

> ### The 'why' game
>
> Consider the following scenario in an informal settlement setting:
>
> ```
> [3-year old Sipho plays in stagnant water] → [gets diarrhoea]
>                                                     ↓
> [Sipho dies on the way to hospital] ← [mother tries to care for him at home giving an enema]
> ```
>
> Starting with the first event circled (that is, Sipho playing in stagnant water), we should ask the question 'why?' and put our response in a circle with an arrow pointing towards the event. There may be a number of reasons for Sipho playing in stagnant water; we should add these to the diagram. It is useful to generate as many reasons as possible. Now for each reason generated, we must ask 'why?' and put our second-generation reasons in circles with arrows pointing to the circles they 'caused'. We should keep on asking 'why?' to each response (i.e. brainstorm) until we run out of ideas.
>
> This process is repeated for each of the events. We may return a few times to earlier 'whys' as we gain momentum and get new ideas. Some of the events have similar causes, so these common causes should be linked with arrows.

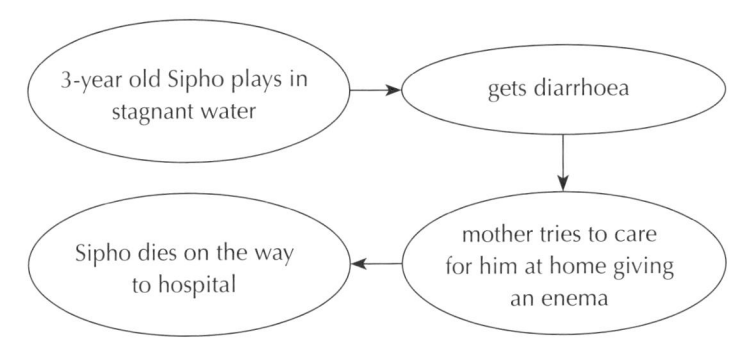

It would be useful for readers to do this exercise before going on to the next paragraph.

Once the 'why?' process has been exhausted, it is useful to present the analysis in a clearer, more systematic way. This can be done by organising factors and causes into larger categories such as political factors, socioeconomic factors, health service factors, disease-related factors and so on. The choice of categories is up to us, but they should flow from the 'reasons' generated in the problem analysis. We should now be able to give a critical analysis of possible reasons why Sipho died. Table 5.1 shows the factors which may have contributed to his death.

In the early planning stage of a research project, we often do not have a series of events to analyse, but a central issue or problem. The same process of asking 'why' can be undertaken in exploring the central problem, for example, the high incidence of unplanned teenage pregnancy or the high HIV transmission rate.

Table 5.1 Factors emerging from the 'why' game that appear to be related to Sipho's death

Environmental factors
- poor housing
- poor (or absent) sewage system
- poor drainage
- poor roads and layout of township
- inadequate water supply
- no recreational facilities (safe and hygienic play areas)

Service-related factors
- no 24-hour health service in the community
- hospital inaccessible
- poor transport system
- poor health education of mothers concerning causes and treatment of diarrhoea
- poor planning, budgeting, and implementation of primary health care policy

Disease-related factors
- water-borne disease
- virulent virus or bacterium
- virus/bacterium induces diarrhoea and vomiting, resulting in dehydration of the child
- if child malnourished, the illness is more severe and compromising to the child
- if untreated, child can die from dehydration

Socioeconomic factors
- high cost of living coupled with low salary or unemployment
- extreme poverty affecting Sipho's life through malnutrition
- low maternal education

Cultural factors
- high fertility considered desirable, thus large family size
- some traditional practices harmful when child has diarrhoea (enema)

Political factors
- maldistribution of land and wealth created and reinforced by past political regimes
- despite the political will to improve the quality of life for all South Africans, change on the ground is slow
- economic constraints exist which prevent the government from rectifying social and economic imbalances in the short term

B | Epidemiological research methods and protocol development

It is important to do part of the problem exploration with colleagues and to consult the literature – outside information and ideas always help us to find further factors and question our own preconceived ideas.

Figures 5.1 and 5.2 below are illustrations of analyses of two health problems which are commonly of concern in South Africa. Note that the same process was undertaken, but that the diagrams represent the end-product after all the messy and challenging work of asking 'why?' has been completed.

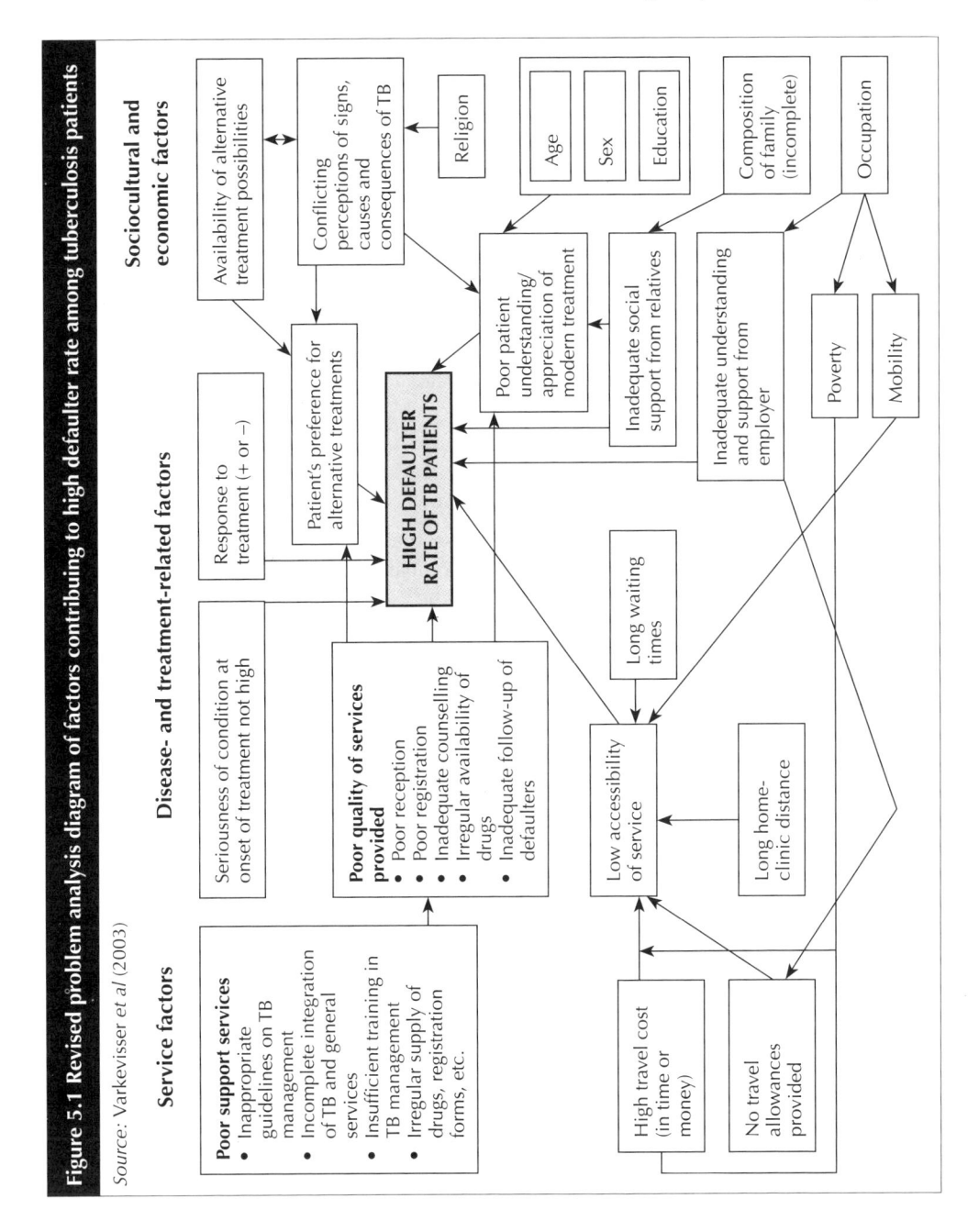

Figure 5.1 Revised problem analysis diagram of factors contributing to high defaulter rate among tuberculosis patients

Source: Varkevisser et al (2003)

Setting objectives for research

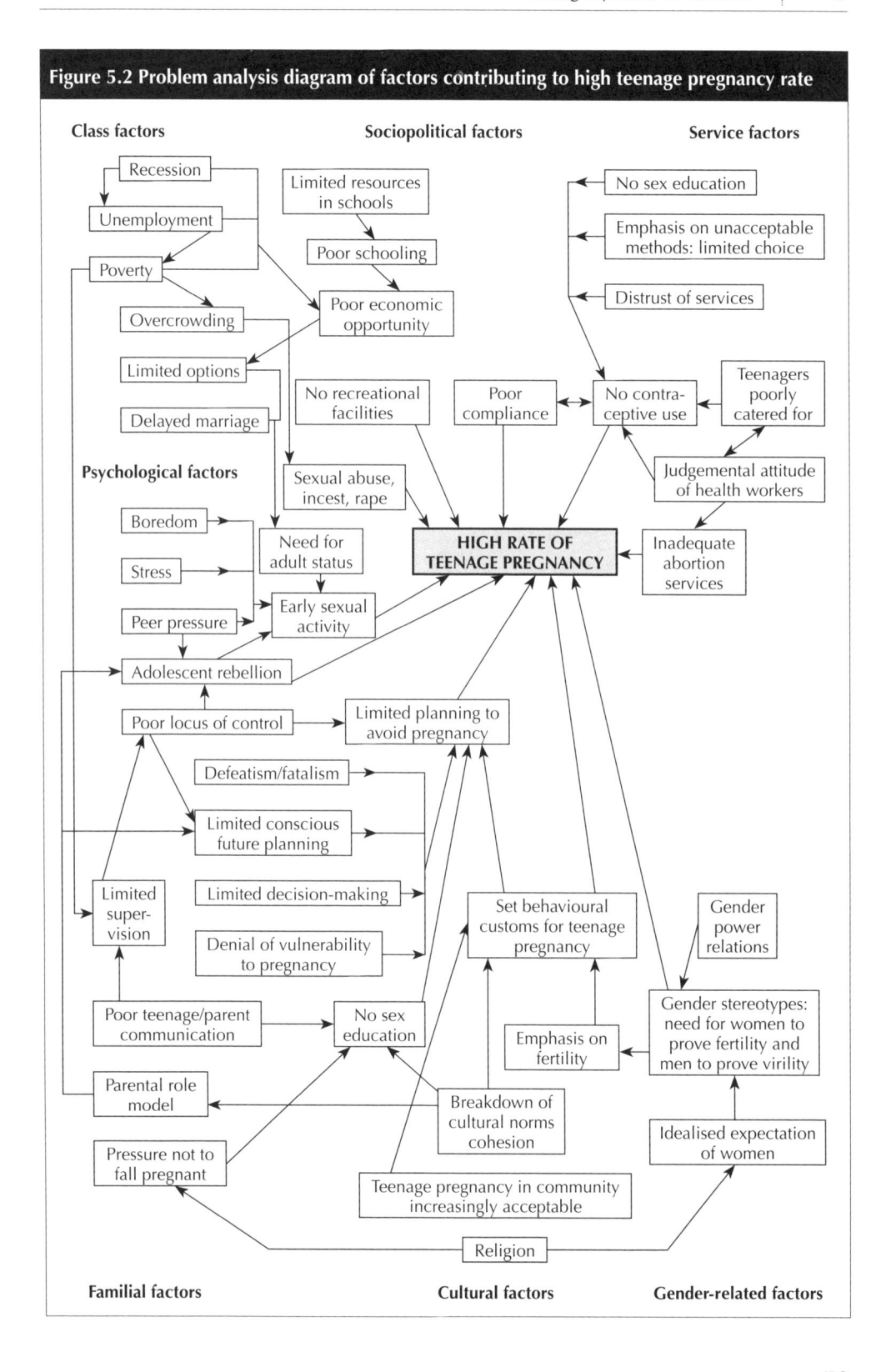

Figure 5.2 Problem analysis diagram of factors contributing to high teenage pregnancy rate

The problem exploration process does not automatically suggest a research topic or question. Instead, it improves understanding of the problem and the multiple factors which influence it. It helps to isolate the component of the problem that the researcher wants to study. The exact research question depends on existing knowledge (including descriptive information about the size of the problem, whom it affects, where and when it occurs), what other studies have been done, what is feasible to do given logistics, money and resources, and the possible usefulness of results yielded by the proposed study. Consultation with people in the field of application – clinicians, managers, decision makers and communities – can enhance the relevance of the research outside the research or academic environment.

Step 2: Explicit statement of the purpose or aim of the study

Once we have explored the central problem fully, we need to decide on and state explicitly the focus or topic of study. This step therefore involves detailing the purpose, aim or intent of the study, including what information the study hopes to gather. The statement of purpose of the study should preferably be no longer than one sentence, but this sentence must state clearly and precisely what the most important contribution of this study will be. The purpose serves as a reference point by which the relevance of each specific objective (see Step 3) will be measured.

The purpose of the study

The purpose is the part of the protocol that many people will read before deciding whether to read the whole protocol. The purpose is not a general statement of the problem; rather it is a specific (not woolly or vague) statement which articulates the main issue being described or the central hypothesis being tested.

Vague statements of purpose lead to vague studies. The purpose is a statement of the exact 'destination' that we want to reach with the study: the methods are the 'road' we will take to get there. Exactness in the purpose requires deep consideration of the problem which motivated the study and a clear decision to restrict the study to one key aspect of the problem or its solution.

We may express the purpose in the form of a statement that is as specific as possible, using action verbs (for example, 'To determine the incidence of diarrhoea among children under five in the summer months in Mamelodi') or in the form of a question (for example, 'What proportion of Mamelodi children get diarrhoea during the summer months?').

Here are some examples of vague versus explicit purpose statements.

Vague purpose statements:
- to study the problem of measles in South Africa.
- to investigate alcohol consumption as a contributor to adult mortality
- to determine the health profile of the Mamelodi community.

Carefully considered purpose statements:
- to study trends in measles notifications in South Africa from 1985 to 2005
- to determine the proportion of adult deaths that are due to alcohol-related conditions in the period 2000-2002
- to determine the nutritional status of children under five years of age in Mamelodi.

In practice, the process of narrowing the focus of study from all the components and aspects of the problem to a clear, definable and achievable purpose is not easy. It is at this stage of the research process that initial contact can be made with experienced researchers, supervisors or tutors who could assist in this process.

Usually, the general problem as defined and explored can give rise to many possible research questions which each needs study. So in order to do full justice to researching the problem, we may need to carry out a number of studies over a period of time, each contributing to the overall understanding of the problem and consequently to the solution.

Generally, in a single study we should attempt to answer only one or at the most two research questions. It is more useful to be able to answer one or two questions well than to provide inconclusive information on a broad range of questions. The researcher needs to be patient and systematic, and humble in recognising that one research project will not solve an entire health problem.

How studies can arise out of exploring a problem

We will use the Sipho scenario described earlier to illustrate how a particular public health problem can give rise to a number of separate studies, each with their own purpose, aim or topic, but still relating to the overall problem described.

Studies arising from the Sipho scenario:

1. To describe the availability of running water, storm water drainage, and water storage practices in the informal settlement.
2. To determine access to and utilisation of primary, secondary and tertiary child health services among mothers of pre-school children in the informal settlement.
3. To determine childhood mortality rates in the informal settlement, by cause, age group and season.
4. To determine prevalence of malnutrition among children under five years in the community.
5. To describe knowledge, attitudes and practices of child caregivers concerning diarrhoea and its treatment.
6. To compare the childhood mortality in communities with and without piped water.
7. To determine the socioeconomic risk factors for diarrhoea.
8. To investigate maternal education as a risk factor for death among children who get diarrhoea.
9. To compare the diarrhoea mortality in a community before and after the introduction of piped water into that community.
10. To evaluate the effect of a community health worker programme focusing on appropriate treatment by mothers of children with diarrhoea.
11. To evaluate the effectiveness of different methods of rehydration in a hospital setting.

The above represent some of the studies emerging from the problem exploration done in this case. If no descriptive information is available and there is therefore a need for numbers and frequencies of characteristics related to the problem, we should undertake one of the first five studies. If there is enough basic information, but a need to understand more about what may be contributing to the problem, we should undertake studies asking questions similar to numbers 6, 7 or 8. If there is good understanding of the causes of the problem, then we should carry out studies to evaluate interventions designed to reduce the problem (numbers 9 to 11).

Step 3: Setting specific objectives (or study hypotheses)

One should start by breaking down the purpose or aim of a study into clear, mutually exclusive objectives which are logically connected. To a large extent, these determine the subsequent planning of the study. Objectives indicate the specific information the study must yield and the detailed research questions that must be answered. They are often stated in operational terms which can be applied in practice. They are also commonly phrased in measurable terms (in such a way that the answer is a number or rate) that are clear and unambiguous. Specific objectives identify the individual components of what will be achieved (but not how it is to be done; that is left for the methods section of the protocol).

Descriptive studies usually set out to describe characteristics of the group being investigated, and the statistical goal is usually simple data description or estimation of a characteristic in the study population (see Chapter 7). For example, in a study of the reproductive and occupational health of female street vendors in Johannesburg, the specific objectives were to describe the demographic profile of the vendors (age, education, region or country of birth), the occupational profile (percentage self-employed, type of work, income, occupational risks), fertility, contraceptive use, prevalence of occupation-related conditions, satisfaction with work environment and experience or threat of theft, physical or verbal abuse (Pick *et al*, 2002).

In analytical studies, the objectives are to examine associations between risk factors and disease and to seek new knowledge on the cause(s) and natural history of diseases or conditions. Finally, intervention studies attempt to determine if a specific intervention is associated with an improvement (or deterioration) in health status. Analytical and intervention studies therefore always involve hypotheses or predictions of a relationship between a factor (or factors) and the outcome under study. The hypothesis or prediction is statistically tested after relevant information has been collected and analysed, and the hypothesis is either rejected or not rejected.

What is the research hypothesis?

The research hypothesis or question is the prediction or supposition which motivates the study. Once we have framed the question or hypothesis, we should state the hypothesis in such a way that it can be tested by appropriate statistics once the data have been gathered. This final statement of the hypothesis is called the statistical hypothesis, a statement in mathematical terms. For example, we would frame the research question: 'Is there an association between educational level and food hygiene practice?' in statistical terminology to enable us to use the appropriate statistical test to test for a difference in median educational level. The statistical hypothesis is typically stated as one of no difference – the so-called *null hypothesis*. In this case it would be 'there is no difference in the median education level of people who practise "good" versus "bad" hygiene'.

Step 4: Implementation objectives

It is important to link research to policy and action. The protocol should state what will be done with the research results and describe strategies to ensure that the results are appropriately communicated. This links with 'why' the study is being done. Decision-makers, service providers, and possible benefactors should be consulted early to clarify the implementation objectives of the study, and to try to ensure that results are more likely to be read and acted upon appropriately.

Conclusion

Exploration of the problem motivating the research helps the researcher to get both a broad and a critical view of the issues related to the central problem identified. Setting objectives for the study is an important (and often difficult) part of the research process, as it helps to focus the study by describing exactly what it hopes to achieve. It helps to break the study into different steps, and acts as a guide during the design of the methods and all subsequent parts of the project.

EXAMPLE 5.1

Setting research objectives: high death rate of children like Sipho

Step 1: *The problem* (what is motivating the study?)

Sipho's death which was explored at the beginning of the chapter (see Table 5.1).

Step 2: *The purpose or aim of the study* (overall topic of a particular study, chosen from a number of possible topics)

To identify risk factors for diarrhoea and diarrhoea mortality among pre-school children (under the age of six years) in Khayelitsha, Cape Town.

Step 3: *Specific objectives* (specific information the study will yield, linked to the purpose or aim)

To ascertain which of the following factors are associated with diarrhoea and diarrhoea mortality:
- Factors related to water: distance to nearest tap, quality of water used.
- Personal factors: mother's hygiene practices, mother's level of education, mother's knowledge of causes and prevention of diarrhoea and dehydration.
- Environmental factors: method of water storage, location of toilet, site of refuse disposal.
- Socioeconomic factors: availability of sugar and salt for oral rehydration solution, ability to afford transport to health services.
- Health service factors: distance from home, opening times, cost of services, consultation of traditional healer.

Step 4: *Implementation objectives*

To make recommendations for interventions targeted at reducing the incidence of and mortality as a result of diarrhoea, based on the results of the study.

Reference:

Adapted from Vundule, C. 1994. *A study on the risk factors for diarrhoea in Khayelitsha, a peri-urban settlement area in the Western Cape.* Epidemiology research report, Department of Community Health, University of Cape Town.

EXAMPLE 5.2

Setting research objectives: interventions regarding safe sex

Step 1: *The problem* (what is motivating the study?)

There is an Aids epidemic worldwide and particularly in Africa. The concurrent existence of HIV and sexually transmitted infections (STIs) renders infected individuals more infective to their sexual partners. In addition, both conditions are transmitted mainly through unprotected sexual activity. Their prevention requires interventions that increase knowledge and awareness of the disease and its causes, cultivate attitudes and social norms that are conducive to healthy and preventive behaviours, and increase the intention to practise such behaviours.

Step 2: *The purpose or aim* (overall topic of a particular study, chosen from a number of possible topics)

Given the above problem, some of the following purposes or aims could be appropriate for the study:
- to determine the behavioural practices related to STIs and Aids (in different target groups)
- to investigate psychological factors associated with sexual behaviour change (in different target groups)
- to determine access to condoms (in different target groups)
- to evaluate safe sex education techniques/programmes
- to determine difficulties in implementing new safe sex education programmes
- to determine factors related to the receptiveness (of different groups) to safe sex health education programmes.

Step 3: *Specific objectives* (specific information the study will yield, linked to the aim)

Assume that the aim chosen for study relates to evaluating safe sex education programmes/techniques:

To test the hypothesis that a single reading by secondary school students in Kwazulu-Natal of a print media intervention called *Laduma* will lead to a change in their knowledge and behaviour regarding STIs and safe sex.

The following specific objectives may be stated:
- to test for an increase in knowledge about STIs after reading *Laduma*
- to test for a more positive attitude towards safe sexual behaviour (abstinence and use of condoms)
- to test for more communication about safe sexual behaviour with partners, parents and peers
- to test for increased intentions to practise safe sexual behaviour.

Step 4: *Implementation objectives*

To make recommendations to education authorities concerning health education in schools regarding sexual behaviour, specifically as to whether the intervention is worth implementing or not.

> *Reference:*
> James, S, Reddy, P, Ruiter, R, Taylor, M, Jinabhai, C, Van Empelen, P & Van Den Borne, B. 2005. The effects of a systematically developed photo-novella on knowledge, attitudes, communication and behavioural intentions with respect to sexually transmitted infections among secondary school learners in South Africa. *Health Promotion International*, 20(2):157–65.

References used in this chapter

Pick, WM, Ross, MH & Dada, Y. 2002. The reproductive and occupational health of women street vendors in Johannesburg, South Africa. *Social Science and Medicine*, 54(2):193–204.

Varkevisser, CM, Pathmanathan, AB & Brownlee, A. 2003. *Designing and conducting health systems research projects.* 2nd rev ed. Amsterdam: KIT Publishers; Ottawa: International Development Research Centre. Reprinted with permission of IDRC.

Werner, D & Bower, B. 1991. *Helping health workers learn.* Palo Alto: Hesperian Foundation.

6

Literature review

Jimmy Volmink

> **OBJECTIVES OF THIS CHAPTER**
>
> The objectives of this chapter are:
> - to describe the different functions that a literature review can serve
> - to provide guidelines on how to conduct a literature review
> - to outline some important issues in writing up the findings of a literature review.

Introduction

> **Review of literature**
>
> Review of literature is the process of taking stock of existing knowledge in order to make informed choices about policy, practice, research direction and resource allocation (Chalmers, 2003). A literature review usually forms part of a research protocol, thesis, grant application or research publication, but may also be a stand alone activity.
>
> As the name suggests a literature review is a 're'-view or 'further look' at what has previously been written on a particular subject. Ideally, it should not be merely a summary of previous findings but should involve a critical examination and synthesis of existing reports. A literature review is therefore intended to convey to the reader the current state of knowledge on a given subject along with the strengths and limitations of the underlying research. Literature reviews are sometimes referred to as 'research syntheses,' 'overviews,' or 'secondary research.' Recently, a distinction has been drawn between reviews that employ informal, subjective methods ('traditional reviews') and those that use more explicit and reproducible methods to collect and interpret information ('systematic reviews') (Egger *et al*, 2001).

Functions of literature reviews

A literature review can serve a number of different functions (Chalmers, 2003; Egger *et al*, 2001).

1. Justification of future research

When researchers (and funders) do not pay sufficient attention to what is already known, research is undertaken on questions that have already been answered. While 'repeating' research in a new context is sometimes justified, unnecessary duplication is unethical because it offers no benefits to study participants (while potentially increasing the risk of harm) and wastes scarce resources. All new research should therefore be justified by means of an adequate review of the literature showing what gaps in knowledge the proposed research intends to fill.

2. Putting new findings into context

Science is meant to be cumulative in the sense that new findings must be related to what has gone before (see Table 6.1 below). This could entail adding to or overturning established knowledge. The results of any new study must therefore be interpreted in the light of existing knowledge.

3. Making sense of research

Readers are often bewildered by the apparently conflicting findings of studies claiming to answer the same question. This variation in study findings can arise from a host of factors including differences in study design, participants, interventions and outcomes as well as various types of error. By evaluating the influence of these factors on the results of primary studies, literature reviews contribute to deciphering and interpreting research.

4. Coping with information overload

The volume of health information has increased massively over the past half century and this trend is likely to continue in the future. Currently some two million articles are published annually in more than 20 000 biomedical journals. In addition, much useful scientific information is located in 'grey literature' (e.g. books, theses, conference abstracts, government and company reports, and other unpublished material) and on the Internet. As researchers, practitioners, policy-makers and other consumers of health information do not have time to read and digest the relevant primary research material in their fields of interest, they rely on literature reviews to keep up to date.

5. Facilitating access to relevant research

Access to research is often haphazard or biased. For instance, it has been shown that studies with 'negative' or 'disappointing' findings are less likely to be published. If they are, they are less likely than 'positive' studies to be published in full, in journals that are widely read, or in English. They are therefore less likely to be cited in reports of subsequent studies. By using comprehensive methods to search for all relevant published and unpublished literature, good literature reviews reduce bias resulting from selective reporting of research.

Table 6.1 The cumulative nature of science

Source: Egger *et al* (2001)

"... If, as is sometimes supposed, science consisted in nothing but the laborious accumulation of facts, it would soon come to a standstill, crushed, as it were, under its own weight ..."

"... Two processes are ... at work side by side, the reception of new material and the digestion and assimilation of the old; and as both are essential we may spare ourselves the discussion of their relative importance ..."

"... The work which deserves, but I am afraid does not always receive, the most credit is that in which discovery and explanation go hand in hand, in which not only are new facts presented, but their relation to old ones is pointed out."

(Lord Rayleigh, Professor of Physics, University of Cambridge, Presidential Address to the meeting of the British Association for the Advancement of Science in Montreal, 1884.)

All research protocols should include a brief literature review. Typically this will serve function 1 above, i.e. to show how the research will answer a question or add to knowledge. When writing up the findings of the research, functions 2 and 3 above apply.

How to conduct a literature review

Format of a literature review

The format of a literature review will depend on the reason for which the review is being undertaken. It may take the form of an overview of research relevant to a broad topic (e.g. studies that report on the diagnosis and management of rheumatic fever) or provide a more focused synthesis (e.g. the most reliable evidence on the effect of BCG vaccine in preventing tuberculosis).

Regardless of the type of literature review, careful thought and planning are required to ensure that a true picture of the underlying research is provided.

In the past many reviewers used subjective and opportunistic methods in synthesising research. There is good evidence that this traditional approach may be biased, leading to false conclusions with potentially serious consequences (Antman *et al*, 1992) (Table 6.2).

Table 6.2 Some shortcomings of traditional reviews

Systematic error (bias) from:
- incomplete literature searches, e.g. only English language studies indexed in one electronic database such as Medline
- selective inclusion of studies, e.g. only those with findings that confirm what the reviewer has found in his/her own studies
- insufficient attention given to study quality e.g. use of inappropriate study designs or studies with flawed methods

Random error (play of chance):
- insufficient attention given to sample size

To address this problem the *systematic review* has been introduced. Systematic reviews apply methods similar to those used in primary research to limit bias and the effects of chance (Chalmers, 2003). (See Table 6.3 below.) In the field of health care, organisations such as the Cochrane Collaboration (http://www.cochrane.org/) (Table 6.4) have long championed their wide-scale adoption as the gold standard for literature reviews. More recently a similar global initiative, the Campbell Collaboration, has started to prepare systematic reviews of the effects of educational, social and legal interventions (http://www.campbellcollaboration.org/).

It is important to realise that conducting a systematic review is not a trivial exercise as it requires appropriate skills, plenty of time and frequently some financial support. Preparing a fully fledged systematic review, as outlined in Table 6.3, will therefore not always be feasible. Nonetheless, the steps provided in Table 6.3 can serve as a valuable guide for anyone who would like to conduct a good literature review. The following

Literature review **6**

Table 6.3 What is a systematic review?

Source: Moher *et al* (1999)

Definition
'A review in which bias has been reduced by the systematic identification, appraisal, synthesis, and, if relevant, statistical aggregation of all relevant studies on a specific topic according to a predetermined and explicit method.'

Steps involved in conducting a systematic review:
1. State the objectives of the synthesis
2. Define eligibility criteria for studies to be included
3. Identify (all) potentially eligible studies
4. Apply eligibility criteria
5. Assess study quality
6. Assemble the most complete dataset feasible
7. Analyse this dataset, using statistical synthesis (meta-analysis) and sensitivity analyses, if appropriate and possible
8. Prepare a structured report of the research

Table 6.4 The Cochrane Collaboration

Source: Cochrane Collaboration (http://www.cochrane.org/)

An international, non-profit organisation that provides an infrastructure for producing up-to-date systematic reviews of the effects of health care interventions.

Cochrane reviews are published electronically and are periodically modified in the light of new data, criticisms, and methodological advances.

---

section presents the key questions to consider before embarking upon a literature review.

1. What question(s) will my review address?

A literature review can address either one question or a few related ones. Given that the review question drives the search for literature, it should not be surprising that the manner in which the question is formulated can have a large impact on the efficiency of the process. Consider the following: 'Is adopting a policy of directly observed treatment good for people with tuberculosis?' A question framed in such an unfocused manner will usually lead to the reviewer finding a large amount of potentially relevant research material and spending many hours sifting through this material in order to find studies that address the question he or she would like to answer.

Application of the 'PICO' method in constructing review questions

Formulating a focused question takes some practice and experience but using the 'PICO method' can be very helpful (Sackett *et al*, 2000). This method requires that at least three of the following components be included in the review question: participants (population), intervention (or indicator), comparator (control) and outcome. The following example illustrates the use of the

> PICO method in constructing the review question: 'In people receiving treatment for clinical tuberculosis (P) does a policy of direct observation of treatment (I) versus a policy of self-treatment (C) lead to different cure and/or treatment completion rates (O)?' The PICO method does not apply only to questions about the effects of interventions. For instance, in relation to aetiology or risk one may ask: 'Are women (P) who smoke during pregnancy (I) compared to women who do not smoke (C) more likely to give birth to children who develop asthma during the first 5 years of Life (O)?'

Formulating a proper review question is perhaps the most important step in conducting a literature review. Regardless of the type of question involved (aetiology, frequency or effectiveness), using the PICO method will make it easier to find answers to the questions in the literature.

2. What criteria will I use to determine study eligibility?

Before conducting the search for relevant studies the reviewer must decide what types of studies will be eligible for inclusion in the review. The 'PICO' method can be used to guide this decision. In addition to the four 'PICO' components mentioned above a decision must be made about whether or not the review will be limited to certain types of study design. For instance, it may be appropriate to limit the review to randomised trials in the case of questions about the effects of an intervention, to cross-sectional studies for estimates of prevalence, or to case-control and cohort studies if the intention is to answer a question about aetiology. (See Chapter 7.)

3. How will I identify relevant studies?

When conducting a systematic review a literature search is conducted that aims to identify as comprehensive a list as possible of primary research articles that meet pre-specified inclusion criteria. However, it may not always be feasible or necessary to conduct an exhaustive search of published and unpublished studies relevant to the review question. For instance, when a student is writing a literature review as part of a study protocol, it would be acceptable for him or her simply to include a reasonably representative sample of all relevant studies. This should provide sufficient information to highlight the most important issues, to comment on the strengths and limitations of previous research, and to contextualise the planned research project.

In all cases, such a protocol should give some background to the problem being researched. If literature on the subject is scarce, the gaps in knowledge can be highlighted by pointing to the few studies that have been done and their limitations. To highlight methodological issues, we could cite studies using similar methods to the one being planned. If the methods used are new or complex, a consideration of what has been written about the validity and reliability of such methods should form part of the review.

Regardless of the type of literature review, it is recommended that a list of potential sources of literature be compiled prior to beginning the search. For practical purposes, laborious, paper-based searching, the mainstay of literature searching in the past, has been replaced by rapid, electronic searching of various bibliographic databases. In the health and biomedical sciences MEDLINE (Medical Literature Analysis and Retrieval System Online) is the best known and most comprehensive source of literature. Compiled by the National Library of Medicine (NLM) in the United States, this database includes records from nearly 5 000 selected publications (mostly English language journals) published from 1966 onwards.

MEDLINE searching

MEDLINE searching is available free of charge via the PubMed search engine which forms part of the NLM's *Entrez* information retrieval system. A MEDLINE or PubMed search yields a list of citations (including authors, title, source, and often an abstract) to journal articles. PubMed includes over 16 million citations from MEDLINE and other life science journals for biomedical articles back to the 1950s. MEDLINE information is also available at a fee through private vendors such as Ovid and Silver Platter.

Bear in mind that MEDLINE is not the only important source of health and biomedical literature. Other popular electronic sources include EMBASE (especially for pharmaceutical studies), CINAHL (studies relevant to the nursing field) and the Cochrane Library (for clinical trials).

Optimal search strategies for finding studies differ for various bibliographic databases. In general they combine subject-specific terms (e.g. smoking, pregnancy) and methodological terms (e.g. cohort studies, case-control studies). The researcher must understand and utilise these strategies in order to perform an optimal literature search. Figure 6.1 presents an actual example of how we might conduct a search in PubMed for studies

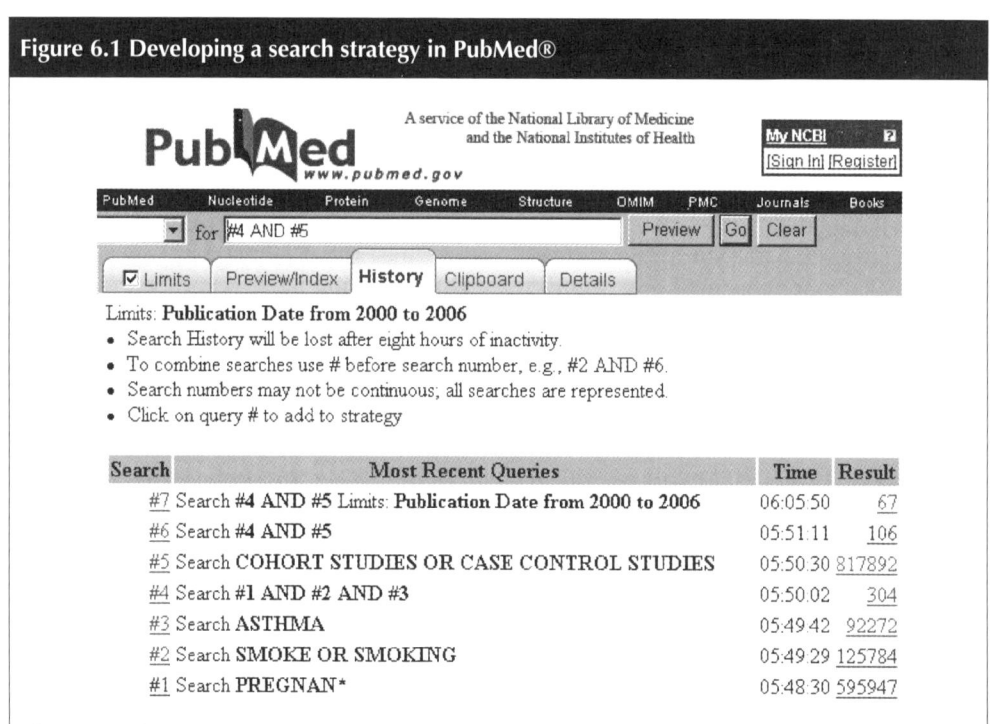

Figure 6.1 Developing a search strategy in PubMed®

Limits: **Publication Date from 2000 to 2006**
- Search History will be lost after eight hours of inactivity.
- To combine searches use # before search number, e.g., #2 AND #6.
- Search numbers may not be continuous; all searches are represented.
- Click on query # to add to strategy

Search	Most Recent Queries	Time	Result
#7	Search #4 AND #5 Limits: **Publication Date from 2000 to 2006**	06:05:50	67
#6	Search #4 AND #5	05:51:11	106
#5	Search COHORT STUDIES OR CASE CONTROL STUDIES	05:50:30	817892
#4	Search #1 AND #2 AND #3	05:50:02	304
#3	Search ASTHMA	05:49:42	92272
#2	Search SMOKE OR SMOKING	05:49:29	125784
#1	Search PREGNAN*	05:48:30	595947

The History function is a good way of combining different searches to maximise your search effiency. The above search strategy shows how you can broaden your search using 'OR' and narrow it using 'AND'. Placing an asterisk (*) at the end of Pregnan* will search for pregnant, pregnancy and pregnancies. Your search can further be limited to publication type i.e. cohort studies and to publication date i.e. 2000 to 2006. Note that PubMed displays the search strategy in descending order.
[Courtesy of Karishma Busgeeth, South African Cochrane Centre, MRC]

that address the question of smoking and pregnancy mentioned in a previous part of this chapter. For further guidance on how to conduct electronic searches we should seek assistance from someone trained in searching the literature, such as a librarian.

4. How will I appraise included studies for validity?

> **Clearing away received dogma**
>
> In his *Treatise on Scurvy* in 1753, the Scots naval surgeon James Lind wrote (Stewart & Guthrie, 1953):
>
> *'As it is no easy matter to root out prejudices, … it became requisite to exhibit a full and impartial view of what had hitherto been published on scurvy, and that in a chronological order, by which the sources of these mistakes may be detected. Indeed, before the subject could be set in a clear and proper light, it was necessary to remove a great deal of rubbish.'*

These words remain apt today as studies still abound in which findings have been seriously distorted by bias. Publication in high impact, peer reviewed journals is no guarantee of the validity of research findings. A literature review should therefore always attempt to evaluate the quality of the included studies with a view to drawing conclusions about the reliability of their results. In a systematic review quality criteria based on the anticipated study designs (see Chapter 7) are pre-specified and applied consistently across studies in order to limit bias in the review process.

Other literature reviews, such as those incorporated in protocols or theses, may use less formal methods, but should also aim to provide the reader with a critical evaluation of the validity of study findings. Where studies of variable quality form part of the review it is important to assess whether the overall conclusions are altered by including poor quality studies.

5. How will I synthesise the study findings?

Data synthesis aims to provide an overall summary of the findings of primary studies while documenting consistencies and differences between studies evaluating the same topic. The reviewer should attempt to explain conflicting findings across studies by evaluating the influence of factors such as study population, interventions and outcomes as well as methodological quality. This can often be achieved by means of a descriptive (narrative) synthesis, but in a systematic review formal statistical techniques *(meta-analysis)* can be used to complement the more qualitative assessment provided in the narrative.

A comprehensive account of the techniques of meta-analysis is beyond the scope of this text. However, a brief explanation of the rationale for meta-analysis and some examples should help the reader understand the concept.

> **The rationale for meta-analysis**
>
> In primary research, study size (and therefore statistical power) is often limited by the available time and money. One problem associated with small studies is that the estimates they yield may be too imprecise to draw meaningful conclusions. (See Chapters 9 and 12.) Meta-analysis is a statistical methodology which allows the reviewer to pool the results of studies that are sufficiently similar thereby increasing statistical power and the likelihood of demonstrating an effect (or association) if one exists.

Literature review | 6

We can illustrate the value of the technique by means of the following example. In 1981, a review published in the *British Medical Journal* stated, '*We still have no clear evidence that (the medication class known as) betablockers improves long-term survival after infarction (heart attacks), despite almost 20 years of clinical trials*' (Egger et al, 1997). None of the existing trials by themselves was large enough to demonstrate conclusively the value of betablockers. However, a meta-analysis of studies published between 1972 and 1990 clearly showed that betablockers reduce the risk of a second heart attack by 22% (Figure 6.2). Later findings revealed that if meta-analysis had been used earlier, unequivocal results could have been obtained as early as 1981, thereby avoiding the need for subsequent studies, saving both time and money.

See Example 6.1 at the end of the chapter for another illustration of a systematic review.

Figure 6.2 Meta-analysis of studies assessing the effects of betablocker therapy on mortality after a heart attack

Source: Egger et al (2001)

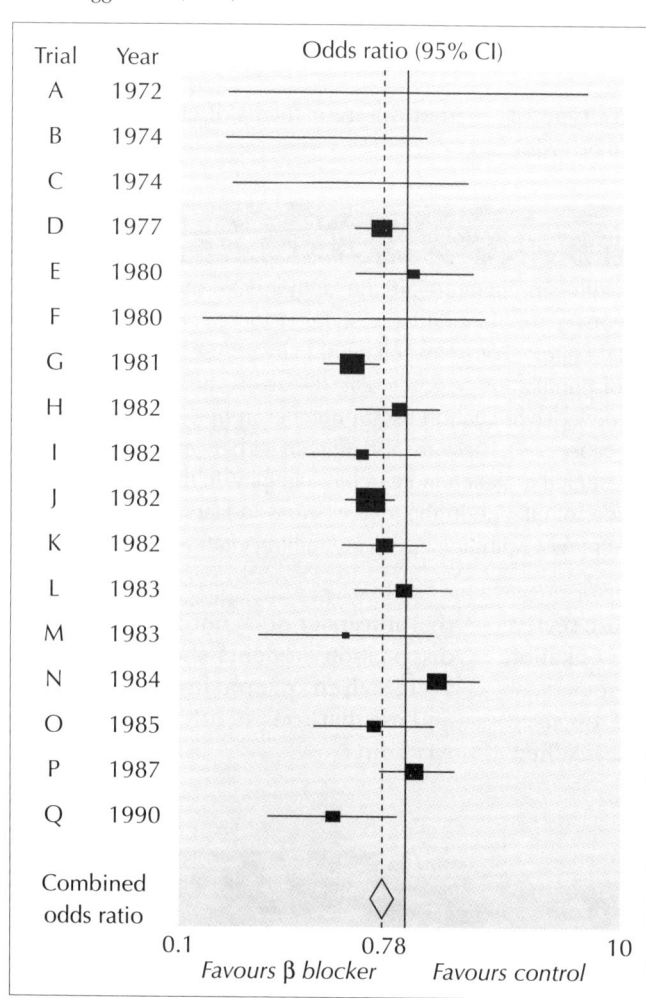

Trial	Year
A	1972
B	1974
C	1974
D	1977
E	1980
F	1980
G	1981
H	1982
I	1982
J	1982
K	1982
L	1983
M	1983
N	1984
O	1985
P	1987
Q	1990

Combined odds ratio

0.1   0.78   10
Favours β blocker   Favours control

Explanation: The first two columns represent the trials that have compared betablockers (a class of drugs) with control (placebo in this case), and the year in which each trial was published. The dark rectangles in the figure represent the odds ratio (a measure of effect) for each trial with the size of the rectangle reflecting the trial size. An odds ratio of less than 1 means that the betablocker reduced mortality. The horizontal line represents the size of the confidence interval (measure of how precise the estimate of the odds ratio was). If the confidence interval crosses the unbroken vertical line (odds ratio = 1), the effect is not statistically significant. Finally, the white diamond marks the 'combined' odds ratio (broken vertical line, = 0,78) with width equal to the confidence interval for all the trials combined. This shows that the use of betablockers results in a statistically significant benefit.

Writing up the literature review

The report of a literature review should clearly communicate the aims, methods, results and implications of the review. Each topic will present its own challenges and the report structure may have to be tailored to the subject area and the information needs of the target audience.

It is important for us to acknowledge all our sources. *Plagiarism* or using other people's ideas and words without acknowledging the source of our information is unethical and if exposed can lead to serious consequences. We can minimise the risk of committing plagiarism by following the simple guidelines provided in Table 6.5.

Table 6.5 Some simple rules for avoiding plagiarism

- Keep track of all your source materials
- Use quotation marks when directly quoting the words used by others
- Use your own words when paraphrasing the ideas of others instead of simply changing the word order or substituting words
- Cite the original source of information or ideas you express in the review

Finally, when we undertake any type of scientific writing, it is important to be aware that different forms of citation exist.

Harvard versus Vancouver citations

The two main types used in the health care literature are the 'author-date' style (also known as the *Harvard style*) and the 'Vancouver footnote/endnote style' (*Vancouver style*) set by the International Committee of Medical Editors. For in-text citation, Harvard uses only the name of the author followed by the year of publication (e.g. 'cardiac disease is the leading cause ...' (Mayosi, 2005)). In contrast, Vancouver style citation uses a number in brackets or superscript (e.g. 'cardiac disease is the leading cause ...'[1]). There are also differences between the two citation styles in how the references are presented in the endnote or bibliography. In the Vancouver style references appear in numerical order of citation in the text, whereas in Harvard they are listed alphabetically. See, for example, http://www.library.uq.edu.au/training/citation/.

Before embarking on the literature review the researcher should determine the citation style required by the university, society, or journal, and this style should be used consistently throughout the review. Where the university does not prescribe a style, dissertation students should choose one style when preparing the protocol and use that consistently throughout their write-up.

Literature review | 6

EXAMPLE 6.1

Systematic review: lay health workers in primary and community health care

Background

Consumers who are not certified health care professionals may be trained to promote health and provide health care services. Lay health workers (LHWs) are widely used to provide care for a broad range of health problems. However, little is known about the effectiveness of LHW interventions.

Review objectives

To determine the effectiveness of LHW interventions in primary and community health care on health care behaviours, patients' health and wellbeing, and patients' satisfaction with care.

Main findings

44 studies were included: 15 were considered to be of high quality and the remaining 29 were low.

- The majority of studies were done in high-income countries [n (number of studies) = 35].
- There was considerable diversity in the targeted health issue and the aims, content and outcomes of interventions.
- This diversity limited meta-analysis to outcomes for five subgroups (n = 15 studies), i.e. to promote the uptake of breast cancer screening, immunisation and breastfeeding promotion and to improve diagnosis and treatment for selected infectious diseases.
- The findings were summarised as relative risks (RR), 95 percent confidence intervals (95% CI) and p-values. These concepts are explained in Chapter 11.
- In comparison with usual care, LHW interventions promoted immunisation uptake in children and adults (three studies: two in children and one in adults; N (number of participants) = 1 942; RR = 1.30; 95% CI 1.14–1.48; p = 0.0001) and LHW interventions improved outcomes for selected infectious diseases, i.e. acute respiratory infection and malaria in children under five years old (three studies; N = 31 116; RR = 0.74; 95% CI 0.58–0.93; p = 0.01).
- LHWs appeared promising for breastfeeding promotion. Four studies investigated the effect up to two weeks post partum (N = 1 662; RR = 1.69; 95% CI 0.91–3.12; p = 0.1). However, significant heterogeneity (variation between studies) existed.
- LHWs were found to have a small effect in promoting breast cancer screening uptake when compared with usual care (five studies; N = 11 316; RR = 1.05; 95% CI 0.99–1.12; p = 0.10).
- For the remaining subgroups (n = 29 studies), the outcomes were too diverse to allow statistical pooling. No general conclusions could be drawn on the effectiveness of these subgroups of interventions.

Implications for practice

The use of LHW interventions is shown to be beneficial in the promotion of immunisation uptake, and in improving the outcomes for malaria and ARI in children. It is recommended that health planners should consider including LHW interventions as a component of health service strategies in these areas. For other health issues, there is insufficient evidence to justify recommendations for policy and practice.

> **Implications for research**
> Rigorous research is needed on the effectiveness of LHW interventions in a wide range of health conditions. More research is also needed on how findings can be transferred to other settings of care and population groups, on methods of training LHWs as well as on the way the interventions are delivered.
>
> *Reference:*
> Lewin, SA, Dick, J, Pond, P, Zwarenstein, M, Aja, G, Wyk, B, Bosch-Capblanch, X & Patrick, M. 2003. Lay health workers in primary and community health care. *The Cochrane Database of Systematic Reviews*, Issue 4, CD004015.pub2, DOI: 10.1002/14651858.

Useful reading

Chalmers, I & Altman, DG (eds). 1995. *Systematic reviews*. London: BMJ Publishing Group.

Useful web sites

Citation styles. [Online]. Available: http://www.library.uq.edu.au/training/citation/. [25 February 2007].

Open learning materials. [Online]. Available: http://www.cochrane-net.org/openlearning/. [25 February 2007].

World Health Organization. *The WHO reproductive health library*. 2004. [Online]. Available: http://www.who.int/reproductive-health/rhl/. [25 February 2007].

References used in this chapter

Antman, EM, Lau, J, Kupelnick, B, Mosteller, F & Chalmers, TC. 1992. A comparison of results of meta-analyses of randomised control trials and recommendations of clinical experts. *Journal of the American Medical Association*, 268:240–8.

Campbell Collaboration: [Online]. Available: http://www.campbellcollaboration.org/. [25 February 2007].

Chalmers, I. 2003. The James Lind initiative. *Journal of the Royal Society of Medicine*, 96:575–6.

Cochrane Collaboration: [Online]. Available: http://www.cochrane.org/. [25 February 2007].

Egger, M, Davey Smith, G & Phillips, AN. 1997. Meta-analysis: principles and procedures. *British Medical Journal*, 315:1533–7.

Egger, M, Davey Smith, G & Altman, DG (eds). 2001. *Systematic reviews in health care: meta-analysis in context*. 2nd ed. London: BMJ Publishing Group.

Moher, D, Cook, DJ, Eastwood, S, Olkin, I, Rennie, D & Stroup, DF. 1999. Improving the quality of reports of meta-analyses of randomised controlled trials: the QUOROM statement: quality of reporting of meta-analyses. *Lancet*, 354:1896–900.

PubMed®. [Online]. Available: http://www.nlm.nih.gov. [18 May 2007].

Sackett, DL, Straus, SE, Richardson, WS, Rosenberg, W & Haynes, RB. 2000. *Evidence-based medicine: how to practise and teach EBM*. Edinburgh: Churchill Livingstone.

Stewart, CP & Guthrie, D (eds). 1953. *Lind's treatise on scurvy. A bicentenary volume*. Edinburgh: Edinburgh University Press.

7
Study design

Chelsea Morroni Landon Myer

OBJECTIVES OF THIS CHAPTER

The objectives of this chapter are:
- to explain the distinction between observational and experimental study designs and between descriptive and analytical study designs
- to describe in detail, with examples, the main study designs used in epidemiological research
- to introduce the measures of association appropriate to each study design
- to list the strengths and limitations of each study design.

Introduction

As outlined in previous chapters, epidemiology aims to determine the occurrence of disease in populations, to identify the causes of or risk factors for disease and to assess the effectiveness of disease control measures. While the term 'disease' is often used for simplicity, in public health a wide range of outcomes may be studied, including injury, health behaviours, health knowledge and even good health.

In this chapter, we discuss the basic study designs used in epidemiology to meet the above objectives. *Study design* refers to the structured approach followed by researchers to answer a particular research question. Study design has also been called the 'architecture' of the study, because the choice of a study design determines how we sample the population, collect measurements and analyse the data. Cost and ethical considerations also influence and are influenced by the choice of study design.

Each of the study designs in epidemiology has its own strengths and limitations. The choice of study design is determined largely by the research question being posed. Epidemiological study designs can be fitted into two broad categories: *observational* and *experimental*. Observational studies can be further classified as *descriptive* or *analytical*.

The most commonly used study designs are listed in Table 7.1, along with their unit of study or observation.

Observational versus experimental studies

Observational studies, whether descriptive or analytical, allow 'nature to take its course'. In other words, the researcher measures (observes) exposure and disease occurrence, but does not intervene. Experimental studies involve intervention on the part of the researcher, who makes an active effort to influence the disease outcome by changing a disease determinant (such as an exposure or behaviour) or through treatment of the disease.

Table 7.1 Common epidemiological study designs

Type of study	Unit of study/observation
Observational studies	
Descriptive studies	
Cohort	Individuals
Cross-sectional	Individuals
Analytical studies	
Cohort	Individuals
Case-control	Individuals
Cross-sectional	Individuals
Ecological	Groups/populations
Experimental studies	
Randomised controlled trials	Individuals
Cluster randomised trials	Groups/populations

Descriptive studies

A descriptive study, which often takes the form of a survey, or a summary of routine data, sets out to quantify the extent of a health problem or the burden of disease in a population. A descriptive study is limited to the description of the occurrence of disease in a population, which may be *prevalence* or *incidence*. For example, in South Africa every year the Department of Health conducts the National Antenatal HIV and Syphilis Seroprevalence Survey. The Department tests a sample of pregnant women attending antenatal services in public sector clinics anonymously for HIV and syphilis. From this survey, the Department of Health is able to determine the *prevalence* of HIV infection and syphilis among pregnant women in South Africa. In another example, all newly diagnosed cases of cervical cancer are documented in South Africa's National Cancer Registry. From this registry, the number of new cases of cervical cancer per 100 000 women per year, i.e. the annual *incidence* of cervical cancer in South Africa, is calculated. Descriptive studies are useful to health service planners in that they provide information that will help them develop appropriate services, allocate resources, decide on priorities and target certain populations (see Chapter 13).

Analytical study designs

In contrast to a purely descriptive study, the goal of an analytical study is to find the causes of or *risk factors* for a disease by assessing whether particular exposures are related to diseases and other health outcomes. An analytical study therefore aims to find the factors that predict or cause disease by examining associations rather than just describing how much disease there is. (Sometimes the term 'descriptive study with an analytic component' is used, particularly in the case of cross-sectional studies, where the main objective is a descriptive one but where the data allow cross-tabulation of exposures and outcomes.)

The results of analytical studies are most simply expressed in the form of a 2 × 2 table. Table 7.2 sets out the general notation for such tables. *Note that the analysis and interpretation of the cells (designated by the letters a, b, c and d) vary according to study design.*

Table 7.2 General form of 2 × 2 table in epidemiological studies

	Have disease or outcome	Do not have disease or outcome	Totals
Exposed	a	b	a + b
Unexposed	c	d	c + d
Total			a + b + c + d

In this chapter, we discuss the basic analytical designs used in observational epidemiology: cohort, case-control, cross-sectional and ecological studies. We further discuss how we may use the findings from such study designs to estimate the association between certain risk factors and the occurrence of disease. Cohort, case-control and cross-sectional studies differ with respect to how individuals are sampled and the order in which exposure and outcome information is collected; for all of these designs the unit of observation and analysis is the individual. In ecological studies, the unit of observation and analysis is a group or population.

In the following discussion we will use the term *outcome* to refer to the health outcome of interest in a study (it could be a disease, death, side effect or complication). We will use the term *exposure* to refer to the exposure of interest in a study, that is, characteristics (risk factors, causes or determinants) that may be associated with the outcome.

The cohort study

A cohort is a group of people who share a certain characteristic and are followed over a period of time. For example, *a birth cohort* is a group of people born during the same period of time. A descriptive cohort study describes the incidence of the outcome in a cohort of people. It can also examine the *natural history* of a disease in a group of patients with the disease.

Design of an analytical cohort study

The goal of an analytical cohort study is to examine a possible relationship between an exposure and an outcome. In a cohort study, also called a *follow-up* study, the researcher begins with individuals who are all free of the outcome of interest (the cohort). The researcher follows both the exposed and unexposed groups through time, and compares the incidence of the outcome in each of the groups. Because the cohort is free of the outcome at the start of the study, the researcher detects new or *incident* cases of the outcome. While only two groups are shown in Figure 7.1, a cohort study may contain more than two comparison groups.

The measure of association that is calculated depends on the type of cohort data, specifically whether the denominator consists of counts (number of persons) or person-time data (e.g., person-years of observation) (see pages 20–23). If counts are used, *risks*, *risk ratios* and *risk differences* can be calculated. If person-time is used, *rates*, *rate ratios* and *rate differences* can be calculated. (See Chapter 11 and 'Useful readings' at the end of this chapter for further explanation of these concepts.)

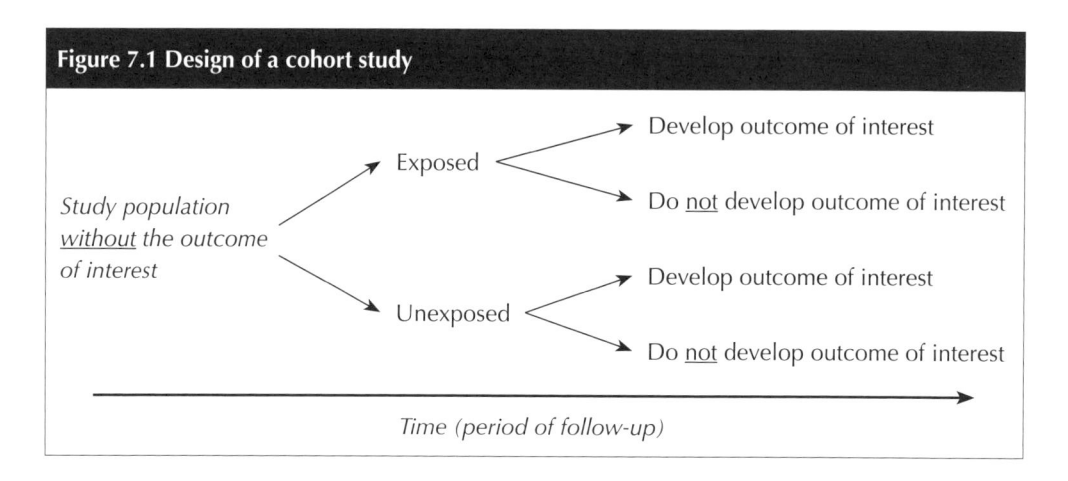

Figure 7.1 Design of a cohort study

Study population without the outcome of interest → Exposed → Develop outcome of interest / Do not develop outcome of interest

→ Unexposed → Develop outcome of interest / Do not develop outcome of interest

Time (period of follow-up)

Example of a cohort study

A cohort study in Durban assessed infant feeding practices and risk of infant HIV infection at 3 months of age (Coutsoudis *et al*, 2001). A total of 549 HIV infected mothers and their infants (who tested HIV negative at birth) were enrolled. These mother-infant pairs were divided into exposure groups with respect to feeding practices, including exclusive breastfeeding (n = 103) and mixed feeding (n = 288) groups. By three months of age, nine of the exclusively breastfed babies and 57 of the mixed feeding babies had developed HIV infection. Table 7.3 shows the 2 × 2 table for this cohort study: note that the uninfected infants are the starting cohort, the outcome is HIV infection, and mixed feeding is the 'exposure' relative to breastfeeding.

Table 7.3 Cohort study calculations

Step 1: Divide study population into exposed and unexposed	Breastfeeding status	Step 2: Follow subjects through time to see if outcome develops		Totals	Step 3: Calculate incidence of outcome in two groups and compare
		HIV infection status at 3 months			
		HIV infected	No HIV infection		
	Mixed feeding	57	231	288	57 / 288
	Exclusive breastfeeding	9	94	103	9 / 103
	Total			391	

> *Risk ratio* = [a / (a + b)] / [c / (c + d)] (see Table 7.2 and Chapter 11)
> = (57/288) / (9/103)
> = (19.8) / (8.7) = 2.28

This result suggests that babies of HIV-infected mothers who receive mixed feeding are 2.28 times more likely to develop HIV infection in the first three months of life than babies of HIV-infected mothers who are exclusively breastfed.

Types of cohort studies

There are two types of cohort studies: *prospective* and *retrospective* (sometimes called *historical*). In a prospective cohort study the researcher identifies the study population at the beginning of the study and observes them through calendar time, recording whether the disease does or does not develop. A retrospective cohort study shortens the time needed to conduct a cohort study as it makes use of historically or previously compiled data.

For example, we may be interested in the relationship between exposure to silica dust and lung disease among people working in the mining industry. Say we do our study in 2006, but find old company records from the 1970s with detailed information on who was employed, the duration of employment and the type of work that they were doing. Using these data sources we can determine who among the company's workers was exposed to silica dust and who was not. The next step is to determine who in the cohort has developed lung disease over the years and who has not. This information could be obtained from surveillance done by the company itself and from applications for compensation for lung disease submitted on behalf of miners after they left the company. This approach is useful when good records are available for exposure and outcome and for conditions in which there is a long period of time between exposure and disease onset.

Note that a cohort study requires that all members of the cohort be followed up through time, including those who have died. Researchers can also use a combination of the two types of cohort studies: exposure ascertained from records in the past (as in a retrospective cohort study) and follow-up and measurement of outcome continued into the future (as in a prospective cohort study).

Strengths of a cohort study

- Knowing with certainty that the exposure preceded the disease is very important when considering the possibility of a causal relationship between exposure and disease. Because the cohort design begins with measuring the exposure of interest among people who are free of the disease of interest and then ascertains the occurrence of the disease over time, the researcher can be confident that the exposure has preceded the disease.
- The risk of developing a disease and incidence rate can be directly measured in a cohort study.
- Cohort studies enable researchers to assess a range of diseases associated with the exposure being studied.

Limitations of a cohort study

- Prospective cohort studies can be long and expensive. To justify a cohort study, it may be necessary for the researcher to establish some prior evidence of an association between the exposure and disease from studies using other designs.
- If the disease being studied is rare, a very large sample is often necessary. A cohort study should be undertaken only when there is likely to be a sizeable incidence of disease.
- Cohort studies are vulnerable to biases from loss to follow-up of participants through time, particularly where there is a long period of time between exposure and outcome. It is therefore necessary to collect contact details of participants and to trace participants who may be lost to follow-up.
- *Information bias* in the reporting of the disease by participants or in the assessment of disease by researchers based on knowledge of exposure status may be a problem in cohort studies. For example, using the silica dust and lung disease example, men who know they were exposed to silica dust may be more likely to report respiratory problems than men who were not exposed. Similarly, medical practitioners may be more likely to investigate for lung disease in people they know have worked on the mines than in patients without such a work history.

The case-control study

Design of a case-control study

In a case-control study, the researcher begins with *cases*, i.e. individuals from an identified population (called the source population) who have developed the outcome of interest, e.g. are diagnosed with a particular disease (Figure 7.2). The researcher then selects a suitable *control group*, i.e. individuals from the source population who do *not* have the outcome of interest. Once cases and controls have been identified, the researcher collects exposure measurements (ideally referring to exposure prior to onset of disease) and compares them between the two groups.

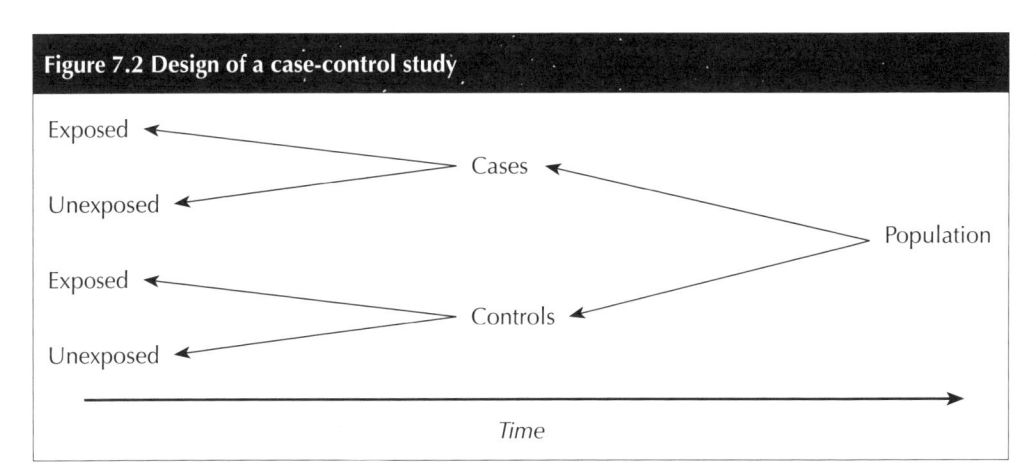

Figure 7.2 Design of a case-control study

```
Exposed   ←
             ← Cases  ←
Unexposed ←
                              ← Population
Exposed   ←
             ← Controls ←
Unexposed ←
                    Time →
```

The odds of exposure in the cases, the odds of exposure in the controls and the *odds ratio* (see Chapter 11) comparing the two are the only measures that can typically be calculated from a case-control study. Note that it is not usually possible to calculate measures such as prevalence and incidence from a case-control study.

Selection of cases and controls

In a case-control study, cases can be selected from many sources, including hospital or clinic patients or disease registries. It is important to note that cases should be new (incident) cases of disease, such as individuals presenting for the first time with a condition of interest. Depending on the condition or disease of interest, selecting cases for a case-control study is usually straightforward. However, the selection of appropriate controls is a major challenge. If we conduct a case-control study and find that there has been more exposure in the cases than the controls, we would like to be able to conclude that there is a positive association between the exposure and disease. The validity of this conclusion depends on whether or not the controls were properly selected.

To select controls, first identify the population that is the source of the cases. Then sample this source population to select controls. Because controls are individuals without the disease of interest from the source population, they should represent people who would have been designated by the study as cases if they had developed the disease. Ideally, controls are drawn from a random sample of people without the disease of interest selected from the same source population from which the cases were selected. However, this is rarely practical, and there are several other sources of controls that are commonly used in case-control studies.

Controls may be selected from non-hospitalised people or hospitalised patients. The use of *hospital controls* is a special approach that is employed when taking a random sample of the source population is not feasible. Hospital controls should be those patients admitted for a range of conditions (a) other than that for which the cases were admitted and (b) which do not have the same risk factors as the disease of interest in the study. (For example, in studying lung cancer cases, controls should not be drawn from patients with chronic obstructive lung disease.) Non-hospitalised controls may be selected from several sources in a community. One feasible option is to select, as a control for each case, a resident of a defined area, such as the neighbourhood where the case lives. *Neighbourhood controls* can be contacted using a door-to-door approach. Another approach is to use a *best friend control*, where the interviewer would ask the case for the name of a friend and contact that friend about participating as a control.

If controls are not selected properly, *selection bias* will result in an invalid answer relating to the exposure-disease relationship. Note that controls are *not* chosen to be the 'same as cases except for the disease'. In particular, controls should be selected without reference to their exposure status.

Matching in a case-control study

If cases and controls differ on characteristics other than the one that is the focus of the study, the researcher may be left with the question of whether the observed association could be due to these other differences between cases and controls rather than to the exposure being studied, i.e. due to confounding (see Chapter 12). Matching is one way of assisting with the control of confounding.

Matching is a process in which we select controls so that they are similar to cases in certain characteristics, such as age, sex, ethnicity, socioeconomic status, and occupation. Matching can happen in two ways: (a) *group or frequency matching* and (b) *individual matching*. In group matching or frequency matching, controls are selected in such a way that the proportion of controls with a certain characteristic is the same as the proportion of cases with that characteristic. So if 30% of the cases are unemployed, 30% of the controls would be unemployed. With individual matching, for each case in the study a control is selected who is similar to the case in certain characteristics. So, if the first case in the study is a 25 year-old black female, the researcher will select a control who is a 25 year-old black female. This type of study results in *matched case-control pairs*. Matching can be useful, but it often introduces complexity into the logistics of a study and the analysis of data, and may in fact not be necessary. For more information, consult an advanced epidemiology textbook.

Example of a case-control study

A case-control study was conducted in Cape Town to assess the relationship between injectable contraceptive use and breast cancer among women (Shapiro *et al*, 2000). Cases were women under the age of 55 years with a first time diagnosis of histologically-confirmed breast cancer presenting to two tertiary hospitals in Cape Town. Controls were women under the age of 55 years without breast cancer, hospitalised at the two tertiary hospitals (for trauma, acute infections, etc.). Four controls were selected for every case. In Table 7.4 the data from this study are presented.

Table 7.4 Case-control study calculations

		Step 1: Identify cases and select controls	
		Breast cancer cases	Controls
Step 2: Determine exposure in cases and controls	Injectable contraceptive use	318	166
	No injectable contraceptive use	1 181	444
	Step 3: Calculate the odds of exposure in two groups and compare using an odds ratio		

Odds ratio = (a / c) / (b / d) (see Table 7.2 and Chapter 11)
= (318 / 1181) / (166 / 444)
= (0.269) / (0.374) = 0.7

Women with breast cancer are 0.7 times as likely (i.e. *less* likely) ever to have used injectable contraceptives as women without breast cancer.

Strengths of case-control studies

- The case-control design enables researchers to assess a range of different exposures associated with a single outcome.
- The odds ratio calculated from a case-control study can be interpreted in a similar way to a rate ratio or risk ratio under certain circumstances (depending on how the cases and controls are chosen, or if the outcome in question is rare). Readers interested in the more technical aspects of case-control studies can consult Gordis (2000). (See 'Useful readings' at the end of this chapter.)

- Case-control studies do not require prospective follow-up of exposed and unexposed participants. This characteristic is especially useful in the study of diseases that occur a long time after exposure, and/or of diseases that are rare, because participants are selected after they become cases (or are chosen as controls), at which point previous exposure is measured. Case-control studies therefore usually require less time and fewer resources than cohort studies.
- Case-control studies are also more efficient than cohort studies in that they involve smaller numbers of participants in utilising all of the cases but only a sample of controls. (Note that a case-control study can be thought of as an efficient form of a cohort study, in which all the cases but only a sample of those who do not develop the disease, i.e. controls, are studied.)

Limitations of case-control studies

- Selection of an appropriate control group, i.e. one that represents the source population, can be very difficult. The selection of the appropriate control group requires careful consideration; an inappropriate control group will result in *selection bias* and the results of the study will be invalid.
- Establishing the correct temporal relationship between exposure and disease is more difficult in case-control studies than in cohort studies, because we determine exposure status in a case-control study after the occurrence of disease in the cases. We must take great care to discern whether the exposure occurred before the onset of disease.
- Some case-control studies are vulnerable to *recall bias*. This is because in case-control studies that rely on interviews for data collection, exposure status is determined after the occurrence of disease in the cases. So reporting of exposure by the cases and controls and assessment of the exposure by the researchers may be influenced by knowledge of disease status. For example, even though there may be no difference in exposure, cases may be more likely to 'remember' and/or report exposures than controls.
- The measure of association that can be calculated from a case-control study is usually restricted to the odds ratio. Because selection into the study is based on disease status, the incidence of disease and absolute measures of association between exposure and disease, such as risk differences, cannot usually be calculated.

The cross-sectional study

Design of a cross-sectional study

Cross-sectional studies (Figure 7.3) can be descriptive or may include an analytical component. Like cohort and case-control studies, the goal of an analytical cross-sectional study is to examine the relationship between an exposure and an outcome. Unlike cohort and case-control studies, a cross-sectional study does not assess and compare occurrence of new (incident) cases of disease in two groups. Rather, it assesses and compares the *prevalence* of disease or exposure across the two groups. Cross-sectional studies are frequently called prevalence studies.

In a cross-sectional study, the researcher usually selects the sample without reference to exposure or disease; often the sample is drawn at random from a defined population. He or she then measures the presence (or history) of both disease and exposure in each participant in the study. Finally, the researcher compares the prevalence of disease among those who are exposed and those are not exposed to determine if there is a difference in the prevalence of disease according to exposure status.

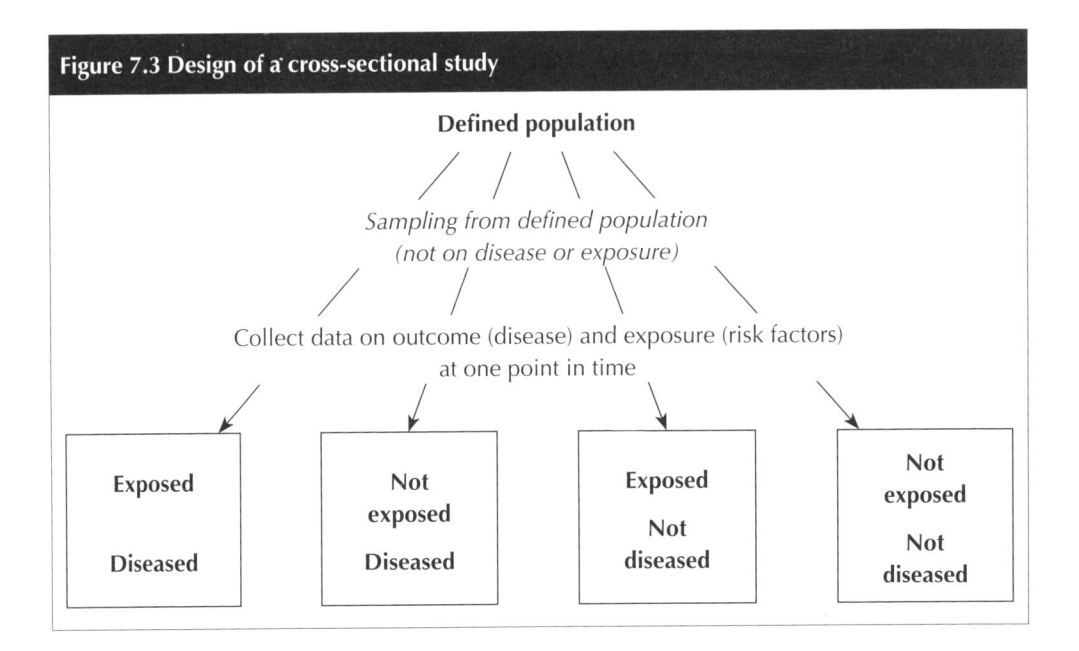

Figure 7.3 Design of a cross-sectional study

Defined population

↓

Sampling from defined population
(not on disease or exposure)

↓

Collect data on outcome (disease) and exposure (risk factors) at one point in time

↓

| Exposed Diseased | Not exposed Diseased | Exposed Not diseased | Not exposed Not diseased |

Prevalence, prevalence ratios, prevalence differences, and *prevalence odds ratios* can be calculated from cross-sectional studies (see Chapter 11).

Example of a cross-sectional study

The 1998 *South African Demographic and Health Survey* collected information on alcohol dependence using the CAGE Questionnaire (a validated four-question screening tool for alcohol dependence) and gender among 13 826 randomly sampled people over the age of 14 years living in South Africa (Parry *et al*, 1998). This is illustrated in Table 7.5.

Table 7.5 Cross-sectional study calculations

	Step 1: Select study sample and determine who has exposure and outcome			
	Alcohol dependent	Not alcohol dependent	Totals	**Step 2: Calculate prevalence of outcome in two groups and compare**
Men	1 587	4 082	5 669	1 587 / 5 669
Women	816	7 341	8 157	816 / 8 157
Totals			13 826	

Prevalence ratio = [a / (a + b)] / [c / (c + d)] (see Table 7.2)
= (1 587 / 5 669) / (816 / 8 157)
= (0.279) / (0.100) = 2.79

The result indicates that South African men are 2.8 times more likely than South African women to be alcohol dependent.

Strengths of cross-sectional studies

- Cross-sectional studies are relatively easy and economical to conduct.
- They are useful for evaluating the relationship between exposures that are relatively fixed characteristics of individuals (such as sex and ethnicity) and outcomes.
- They are useful for assessing the health care needs of populations.
- Cross-sectional studies are often an important first step in assessing the possibility of a relationship between an exposure and a disease, before more costly or difficult case-control or cohort studies are undertaken.

Limitations of cross-sectional studies

- Because prevalence is a mixture of incidence and *duration with* the disease, cross-sectional studies have difficulty distinguishing between factors that cause the disease and those which prolong the period with the disease (e.g. factors making the disease more severe or prolonging life).
- Establishing the correct temporal relationship between exposure and disease is difficult in cross-sectional studies, where the exposure status and disease status are measured together. This is especially so if the disease is chronic, such as diabetes, and the exposure changes over time, such as diet. In such a case, the disease may have led to changes in the diet.
- Compared to cohort and case-control studies, cross-sectional studies therefore provide weaker evidence about causation of disease.

The ecological study

In cohort, case-control, and cross-sectional studies, the units of observation and analysis are individuals. That is, disease and exposure status are determined for each individual in the study. In an ecological study (sometimes called a *correlational study*), the units of observation and analysis are populations or groups of people, rather than individuals. Groups may be neighbourhoods, provinces, countries, etc. For example, Figure 7.4 shows age-adjusted mortality rates by states and level of social trust among state residents in the United States (Kawachi *et al*, 1997). (For more on how social factors influence health, see Chapter 16.) Here, social trust was measured as the percentage of residents who responded affirmatively to the following statement: 'Most people would try to take advantage of you if they got the chance'. High levels of mortality seem to be associated with low levels of social trust.

Strengths of ecological studies

- Ecological studies are simple to conduct because they usually rely on data collected for other purposes. They can stimulate further studies by generating hypotheses.
- Some variables, e.g. income distribution, can be measured *only* at the group level and ecological studies or hybrid studies using such variables may be the only way to examine their influence on health and disease.

- Ecological studies are useful (even essential) where there is very little variation *within* a population in the exposure of interest, e.g. with respect to diet. One would then compare disease occurrence *between* populations (e.g. countries) with different diets.

Limitations of ecological studies

- The findings of ecological studies are often difficult to interpret because the relationship between exposure and disease in each individual is not measured. The relationship between exposure and disease at the population level may not be the same as the relationship between exposure and disease in individuals. Invalid conclusions drawn from ecologic data are referred to as being due to ecological bias, sometimes called the *ecological fallacy*. The ecological fallacy usually arises when confounding factors, operating either within or between the groups under comparison, are not accounted for in study design or analysis.

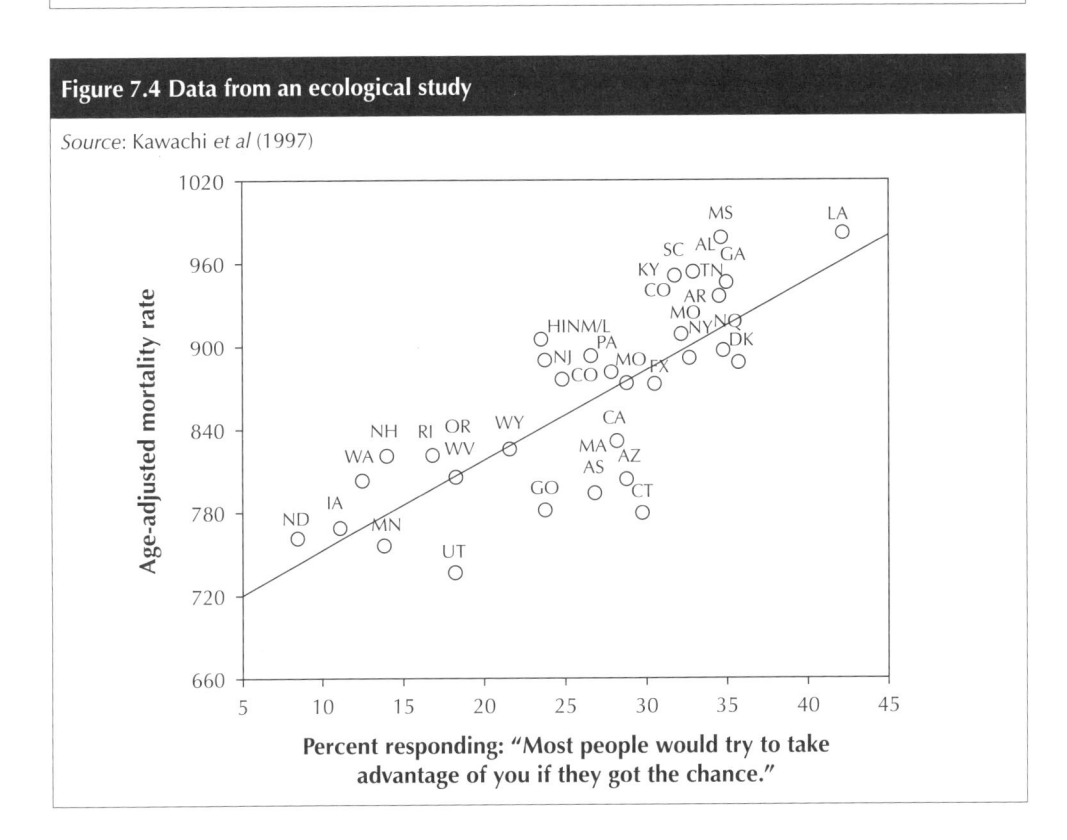

Figure 7.4 Data from an ecological study

Source: Kawachi et al (1997)

Experimental studies

All of the study designs described above are observational: the researcher measures exposure status and compares disease occurrence between groups of exposed and unexposed participants, but does not intervene directly. Experimental studies involve intervention on the part of the researcher as part of a planned prospective study. Experimental studies in epidemiology are therefore also called *intervention studies* because the researcher makes an active effort to influence the disease outcome by changing a disease determinant (such as an exposure or behaviour) or through treatment of the disease. Experimental epidemiology usually involves the study of a preventive intervention (e.g. a vaccine or behaviour change intervention) or therapy designed to reduce the occurrence of disease.

The randomised controlled trial

The most rigorous experimental design in epidemiology is the randomised controlled trial (RCT), in which the researcher randomly allocates eligible people to receive (intervention group) or not to receive (control group) one or more interventions that are being compared. (Do not confuse this type of control group with that in a case-control study). The control group receives either the standard treatment or a *placebo* (an inactive formulation which looks identical to the intervention treatment) if no standard treatment exists. We assess the results of an RCT by comparing the occurrence of the outcome of interest between the intervention and control groups.

RCTs can be conducted among individuals or among groups such as in a community or cluster randomised intervention trial. The latter is becoming increasingly important in public health. In the next section we describe an RCT among individuals to illustrate the key features of this study design.

Design of a two-arm individual randomised controlled trial

An RCT is a prospective study designed to establish a causal relationship between an exposure and an outcome. The researcher begins with individuals who are free of the outcome of interest (Figure 7.5). Participants must meet specified criteria before being considered eligible for participation in the study. These individuals are then randomised to an intervention or a control group. Both the intervention and control group are followed up through time and the incidence of the outcome in each of the groups is compared. The purpose of the RCT is to see if the incidence of the outcome differs between those randomised to the intervention and those randomised to the control group. RCTs also allow researchers to document adverse events associated with the intervention.

Randomisation means that each participant is allocated to one of the two groups in such a way as to have an equal chance of being allocated to either of the groups. (Do not confuse randomisation with *random sampling*: see Chapter 8.) The purpose of randomising participants is to ensure that the groups being compared are equivalent with respect to baseline characteristics, including known risk factors for the disease as well as unknown risk factors and those not measured in the study. Randomisation prevents *selection bias* (that is, it prevents participants, clinicians or researchers from using their subjective judgment to decide into which group to place participants). It also assists with the control of confounding by maximising the chances that the two groups are comparable at the beginning of the study. So, assuming that the randomisation works, the researcher can attribute any differences in disease outcomes at the end of the study to the intervention being tested.

The best practical method for randomisation is a computer-generated random allocation sequence. Methods for ensuring that the random allocation *sequence* is concealed from researchers, clinicians and participants until treatment has been assigned ('allocation concealment'), such as using opaque envelopes, are important. If the random allocation sequence is known before treatment assignment then, for example, clinicians could use the sequence of participant enrolment to place their patients into the groups of their preference. This would be a form of selection bias, and would defeat the purpose of randomisation.

In addition, participants and researchers should be 'blinded'. (See next page.)

B | Epidemiological research methods and protocol development

What is blinding and why do we use it?

Blinding means that the participants and study staff do not know to which trial group an individual has been assigned. Blinding reduces the likelihood of bias owing to differences in perceived response to treatment (sometimes called performance or reporting bias) on the part of participants. It also prevents bias in healthcare provider behaviour and provider or researcher outcome assessment (sometimes called assessment, diagnostic or detection bias). Blinding can also prevent data analysts from knowing trial group assignments until the last possible moment. In 'single-blind' trials only the participant is blinded; in 'double-blind' trials both the participant and the clinicians or researchers are blinded; and in 'triple-blind' trials, the participants, clinicians, researchers and data analysts are blinded. Blinding is not possible in all RCTs and is most important when subjective outcomes such as reported adherence, quality of life and quality of care are being measured. In therapeutic RCTs, blinding often involves using a placebo drug in the control arm that appears identical to the active drug being tested in the intervention arm.

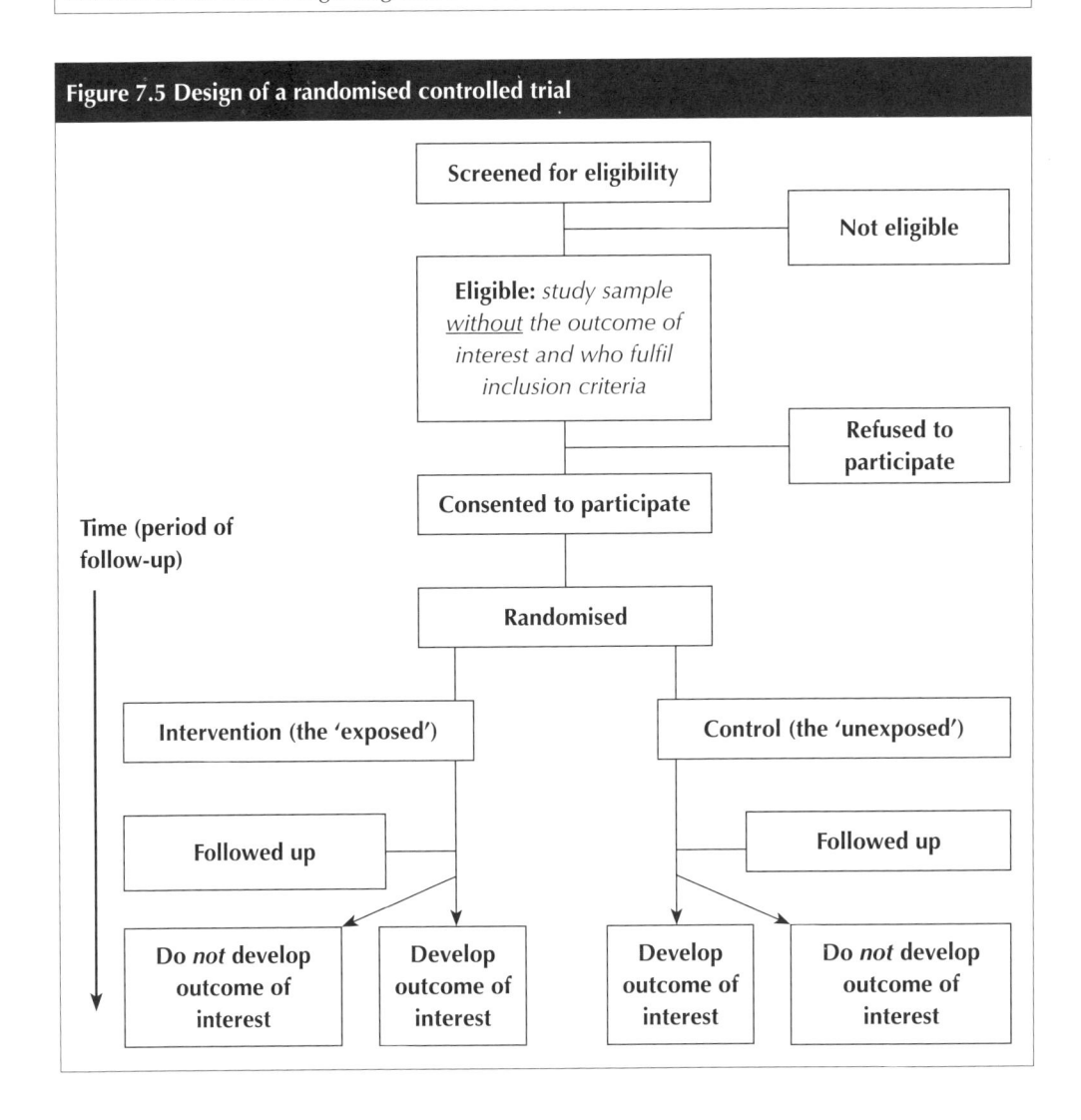

Figure 7.5 Design of a randomised controlled trial

```
                    Screened for eligibility
                              |
                              |──────────────→ Not eligible
                              |
                    Eligible: study sample
                    without the outcome of
                    interest and who fulfil
                       inclusion criteria
                              |
                              |──────────────→ Refused to
                              |                 participate
                    Consented to participate
                              |
Time (period of               |
follow-up)                    |
                         Randomised
                         /         \
            Intervention (the       Control (the
             'exposed')              'unexposed')
                 |                        |
            Followed up              Followed up
               /    \                   /    \
    Do not    Develop          Develop      Do not
    develop   outcome of       outcome of   develop
    outcome   interest         interest     outcome
    of                                      of
    interest                                interest
```

Risks, risk ratios, risk differences and mean differences can be calculated from RCTs (see Chapter 11). Another measure often calculated from an RCT is the *number needed to treat* (NNT). NNT represents the number of people who need to receive the intervention in order to prevent *one* case of the outcome or disease in the intervention group. NNT is important when making decisions about whether or not to implement an intervention that has been shown to be effective in an RCT on a wider scale, especially in resource-limited settings.

Example of a randomised controlled trial

An RCT was conducted in Cape Town to compare successful tuberculosis (TB) treatment outcomes between self-supervision and directly observed therapy (DOT), the 'standard of care' (Zwarenstein *et al*, 1998) (Table 7.6). Patients with tuberculosis were randomised to either self-supervision (n=105) or DOT (n=111) and followed for six months to measure the proportion of patients with successful tuberculosis treatment outcomes in the two groups. Sixty percent of self-supervised and 54% of DOT patients had successful tuberculosis treatment.

Table 7.6 Randomised controlled trial calculations

Step 1: Randomise participants to either intervention or control		Step 2: Follow participants through time to see if outcome develops			Step 3: Calculate incidence of outcome in two groups and compare
		Successful TB treatment	Unsuccessful TB treatment	Totals	
	Self-supervision	63	42	105	63 / 105
	Directly observed therapy	60	51	111	60 / 111
	Total			216	

Risk ratio = $[(a/a + b)] / [(c/c + d)]$ (See Table 7.2)
= (63/105) / (60/111)
= (0.6) / (0.54) = 1.1

Patients who self-supervised their tuberculosis treatment were 1.1 times more likely to achieve successful tuberculosis treatment after 6 months compared to patients who had DOT. In other words, for practical purposes, self-supervision was 'equivalent to' DOT.

Cluster randomised trials

A cluster randomised trial is an RCT in which groups of people, facilities or entire communities are assigned to certain interventions. A brief example is given below. This design is discussed in greater detail in Chapter 25.

Strengths of randomised controlled trials

- Of all study designs, RCTs can provide the strongest information about the effectiveness of interventions.
- An RCT has the potential to prevent confounding and selection biases that are common to observational studies. An RCT can therefore better isolate the effect of a single exposure or intervention on a particular disease outcome.
- Because the exposure or intervention is controlled by the researcher, the researcher can be assured that the exposure preceded the outcome. This is important for establishing with confidence a causal relationship between the exposure and the outcome.
- Blinding can be used to reduce reporting and assessment or detection biases associated with participant and researcher knowledge of the study group to which a participant has been allocated.

Limitations of randomised controlled trials

- For ethical reasons, RCTs cannot be used to test hypotheses about whether certain factors cause disease or about the effect of harmful exposures (although they can test the effect of removing potentially harmful exposures).
- Even for beneficial interventions, RCTs raise many ethical problems, which have to be dealt with before, during and after the trial.
- RCTs are vulnerable to biases from loss to follow-up, particularly if the period of follow-up is long. As in cohort studies, efforts must be made to minimise the chance of loss of participants through time.
- RCTs tend to be complex, time-consuming and expensive.

A cluster randomised trial was conducted in Rakai, Uganda, to test whether mass sexually transmitted infection (STI) treatment reduces incidence of HIV infection (Wawer et al, 1999). Fifty-six communities were grouped into 10 clusters and the clusters were randomly assigned to the intervention (mass STI treatment every 10 months, of all adults in the community regardless of STI symptoms or laboratory results) or control arm (no mass STI treatment). Participants in both arms who were free of HIV infection at the start of the study were followed for 20 months and HIV incidence in the two arms was compared. At 20-month follow-up, the incidence of HIV infection was approximately 1.5 per 100 person-years in both groups (rate ratio 0.97). No effect of the STI intervention on the incidence of HIV infection was observed.

Quasi-experimental study designs

Experimental epidemiological studies also include *before-after* studies. In a before-after study, measurements on an outcome of interest are made before and after some intervention in a single group of individuals. These types of study designs are common as they correspond to programme evaluation activities frequently linked to public health interventions. Such studies are considered *quasi-experimental* since there is no random allocation to intervention: all participants receive the intervention, and the comparison is based on time (before versus after). For example, researchers may measure knowledge of HIV/Aids among school children before and after an HIV/Aids education programme in a single school. They would then compare the before and after measurements to determine whether the intervention had changed children's knowledge of HIV/Aids. This type of study, and other quasi-experimental designs, can have significant shortcomings and therefore provide weaker evidence than RCTs. In the example of HIV/Aids education, let us say the HIV/Aids education programme was conducted in the school over a six-week period. During this period there may have also been community activities that increased the children's knowledge of Aids other than the school education programme. Without a comparable control group that did not receive the intervention and in whom the researcher can determine if any changes in knowledge occurred, it is difficult to evaluate the effect of the intervention. It is therefore advisable to have a control group even if there is no randomisation.

Conclusion

Each of the study designs in epidemiology has its own strengths and limitations. The choice of study design is determined largely by the research question being posed and the resources available to the researcher. It is possible to answer some research questions by more than one study design. When this is the case, the researcher needs to consider other issues such as study cost and funding, availability of data, ethical considerations and ability to control likely biases. Efficiency, i.e. getting the information or answer we seek at least cost, will always be an important criterion.

Useful readings

Beaglehole, R, Bonita, R & Kjellstrom, T. 1993. *Basic epidemiology*. Geneva: World Health Organization.

Friedman, LM, Furberg, CD & Demets, DL. 1998. *Fundamentals of clinical trials*. 3rd rev ed. New York: Springer-Verlag.

Gordis, L. 2000. *Epidemiology*. 3rd rev ed. Philadelphia: WB Saunders Company.

References used in this chapter

Coutsoudis, A, Pillay, K, Kuhn, L, Spooner, E, Tsai, WY, Coovadia, HM & South African Vitamin A Study Group. 2001. Method of feeding and transmission of HIV-1 from mothers to children by 15 months of age: prospective cohort study from Durban, South Africa. *AIDS*, 15(3):379–87.

Department of Health. 2005. *National HIV seroprevalence survey of women attending public antenatal clinics in South Africa 2004*. 15th Annual Report. Pretoria: South African Department of Health.

Kawachi, I, Kennedy, BP, Lochner, K & Prothrow-Stith, D. 1997. Social capital, income inequality and mortality. *American Journal of Public Health*, 87(9):1491–8.

Parry, CD, Pluddemann, A, Steyn, K, Bradshaw, D, Norman, R, & Laubscher, R. 2005. Alcohol use in South Africa: findings from the first demographic and health survey 1998. *Journal of the Study of Alcohol*, 66(1):91–7.

Shapiro, S, Rosenberg, L, Hoffman, M, Truter, H, Cooper, D, Rao, S, Dent, D, Gudgeon, A, Van Zyl, J, Katzenellenbogen, J & Baillie, R. 2000. Risk of breast cancer in relation to the use of injectable progestogen contraceptives and combined estrogen/progestogen contraceptives. *American Journal of Epidemiology*, 151(4):396–403.

Wawer, MJ, Sewankambo, NK, Serwadda, D, Quinn, TC, Paxton, LA, Kiwanuka, N, Wabwire-Mangen, F, Li, C, Lutalo, T, Nalugoda, F, Gaydos, CA, Moulton, LH, Meehan, MO, Ahmed, S & Gray, RH. 1999. Control of sexually transmitted diseases for AIDS prevention in Uganda: a randomised community trial. Rakai Project Study Group. *Lancet*, 353(9152):525–35.

Zwarenstein, M, Schoeman, JH, Vundule, C, Lombard, CJ, & Tatley, M. 1998. Randomised controlled trial of self-supervised and directly observed treatment of tuberculosis. *Lancet*, 352:1340–3.

8

Population and sampling

Gina Joubert   Judy Katzenellenbogen

> **OBJECTIVES OF THIS CHAPTER**
>
> The objectives of this chapter are:
> - to define the study population
> - to discuss the need for sampling
> - to describe random sampling techniques and their appropriateness in different circumstances
> - to discuss sampling bias
> - to outline issues to consider when choosing a sample size.

Study (target) population

When conducting a study, it is important to define clearly the group about which we want to gather information and draw conclusions. This group, called the study (target) population, should be clearly defined in respect of person, place and time, as well as other factors relevant to the study. For example, if we want to study the use of maternal health services in Kimberley, the study population is defined as 'all women of child-bearing age (15 to 49 years)' (person), 'resident in Kimberley' (place), 'at the time of the study' (time).

Researchers who want to determine some characteristic of members of a community often decide to conduct the study on clinic attenders (for example, HIV status of antenatal clinic attenders), since they are community members who can be reached with little effort. Clinic attenders are, however, not representative of the general population, since those who attend the clinic usually differ from community members who do not. In such a study the study population is clinic-attending community members, not all community members.

Inclusion and exclusion criteria need to be stated for the study population, for example, that the participants must be able to read and write certain languages. If an inclusion criterion is stated as above, it is not necessary to specify again that persons who cannot read or write the specified languages are excluded.

The sample

In descriptive and cross-sectional studies, the aim of the study is to describe some characteristic(s) of a population. The sample should therefore be representative of the study population. The focus on the representativeness of samples in these studies is in contrast to case-control, cohort and experimental studies, in which the emphasis is on comparing groups. These groups need to be comparable to each other with respect to factors other than the exposure and outcome under investigation. In Chapter 7, we discussed methods to select cases and controls to ensure that cases and controls are comparable. We also described the technique of randomisation in trials to ensure comparability between intervention groups. Sampling as discussed in this chapter is relevant mainly to descriptive and cross-sectional studies.

The nature of sampling

If the researcher wants to investigate the use of maternal services in Kimberley, for example, does he or she need to interview everyone in the study population? It would be a cumbersome, expensive and almost impossible task. Besides not being practical, it is not necessary to study all individuals in the study population. Rather, a sample (subset or subgroup) of individuals can be studied closely, ensuring that good quality information is obtained. If done properly, sampling is in fact more cost-efficient in getting the information we want than studying everyone. The way in which a sample will be selected must be described clearly in the protocol so that readers can judge how representative the sample is. Scientific sampling methods have been developed to ensure that samples are representative of the study population.

Random sampling

Random sampling (not to be confused with *haphazard* or arbitrary sampling!) is a specific selection technique which can ensure that the sample is representative of the population. This is also known as *probability sampling*, since each individual in the study population has a probability (*known* chance) of being included in the sample. While the researcher controls the sampling process, he or she has no control over exactly which individuals are selected. In the end, whether an individual is selected or not is determined purely by chance and not by the choice of the investigator.

In the discussion that follows, it will be assumed that information is required on individuals. If, however, information on households (water and sanitation access, household income, density) is needed, random samples of households could be similarly drawn.

Sampling frame

To be able to do random sampling, a *sampling frame* is needed. This is a list or some representation (for example, a map) of the study population, either of individuals or of groups of individuals (for example, households or villages), depending on the specific type of random sampling used. The items on the sampling frame are called *sampling units*. It is important that the sampling frame should contain all the individuals in the study population: a sample can be representative only if the original frame is complete. Table 8.1 is an example of a section of a sampling frame consisting of medical doctors listed in the Bloemfontein telephone directory. It is unlikely that a doctor practising in Bloemfontein will not be listed in the telephone directory. It is, however, often difficult to get a good sampling frame from which to sample for certain studies. For example, where would we get a sampling frame for selecting households in a large informal settlement? In townships or peri-urban areas, there are often no reliable maps to use as sampling frames. It is then necessary to explore other possibilities, such as aerial photographs or hand-drawn maps to use as a sampling frame. Figure 8.1 shows a hand-drawn map of part of Khayelitsha (Pick *et al*, 1990).

Table 8.1 Medical doctors listed in the Bloemfontein telephone directory

Africa MK
Albertse HW, Ear, Nose and Throat Specialist
Aldrich GW
Badenhorst L, Pathologist
Badenhorst OA, Orthopaedic Surgeon
Baloyi MP
Bam EJ, Dermatologist
Barnard E

Basson JI, Radiologist
Bester FCJ, Physician
Beyers CF, Paediatrician
Bohme FTS, Radiologist
Boltman C
Bonnet HJ
Bonnet ML, and so on

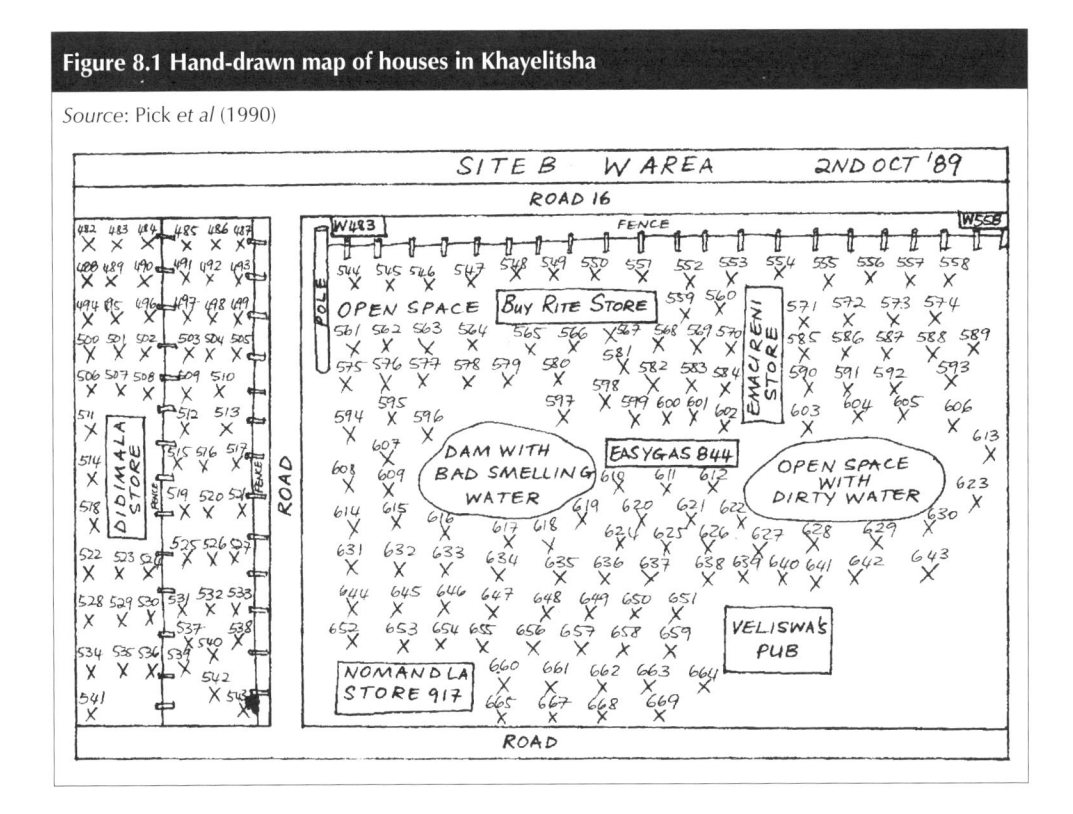

Figure 8.1 Hand-drawn map of houses in Khayelitsha

Source: Pick et al (1990)

Simple random sampling

In simple random sampling of individuals, the sampling unit is an individual and each individual in the population has an equal chance of being selected for the sample. The researcher has to draw up a complete list of all individuals in the population and each individual has to be given a consecutive number. To choose a simple random sample of medical doctors in Bloemfontein in order to investigate their knowledge of emergency services, one would make a list of all doctors and consecutively give each doctor on the list a number (Dr Africa is number 1, Dr Albertse number 2, and so on). In the case of a simple random sample of households having to be selected in the mapped area, each house is allocated a number, as shown in Figure 8.1.

Population and sampling

To select those who are to be included in the sample, random numbers must be drawn. This can be done by drawing numbers from a hat, using an existing table of random numbers (see Appendix II), or by generating random numbers on the computer (see Chapter 14 for an example using Excel). If we wish to select a sample of 20 from a population of 80, the individuals whose numbers correspond to the first 20 random numbers drawn between 1 and 80 will be included in the sample (see Table 8.2). Random number tables such as the one in Appendix II appear in statistics and epidemiology text books, and usually consist of numbers with up to 6 digits. If the population size consists of 4 digits (for example the population consists of 2 000 members), the first 4 digits (or the last 4 digits) of each number in the random number tables are used.

Table 8.2 How to draw a simple random sample

The following example describes the drawing of a sample of 20 individuals from a population of 80 using a random number table.

Give every individual a number (80 individuals).

Use a table of two-digit random numbers (see table alongside). Close your eyes and put your pen on one of the numbers in the random number table, for example 45. This will be your starting point. Start with the selected number and choose a direction (up, down, left or right). We have chosen downwards. When you get to the bottom of a column, move to the top of the next column. Record the consecutive numbers that appear in the table, moving in the chosen direction until you have selected 20 numbers which lie between 1 and 80. Any number above 80, and numbers which have already been selected, are ignored.

RANDOM NUMBER TABLE

25	19	64	82	84
23	02	41	46	04
55	85	66	96	28
68	45	19	69	59
69	31	46	29	85
37	31	61	28	98
66	42	19	24	91
33	65	78	12	35
76	32	06	19	35
43	33	42	02	59
28	31	93	43	94
97	19	21	63	20

Stratified random sampling

If we have some knowledge that certain relevant strata (subgroups) of the population differ with regard to the measurements being made, we would want these strata to be represented adequately in the sample. For example, new residents of peri-urban informal settlements may be at highest risk for disease. Although they may form only a small proportion of the study population, they can be chosen as a distinct stratum. In the case of the medical doctors, some are general practitioners and some are specialists, and they may have different levels of knowledge about emergency services. The study population should therefore be divided into these strata which should be mutually exclusive (that is, no individual should fit into more than one stratum) and collectively exhaustive (that is, every individual should have a stratum to fit into). A simple random sample of individuals is then selected from each stratum. This is called *stratified random sampling*.

It is therefore necessary to have a full list of the individuals in each stratum. Typical strata are age groups, sexes, geographical areas or social class categories, information which is available *before* we start drawing the sample. Strata should be selected so that the variation of the characteristic of interest between strata is maximised and variation within strata minimised. There should therefore ideally be little difference with respect to the characteristic of interest within a stratum, and large differences between strata (see Table 8.3 below).

Often the number of individuals selected from each stratum is *proportional* to the size of the stratum in the study population. This is called *proportional stratified sampling* or sampling proportional to size. In the example of the medical practitioners in Bloemfontein, if 40% of the doctors are specialists, then 40% of the sample must be drawn from the list of specialists. The results of the specialists and the general practitioners are then combined to get the result of the group overall.

However, equal numbers can be chosen from each stratum to facilitate comparisons between strata even if the strata are of different size. This is often needed when there are some very small strata, which, if subject to proportional sampling, would not result in enough sampled individuals to allow statistical comparison. If strata are not chosen proportionately to their size in the study population, the researcher has to adjust or weight stratum-specific results proportionately when combining them to obtain overall results (see Appendix I on standardisation).

Simple random sampling and stratified random sampling are easy to apply in, for example, a school, where full class lists can be obtained and pupils can be grouped in strata according to sex, age or grade.

Cluster random sampling

If we wish to study households in a metropolitan area, it may be cumbersome to use simple random sampling where each household is given a unique number and selected households are dispersed over a large area, requiring much traveling. In such situations, *cluster sampling* may be considered.

Drawing a cluster sample

In cluster sampling, the study population is first divided into groups or bunches (clusters) of a certain size. So, for example, the map could be divided into city blocks. Typical clusters are schools, city blocks or villages. Clusters (and not individual units) are then numbered consecutively and clusters are then selected using simple random sampling. All individuals, or a random sample of the individuals in the selected clusters, are included in the sample.

This method is convenient in studies involving large geographical areas. In rural research, villages are often treated as clusters. A full list of villages is drawn up, a sample of villages is drawn using simple random sampling, and individuals within these villages are included in the sample. Considerable savings are made in this way in respect of time, personnel, and transport.

One of the most frequently used forms of sampling is *stratified cluster sampling*. In a study (Yach *et al*, 1987) which aimed to estimate the infant mortality rate in a rural area of the Eastern Cape, strata were defined in respect of village type: urban, traditional, resettled and 're-resettled'. All villages were classified into one of the strata and villages (the clusters) were then chosen randomly from each stratum. In small villages, all households were included in the sample. Large villages were further divided into clusters, some of which were then randomly selected. Within a household, all women of the specified age group were studied. This is an example of *multistage sampling*: sampling took place at various stages or levels: villages were first selected according to type of village, and thereafter clusters of households within a selected village were chosen.

Disadvantages of cluster sampling

Cluster sampling does have disadvantages. If the characteristics being measured are varied (heterogeneous) within each cluster (for example, people in the cluster use a range of food preparation methods), then the clusters would be representative of the population. The results obtained from the cluster sample would be similar to (as precise and unbiased as) those from a simple random sample, and the cluster sample would be easier to study than a random sample. But as people in the same cluster would tend to be similar to one another (homogeneous, for example, with respect to food preparation methods) and different from people in other clusters, the cluster sample could end up being statistically less efficient than a simple random sample. In addition, results could be biased. It is therefore suggested as a rule of thumb that the sample size of a cluster sample should be *at least double* that of the corresponding sample size in a study using a simple random sample. Additionally, many clusters with few individuals per cluster should be chosen, rather than few clusters containing many individuals. Furthermore, it is important that the statistical analysis takes the cluster design (an example of a 'design effect') into account.

Table 8.3 outlines the main differences between stratified and cluster sampling since students often confuse these techniques.

Table 8.3 The differences between stratified and cluster sampling

Characteristic	Stratified sampling	Cluster sampling
Desired *internal* relationship	Subjects in same stratum similar to one another regarding the stratifying factor (homogeneous)	Subjects in same cluster different from one another regarding the factors of interest (heterogeneous)
Desired *external* relationship	Different from other strata	Similar to other clusters
Rationale	Ensure representative sample Enable stratum specific estimates	Efficiency (of access to subjects), i.e. maximum information for least cost May be only way of access to subjects
Statistical	Need to ensure appropriate weighting in calculating overall estimate	Allow for design effect: increase sample size and/or allow for in analysis

Systematic random sampling

Systematic random sampling is often done intuitively. A teacher may choose the child in every third desk to go to see the school nurse, or a nursing manager may go through every fifth patient's file to see what kind of patients come to a clinic.

In systematic sampling, individuals are selected at fixed intervals from some list or ordering, for example, a queue. In the example of the medical practitioners, every tenth doctor may be selected from the list. Similarly, every third house may be selected from the map. In systematic random sampling, the first participant is chosen at random using a random number.

An advantage of systematic random sampling is that the complete population need not be known before we start to select the sample. For example, one could aim to select a random sample from the admissions to a hospital as people are admitted. The procedure is random, since the first patient is selected at random. Each nth individual after the starting point is then selected.

Choosing a systematic sample

If the population size is known, the strategy depends on the number in the population and the size of the sample. If one would like to draw a systematic sample of 20 individuals from a population of 80, the sampling interval is 80/20 = 4, that is, every fourth person will be selected. To determine the random starting point we have to select a random number within the first *sampling interval*, in this case between 1 and 4.

It is important that the list or queue is not ordered according to some system or cyclical pattern. If street blocks consist of five houses each, of which the two corner houses are bigger than the others, a systematic sample of every fifth house would not give a representative sample. Systematic sampling is particularly useful if a sample of patient records has to be selected.

Non-random sampling

Various types of non-random sampling exist. These include the following:
- haphazard (or convenience)
- quota
- consecutive
- volunteer
- snowballing
- targeted; and
- purposive.

These are not exclusive (or even well-defined) types and they overlap in practice.

Haphazard or convenience sampling: This refers to selecting people who are easily available to participate, for example, patients in the waiting room of a clinic on the morning that the researcher visits. This will almost always introduce bias.

Quota sampling: The interviewer is given a description of the types of people who should be interviewed and the number needed of each type. The selection of individuals is left to the interviewer and there is no attempt at randomness.

Consecutive sampling: Consecutive persons are included in a sample until a certain number have been studied. For example, to study the prevalence of major depression in a rural community, all patients attending the clinic in the community during one calendar month could be included in the sample. As stated before, those visiting the clinic may differ from those who do not visit the clinic. In addition, the prevalence of the disease during December may differ from that during July. To address the problems of seasonal variation, we may decide rather to study a sample of patients attending the clinic throughout the year, including the first ten patients each morning. However, the patients arriving first in the morning may differ from those who come later. For example, those who are employed probably visit the clinic before work, and may be less likely to have depression than the unemployed, who come later in the day. These are examples of bias (see below) to which non-random samples are particularly prone.

Volunteer sampling: People take part in a study in response to an advertisement or call for participants and are not selected according to a sampling method. Volunteers may be those who are particularly interested in the research topic or are concerned about their health or who need the financial incentive offered. They are therefore not representative of the larger group they come from.

Non-random sampling is generally not recommended in quantitative studies, since the level of representativeness is questionable and inferences (generalisations) can consequently not be made about the study population. Most statistical procedures also assume that samples have been randomly drawn.

There are, however, situations where non-random sampling is useful and the only way open to the researcher. In studying rare diseases, it is difficult to locate sufficient cases in a community-based random sample. Thousands of people may have to be screened at great cost before a handful of cases are found who can be interviewed.

Snowballing (or *networking*): This is a sampling technique whereby each case is asked to name all other people he or she knows with the disease. By following up these people and obtaining further names from them, a sample is collected. Similarly, members of a community could be asked to name all the people they know with the disease. Clearly, this sample could be biased, since the most isolated cases may not be mentioned by anyone and may therefore not be included. The cases could also form separate non-overlapping networks which would mean that networking would lead only to cases belonging to one network, which may be very different from the others.

Targeted sampling: A similar approach has also been used to reach so-called 'hidden' populations: hidden because their activities are clandestine, for example, intravenous drug users or sex workers. Many studies on drug usage have been done by studying random samples of drug users who present at some institution (drug treatment programmes, criminal courts), but those presenting could be vastly different from those who do not. The sampling technique called 'targeted sampling' has been developed to reach members of 'hidden' populations in the community through a combination of techniques such as networking and key informants (Watters & Biernacki, 1989).

Purposive sampling: If the researcher wishes to form a focus group for discussion or do in-depth interviews on a topic (see Chapter 26 on qualitative methodology), it is acceptable (and indeed desirable) not to select a random sample. This form of sampling allows for selection of key or typical individuals from the spectrum in which we are interested. Issues which emerge in the interviews or discussion could be explored further in quantitative studies using representative samples.

Sampling bias

Bias occurs if the sample is not representative of the study population, that is, if the individuals in the sample differ systematically from the study population. By using random sampling techniques we aim to minimise bias. However, bias can occur even if random sampling is used. If the sampling frame used is not a full list of the study population, we may obtain biased results. For example, using telephone directory entries as the sampling frame for a city's inhabitants would lead to a biased sample consisting only of those people who have landline telephones and listed numbers. They would probably differ demographically from those who do not have landline telephones or prefer to have unlisted telephone numbers.

Even if the researcher has a complete list of the study population, it may be difficult to locate certain people for interviewing. If the interviewer conducts a community survey by visiting homes during the day, it is likely that children, the elderly, and unemployed people will be at home. Special attempts have to be made to reach the employed people who were selected to be in the sample, by going back in the evening or over a weekend. An individual cannot be excluded from the sample just because he or she is not at home at the time of the interviewer's visit. Furthermore, such an individual should not be replaced by a 'similar' person who happens to be available. The person who is at home in the afternoon may be very different from the one who is not.

People may also refuse to participate. Especially in postal surveys where respondents have to return completed questionnaires by mail, the initial response rate can be very low. In postal surveys an attempt should be made (such as second and third mailings, incentives for participation) to increase the response rate.

Response rate

Variations from the intended sample, whether because subjects are inaccessible or decline to participate, should always be carefully recorded. We should be able to account for the exact numbers approached and those unavailable or declining. In any study where the response is less than 100% (the ideal, but a response rate of above 80% would also be acceptable), attempts should be made to obtain demographic information on the non-respondents or on a random sample of the non-respondents. In this way, we could investigate whether the respondents and non-respondents differ in any substantial way, consequently introducing bias in the results. In writing up a study, response rates should always be reported.

Sample size
(to be read with Appendix IV)

If the researcher is dealing with a small study population, for example all the grade 12 pupils in a specific town, there should be no need to sample and the entire population can be studied. When the size of the study population is so large that the researcher has to select a sample from the study population, the question is how big a sample should be selected. An unnecessarily large sample entails wastage and can lead to problems since it may be difficult to closely supervise the collection of a huge amount of information. On the other hand, if a study is done on a sample which is too small, the results produced will be neither useful nor conclusive, and time and money will have been wasted.

For example, if a study is done to determine the prevalence of asthma in a community, a sample size of 10 may yield two asthmatics, giving a result of 2/10 = 20%. Had one additional asthmatic been identified, the percentage would have been 30%. Likewise, if one fewer had been identified, the percentage would have been 10%. These results are clearly very 'unstable' – one extra case swings the percentage tremendously. If the sample size had been 200, 40 cases would have yielded a 20% prevalence, but one or two extra cases (41/200 or 42/200) would hardly have affected the percentage. So the larger sample size has yielded a result that is much more stable and reliable.

The sample size need not be a specific percentage of the study population. Formulae exist for calculating the 'correct' sample size needed (see Appendix IV), but the researcher has to be able to provide some information before these formulae can be applied. If the study sets out to estimate the prevalence of a certain characteristic, the researcher has to have an idea in advance of what the prevalence is likely to be (2%, 20% or 50%). If the aim is to estimate the level of a certain variable, for example, blood pressure, we have to consider the expected level and variability of the characteristic. Similarly, if the difference in risk in two groups is to be estimated, some idea of the expected difference is needed. Such information can be obtained from a pilot study or from the published results of previous studies.

In addition, we have to consider how *precise* or *stable* we want the sample estimates to be. The more stable the estimate must be, the larger the sample size needed. For example, if we expect the prevalence to be 30%, and would like to be 95% sure that the sample estimate is within 5% of the true population value, a sample of 323 is needed. To be within 10% of the population value, we would need only 81 subjects, but at the cost of less certainty.

If the study sets out to determine the significance of a difference between groups or the association between factors, the researcher has to specify how large a clinical or 'public health' difference or association needs to be detected as statistically significant. For example, if a difference in blood pressure of 10 mm Hg (pre-defined as an important difference, clinically or from a public health perspective) has to be detected as statistically significant, a smaller sample will be required than if a difference of 5 mm Hg has to be detected as statistically significant. On the basis of knowledge of the subject matter, the size of the important or relevant difference has to be decided on in advance. In a large sample, a difference of 2 mm Hg may be detected as statistically significant, but this may not be significant from a clinical or public health perspective.

For further discussion on clinical significance, statistical significance and sample size, see Chapter 11 and Appendix IV.

Time, staff and cost constraints are important factors influencing the sample size chosen. The researcher can collect a sample only if the size is practically feasible. The size of the study population and the duration of each interview or examination must be taken into account to determine what is practically feasible. It is usually necessary to get the help of a statistician or epidemiologist in order to calculate the formula-based sample size. The researcher will be left with the decision as to whether the study is worth doing if the size which is practically feasible differs greatly from the one which has been theoretically calculated.

The importance of design effect

Most formulae for calculating sample size assume that simple random sampling will be used. One should therefore discuss with the statistician or epidemiologist which sampling strategy one intends to use (for example, cluster sampling), so that the sample size can be adjusted. The *design effect* of a particular sampling method indicates how the sampling design influences the precision of the estimates obtained, using simple random sampling as the benchmark. A design effect of 1 means that the estimates are as precise as those obtained from a simple random sample, whereas a design effect larger than 1 indicates that the estimates are less precise than that of a simple random sample. By estimating the design effect in advance, one can determine how the sample size should be adjusted to maintain a desired level of precision.

To obtain good estimates for prevalences in subgroups (for example, in different age groups), one needs adequate sample sizes in *each* subgroup. If a sample size has been calculated to give an overall estimate of a certain precision, it will not yield subgroup-specific estimates of the same precision. One needs a larger sample to make these subgroup estimates precise.

Many studies set out to calculate the prevalence or level not of one variable but of many. For example, in a community survey to investigate various possible risk factors for heart disease (for example, smoking, alcohol usage, obesity, cholesterol levels), none of the risk factors can be said to be the one of prime interest. In this case, formulae based on the level and variability of a single variable are not useful, and one will need to consult a statistician or epidemiologist to help decide on a sample size which would give meaningful results.

Conclusion

Sampling is done in order to study a subgroup of a population while being able to make generalisations to the population from which the group was drawn. Random sampling is used to maximise the chances of selecting a group of representative subjects. This requires a sampling frame and a highly specific procedure which provides randomness in the selection. Often a simple sampling strategy will suffice, but in other cases more complex sampling strategies are required and a statistician should be consulted.

EXAMPLE 8.1

Selecting school children at school and in the community

The following two studies were both aimed at selecting school aged children, but in the first study children were selected at school, whereas in the second study they were selected in the community. The two studies therefore used different sampling frames and selection methods.

Selecting schoolchildren at school

The aims of the study were:
- to document the prevalence of use of cigarettes, alcohol, and cannabis among high school students in Cape Town; and
- to investigate whether use of these substances was associated with a set of hypothesised psychosocial correlates.

'The study population was all students in Grades 8 and 11 attending public schools in Cape Town, South Africa. Schools were stratified by postal code groupings, and 39 schools were selected in such a way that the proportion of the selected schools in a selected stratum was directly proportional to the number of students in that stratum. Within each stratum, the selection probability of a school was proportional to the number of students in that school. Forty students were then randomly selected from the combined class list of two randomly selected classes from each participating grade. An additional five students were selected as replacements for absentees. A maximum of five absent students were replaced.'

Reference:
Flisher, AJ, Parry, CD, Evans, J, Muller, M & Lombard, C. 2003. Substance use by adolescents in Cape Town: prevalence and correlates. *Journal of Adolescent Health*, 32(1):58–65.

Selecting school-age children in the community

The objectives of the study were:
- to determine the proportion of school-age children from a South African township who were not attending school
- to compare the prevalence of mental and physical health problems and indicators of economic hardship between school attenders and non-attenders.

'The investigation was undertaken at Sites B and C in Khayelitsha, an informal settlement on the outskirts of Cape Town, with a population of approximately 92 000. Residents live in serviced or unserviced areas, which differ economically. Serviced areas have piped water and water-borne or bucket sewerage. No such services are available in unserviced areas. All schools were within the serviced areas. Half the sample was drawn from each of serviced (n=249) and unserviced areas (n=251).

'The researchers undertook a multistage sampling procedure. They randomly selected six roads from 18 main roads in the area, identified by aerial photographs and street maps. They visited every fifth dwelling on one side of each road from a random starting point until they had obtained a sample of approximately 250 children from each area. If no adult informant was present, three return visits were made to each dwelling before removing the dwelling from the sample. When more than one eligible child lived in a dwelling, the subject was selected using a table of random numbers.'

Reference:

Liang, H, Flisher, AJ & Chalton, DO. 2002. Mental and physical health of out of school children in a South African township. *European Child and Adolescent Psychiatry*, 11:257–60.

Useful reading

Scheaffer, RL, Mendenhall, W & Ott, RL. 2005. *Elementary Survey Sampling*. 6th ed. Duxbury Resource Centre.

References used in this chapter

Pick, WM, Cooper, D, Klopper, JML, Myers, JE, Hoffman, MN & Kuhn, LA. 1990. A study of the effects of urbanisation on the health of women in Khayelitsha, Cape Town. *Working paper no 1: rationale and methods*. Cape Town: Department of Community Health, University of Cape Town.

Watters, JK & Biernacki, P. 1989. Targeted sampling: Options for the study of hidden populations. *Social Problems*, 36(4):416–30.

Yach, D, Katzenellenbogen, J & Conradie, H. 1987. Ciskei infant mortality study: Hewu district. *South African Journal of Science*, 83:416–21.

9

Data collection and measurement

Judy Katzenellenbogen   Gina Joubert

> **OBJECTIVES OF THIS CHAPTER**
>
> The objectives of this chapter are:
> - to describe and evaluate different types of instruments for epidemiological measurement
> - to outline steps in compiling a questionnaire or data capture form
> - to describe ways of investigating the quality of the data collected
> - to outline ethical, language and supervisory issues in measurement.

Introduction

The collection of information for a study is called *measurement*. It is the process by which values are obtained for the characteristics of individuals being studied. Whether we want to study children's weights, compliance with treatment, illness rates in a community, or women's attitudes towards contraception, we need to measure some characteristics. These characteristics are called *variables*.

Measurement instruments

Measurement can be done by a variety of means:
- with instruments (a scale, thermometer, blood tests)
- by questioning (by interviewer or self-administered questionnaire)
- by the use of documentary sources (such as hospital folders, clinic reports)
- by direct observation.

There is usually more than one method of collecting the desired data. In practice, a combination of measurement instruments is often used. Information gathered may consist of replies to questions asked of respondents as well as measurements made by the researcher or interviewer. For example, one may obtain information about the prevalence of hypertension by measuring blood pressure with a sphygmomanometer (instrument), by asking subjects whether a doctor has ever told them that they have high blood pressure (interview), or by referring to medical records (documents).

The most appropriate type of measurement instrument to use depends on:
- the population under investigation
- the type of information needed
- the environment of data collection
- the type of observer or interviewer
- the time, money and human resources available.

Review of records

Much potentially useful health-related information is collected routinely as part of patient care, for example, for each patient who visits a clinic. Detailed information may be available for long periods, although the format, completeness and accuracy may be compromised because the information was recorded by a range of different people for clinical and not research purposes.

Questionnaires

Questionnaires are commonly used in epidemiological surveys and will receive closer attention in this manual than other methods of measurement. Even when questionnaires are not used in a study, the information gathered has to be recorded on a data capture sheet. Many of the issues in questionnaire design also apply to the data capture sheet. On some occasions, data can be entered directly into computers in the field.

A questionnaire is a list of questions which are answered by the respondent, and which give indirect measures of the variables under investigation.

Questions can be asked in different ways – by self-administration or by interview.

Self-administered questionnaires: These require the respondents to fill in the questionnaire by themselves. In most instances, the respondent reads the questionnaire independently, but at times the questions may be read out one at a time and answers filled in by the respondent in a structured manner. An interviewer may stand by to assist with any problems that may arise. Self-administered questionnaires may be completed in groups (for example, in a class) or posted to respondents. The latter is called a *postal questionnaire*.

In all these circumstances, the questionnaires have to be extremely clear and well laid out, since untrained people will be completing them.

Structured interviews: The interviewers follow a clearly structured format to prevent them from placing their own interpretation on the questions. Interviewers ask questions in a standard way, with the same probes and clarifications for each respondent, and they also record the verbal responses of participants in a uniform way. This standardisation increases the reliability of the information obtained (i.e. getting the same response on repeated measurement).

Unstructured interviews: In an unstructured interview, an interviewer has a set of guide questions or themes that must be covered during the interview. The sequence, wording and approach used depend on the interview situation. The respondent is therefore given much more freedom to express thoughts and opinions. The interviewer tries to achieve the study aims without imposing a structure on the respondent. Reliability decreases with the subjectivity of the unstructured interview, and interviewers therefore need to have specific skills and experience for these types of interviews. (See Chapter 26.)

Each method of questioning has advantages and disadvantages, and the methods chosen for the project must be practical and appropriate for that project. Table 9.1 outlines some advantages and disadvantages of the methods discussed above.

Steps in questionnaire development

The following steps provide a guide to developing our own questionnaire.

Step 1: List the variables to be measured

Questionnaires should be concise and carefully thought out. Variables to be collected should be within the scope of the study, keeping the length of time to complete the questionnaire within reasonable limits. First make a short list of variables based on the study objectives stated in the protocol, ensuring that only essential issues are covered. Only questions necessary for achieving the specific objectives should be included. Basic demographic information such as age, gender and measures of socioeconomic status are of value in most studies.

Table 9.1 Advantages and disadvantages of different methods of data collection

Advantages	Disadvantages
Review of records	
• Little expense collecting the data	• Format cumbersome as data were recorded for non-research purposes
• Allows historical comparison	• Data often incomplete
• Can be quick (although time often underestimated)	• Variables inconsistently defined and recorded by different people at different times
• Data cannot be influenced by the project	• Limited variables available
Individual interviews	
• Personal contact can facilitate response and quality information	• Time-consuming and expensive
• Respondent need not be literate	• Interpersonal factors (e.g. respondent's suspicion) may interfere with data collection
	• Interviewer variation affects data quality
Telephone surveys (a special type of individual interview)	
• Can cover wide area	• Exclude people with unlisted number or no phone – introduce bias
	• Non-verbal cues absent: affects communication
	• Questionnaire needs to be short, thereby limiting information
	• Suspicion aroused when call received at home
Self-administered questionnaires	
• No inter-interviewer variation	• Respondent must be literate
• Can be anonymous	• Little control over data quality and form completion
• Generally less costly and time-consuming	• Questionnaire must be very clear and well laid out
Postal questionnaires (a special type of self-administered questionnaire)	
• Can cover wide geographic region	• Limited to respondents who have fixed contactable addresses
	• Generally low response rate (<30%)
	• Unsure who filled in the questionnaire

Standardised questionnaires

It is necessary to allow adequate time to develop a questionnaire methodically and thoroughly. As a questionnaire may already exist for all or some of the variables under study, it is useful to review the literature and websites to determine if a *standardised* questionnaire is available. Making use of standardised questionnaires avoids unnecessary effort in designing a new questionnaire and facilitates the comparison of findings between studies. Check whether these standardised questionnaires have been validated. Standardised questionnaires should also be checked for their suitability to the South African situation as they may need adaptation in language and method of administration. Some items may need to be reviewed for appropriateness. Useful web sites and books for accessing standardised health questionnaires are listed at the end of this chapter.

Step 2: Formulate the questions and answer options

Phrase questions carefully

- Questions should be simple, concise, and very specific. Make sure that there are no ambiguities. The respondent should know exactly what is being asked.
- Try to avoid double negatives in questions, such as 'Were the clinic staff not discourteous to patients?'
- It is better to ask one question at a time. 'Were the clinic staff helpful and the clinic clean and comfortable?' contains three questions. Break questions up into component parts to avoid confusion.
- Avoid questions which suggest to the respondent the answer that is expected or wanted (*leading question*). For example, 'Do you think smoking is bad for your health?' versus 'What is your attitude towards smoking: do you think it is good for one's health, bad for one's health or that it has no effect on one's health?'
- Avoid *loaded questions*, that is, questions that lead to specific associations or emotional reactions. People differ as to the types of questions that they perceive as loaded (which could be sensitive or threatening). Examples of sensitive characteristics may include income, race, alcohol use, sexual practice, and psychological stress.
- Find out from potential respondents in a pilot study whether the questions are meaningful to them and how to phrase the questions to ensure that they are understandable and acceptable. Always keep the target population in mind when formulating questions. Local slang may enhance the suitability of the questionnaire. Avoid technical language if the target population consists of lay people.
- Keeping the target population in mind, avoid questions that require interpretation influenced strongly by education, culture and language, for example: 'Do you eat three balanced meals a day?'

Develop questions which will elicit the variables you want to measure in the best way possible

At times, one variable may need a series of two or three questions to capture the true characteristic. This is the case with complex or composite variables that have a number of components, for example, socioeconomic status or household density. In the latter case the characteristic requires the number of individuals in a household to be divided by the number of rooms in the house.

Decide on the answer options

Questions are *open-ended* if the respondent can reply in whatever way he or she chooses, for example, 'What is your opinion on the use of oral contraception?' The alternative is to have *closed questions* where the answer is either 'yes' or 'no', a number, or a choice of one of a group of predetermined answer categories.

Closed questions encourage quicker, more standardised data collection, but may limit responses or inhibit the respondent. At times, a question may be asked in an open-ended way, but the answer may be placed into a predetermined category when recording the response to the question.

For example:
Question: 'What is your opinion about the use of oral contraceptives?'
Actual response: 'They disturb the hormones in my body and don't work.'
Recorded response:
(i) approved (ii) disapproved
(iii) indifferent.

Closed question categories should be *mutually exclusive* (that is, no overlap of categories) and *exhaustive* (that is, they should cover all possibilities). One should always allow for an 'other' category where the interviewer specifies the answer when recording.

For example:
What language do you speak at home?
1. Zulu
2. Xhosa
3. Sotho
4. Tswana
5. English
6. Afrikaans
7. Other (specify....................)

Questionnaires usually have a mixture of open- and closed-ended questions. Respondents may need to indicate on a scale of 1 to 4 or 1 to 6 (called a Likert Scale) what their attitudes towards some issues are.

For example:
Please indicate your opinion on the following statement by circling the appropriate number along the line:

A cure will be found for Aids within the next five years.

Strongly agree					Strongly disagree
1	2	3	4	5	6

In general, it is advisable to have an even-numbered scale to avoid excessive selection of the middle value. The greater the number of values provided, the greater the tendency among respondents to avoid extreme values. It is therefore not advisable to offer too wide a scale. Researchers should ensure that the scale is balanced; that is, that there are as many positive as negative categories.

Step 3: Decide on the organisation and structure of each question

- Design the recording procedure with the interviewers or recorders of information in mind.
- Consider whether any questions need introduction or explanation.
- Decide whether to accept multiple responses or not (for example, in the question about what language is spoken at home, is only one language acceptable or can more than one be circled?).
- Certain questions may apply only to some of the respondents, and one should therefore 'funnel' them. The questions for the 'select' group should be put into a block clearly labelled so that these questions are asked only of suitable respondents, or are answered only by suitable respondents. The following example of such a 'stem and branch' question funnels the questions twice, first selecting only females (the stem), and then selecting only those who are not menstruating (the branch).

Females only:
Do you still get your periods?
1. Yes
2. No

If no:
Did your periods stop:
1. Naturally
2. Due to surgery
3. Due to radiation or chemotherapy
4. Due to injectable contraception
5. Other (specify)..........................
6. Unknown

- Some items require a prompt, that is, a question or statement which triggers a response without suggesting what the answer should be. Determine if such prompts are required and if so, how and when.

There is the danger that a respondent will give a negative answer when they should not have ('false negative'). To avoid this, the interviewer could ask from a list prompting the respondent. The answers are divided into categories which make it clear which responses were prompted and which were not. Using the example of contraceptive use: Have you ever used any type of birth control or family planning? Yes/No

If yes:
Which methods have you used?

	Unprompted	Prompted
1. Birth control pills	1. Yes 2. No	1. Yes 2. No
2. Injections	1. Yes 2. No	1. Yes 2. No
3. Intra-uterine device	1. Yes 2. No	1. Yes 2. No
4. Diaphragm	1. Yes 2. No	1. Yes 2. No
5. Foam, jelly or cream	1. Yes 2. No	1. Yes 2. No
6. Condom	1. Yes 2. No	1. Yes 2. No
7. Sterilisation	1. Yes 2. No	1. Yes 2. No
8. Partner's vasectomy	1. Yes 2. No	1. Yes 2. No
Other (e.g. withdrawal) Specify:	1. Yes 2. No	1. Yes 2. No ....

- It is important to train interviewers to use and record prompts in a uniform way. Decide if or how more than one response will be recorded.
- At times, a question may require that the interviewee be shown an example or picture to choose from, for example, a brand of pills or a food model.

Step 4: Determine the sequence of the questions

Plan the sequence of the questions carefully to ensure logical flow. Basic demographic information is usually unthreatening and is often asked first. Sensitive questions are usually put later in the questionnaire, so that some trust has been built up by the time they are asked. In addition, if subjects refuse to answer these sensitive questions, the interviewer has at least collected some information. Questions which reveal the specific objectives of the study might also need to be kept until last to avoid influencing the answers to earlier questions.

Step 5: Plan the layout and design of the questionnaire

Visual presentation

The visual presentation and lay-out of the questionnaire should be as clear as possible so that errors can be minimised. Here are some guidelines to follow:
- type the questionnaire neatly without spelling mistakes – use a spell-checker and/or have it proof-read
- ensure good visual spacing (double spacing with reduced print often works well)
- use highlights if needed
- indent intelligently
- print without smudges
- make neat blocks (on computer or using a stencil) for ticking answers or filling in numbers
- provide enough space for answers to open-ended questions
- different colour paper may be used for the different sections of the interview or for different subgroups of respondents, for example, household information on white, demographic information on green
- visual markers such as arrows and blocks can make administering the questionnaire easier, particularly for stem and branch questions.

Introductions, instructions and consent

- If no interviewer or researcher is present when the respondents complete the questionnaire, a covering letter should be provided giving a short description of the project and details of the researcher, including name, affiliation and contact information.
- Ethics committees may require signatures from the respondents that confirm that they were fully informed and consented to participation in the study.
- Clear instructions to the respondent or interviewer must appear at the top of the questionnaire, for example, *Mark your choice by putting X in the appropriate box.*

Identification information on forms

The questionnaire or data capture form of each participant should have a unique identifying number. These numbers start from 1 and are given consecutively as participants enrol. They assist in tracking data errors or queries that may be picked up during the analysis (see Chapter 10). To ensure confidentiality of information, the researcher can keep a separate list of identification numbers linking them to names and surnames or hospital files. If names and personal details are recorded on a separate removable sheet, it is imperative that the subject identification number appears on both this sheet and the questionnaire, for linkage.

If there is more than one interviewer, interviewers' names or codes should appear as part of the identification details on the questionnaires administered by them.

Step 6: Consider the scale of measurement of the variables

In considering the process and means of measurement, an awareness of the *scale of measurement* of the variables (see Chapter 10) helps the researcher to plan adequately for the analysis stage. For example, when collecting information on heights, physical measurements are done and recorded. Here the observations have numeric meaning, and an average can be calculated. However, when collecting information on sex, each observation is categorised as male or female, and the number of observations in each category is counted. Here we cannot find an 'average' sex: we have to calculate the percentage of observations in each category. An understanding of the scales of measurement is important, as different statistical methods are suitable for different types of variables.

Step 7: Consider what coding needs to be done after data collection

Some tips on coding

Before the raw information can be analysed quantitatively it must be prepared for analysis. The process by which the information is converted into numbers or categories is called coding. So, for example, if male = 1 and female = 2, all the respondents who are male have a number 1 recorded for the variable 'gender'. Note that for the variable 'gender' the code '1' is merely a category, but for the variable 'age' the code '1' would have numeric meaning. If one chooses to use codes such as 'm' for male and 'f' for female, one must be consistent in using capital letters or small letters throughout. Long words should not be used as codes since typing errors will complicate the analysis.

Every variable collected must have set values with which to code responses. This is easy for variables which measure characteristics, such as weight and height, but gets more cumbersome when open-ended questions have to be given codes. These open-ended questions should, where possible, be given codes before the study so that responses can be coded rapidly. In practice, many researchers allocate codes to these more qualitative questions only once they see the types of responses that have emerged. They then allocate codes to the broad themes that emerge in the data.

Coding is an important, often time-consuming task during the data-collection phase. Adequate time should be allocated to this process, and money budgeted to pay coders. The task can also serve as a form of supervision and checking to assess the quality of the data. Sometimes, if mistakes are found while still in the field, interviewers can return to the respondents to check or correct the errors.

Step 8: Consider the means of data analysis

The design of the questionnaire or the data capture sheet must be discussed with the person(s) who will do the analysis, since the design must take into account how the data will be analysed. There are several possibilities.

Analysis by hand: A data capture sheet (Figure 9.1) can be made, with variables listed vertically and each record running horizontally. Information is filled into each space. From such a listing, the researcher can easily do simple counts of certain variables, for example, the number of males in the group. Cross-classification (for example, how many of the males compared to the females have high blood pressure?) may be rather cumbersome, however.

Analysis by computer: Computer analysis of data using statistical software is by far the quickest and most accurate way of obtaining results. A suitable data capture software program (for example, Excel, Access or Epi Info) needs to be selected. A well-designed questionnaire assists transfer of information onto the computer.

If the data analysis is being done within a big institution, data typists may be available to type the information into the required format. If you hire outside data typists, they should be experienced if possible and you should monitor the output carefully. Double entry of data (which means that the data are typed independently by two data typists and the two sets compared for discrepancies) should be done to minimise typing errors.

Figure 9.1 Data capture sheet

Observation	Age	Sex	BP	Height	Weight	R_x	Hospital
1							
2							
3							
4							
5							
6							
7							
8							
9							
10							
11							
12							
13							
14							
15							
16							
17							
18							
19							
20							
21							
22							
23							
24							
25							

Usually all answers are given numeric codes for ease of transfer (for example, male = 1 and female = 2).

Data are usually typed into an Excel spreadsheet or into a text file with the information belonging to a particular respondent entered across a number of columns in a single row, and information regarding different respondents in separate rows below one another. To be able to type data into text files, there must be blocks for coding along the right-hand margin of the questionnaire. Only coded information may be placed in this space (usually marked 'For official use only') and this information is then typed into the computer by data typists. Each coding block has a unique number. The coding blocks start from 1 and are numbered consecutively. The coding block numbers allow the typists to find their way around the questionnaire and allow the computer to read in specific blocks as specific variables. See Figure 9.2 for an example.

Data collection and measurement

Figure 9.2 Coding of data

Mark the appropriate block with a X or write your answer in the space provided

For Office Use

☐☐☐ 1–3

1. Date questionnaire is completed (dd/mm/yy) ....../....../......

   ☐☐☐☐☐☐ 4–9
   d d m m y y

2. What is your gender?

   | Male (1) | Female (2) |

   ☐ 10

3. What is your age? .... years   ☐☐ 11–12

4. What is your occupation? ....   ☐☐ 13–14

5. What is your highest school qualification? ....   ☐☐ 15–16

6. What is your home language?

1	Sesotho
2	Setswana
3	Afrikaans
4	English
5	Xhosa
6	Zulu
7	Other, specify ....

   ☐ 17

7. Which of the following languages do you speak? (More than one can be marked.)

1	Sesotho
2	Setswana
3	Afrikaans
4	English
5	Xhosa
6	Zulu
7	Other, specify ....

   ☐ 18
   ☐ 19
   ☐ 20
   ☐ 21
   ☐ 22
   ☐ 23
   ☐ 24

Advantages of modern technology ...

Micro hand-held computers are portable computers which allow for entry of data at the point of data collection. The interviewer types in values into a pre-programmed format, circumventing the need for filling in questionnaires and coding. This method also allows for the rapid analysis of data so that interim results are available immediately, and monitoring of fieldwork is made easier. Back-up plans for possible technical problems such as power or battery failure must be in place to avoid loss of information in the field. Make computer copies of the collected data in case the information is destroyed or lost.

Step 9: Pilot ('pretest') the questionnaire

A pilot study is a test run of aspects of the main study. In developing a questionnaire, a series of small pilot studies is needed to refine the instrument. Pilot studies require an in-depth look at the questionnaire with the aim of improving its quality. Usually only a few subjects are chosen per pilot study, for example, 5 to 20 individuals.

Testing the questionnaire

In the early stages of developing the questionnaire, rudimentary questions can be tried out on colleagues and friends in order to investigate the wording and the clarity of the questionnaire. Glaring problems should be picked up at this stage. Later pilot studies should be conducted on groups that are increasingly similar to the target population. For example, if the study hopes to determine the immunisation coverage of pre-schoolers in a particular community, the pilot studies could take place at the paediatric outpatient department of a teaching hospital, then at a day hospital covering a similar population, and lastly using a small community sample. At first the researcher must be active in the pilot, but later the questionnaire should be administered by interviewers similar to those to be used in the main study.

During the pilot study, the interviewer records words and sentences that are not understood and questions that require prompting or explanation. There should be space on the questionnaire to write down the respondents' reactions to certain questions, especially sensitive ones. Open-ended questions will generate a variety of responses, which can be used to determine the options for the main study or the codes to be used. Common responses will be chosen as the categories that will appear on the final questionnaire or coding sheet. Logistical data, such as the time taken, should also be recorded.

At the end of the pilot interview, the respondent may be asked how he or she felt about the nature, style and timing of the questions. Such feedback could be crucial for revision of the questionnaire or study procedures used in the main study.

Step 10: Make necessary changes

After the pilot study, debrief the interviewers fully and note their comments. Address as many of the shortcomings as possible, so that the final questionnaire benefits fully from the feedback.

The training of the interviewers for the main study also doubles up as a final pilot as interviewers often pick up logistical and other problems with the data collection process. In order to benefit from their input, make sure that there is enough time between the interviewer training and the start of the study to make the final necessary changes. There is an added benefit in that the interviewers' contributions makes them part of the questionnaire design team.

Remember to check and recheck coding block numbers.

Quality of the data collected

If the results are to be sound, the quality of the information collected needs to be good. The first, rather intuitive, way of checking data quality is to review issues concerning the data collection process and the respondents. The second is a more formal evaluation of measurement error.

Review of issues concerning data collection process

Before full analysis of the data, it is useful to extract information which can give a sense of how and from whom data were obtained. Three types of data are useful for this purpose.

Information indicating the extent of missing data: Data may be missing because of failure to locate an individual, non-co-operation of an individual (either by refusal to participate or refusal to answer specific questions), illegible entries, or lost records. The extent of missing data should be reported by cause when writing up the study results. This means also that interviewers must record every approach to potential participants. The total number of persons approached make up the denominator for response rate calculations.

Data on the characteristics of respondents: Different types of respondents may respond differently to the study or particular items. Record the respondents' age and sex, status in the home, and other relevant variables.

When information on a particular person is being collected, that person is called the index person. Self-reporting by the index person is desirable in most cases, although in some situations, for example, in the case of children or persons in a coma or with intellectual disability, proxy responses may be necessary. A proxy response means that someone else responds on behalf of the index person. In such cases, it is important to record the relationship of the proxy respondent to the index person.

Data on the setting in which the information was collected: The environment in which data collection takes place can influence the data. It may be important to note the time, place, and even the temperature, as such details may influence the quality of the data. The interviewer may record a subjective assessment of the interview and the quality of the information provided. On this basis, some interviews or items may be excluded from the analysis.

Formal evaluation of measurement error: reliability and validity

Data are only as good as the measurement instruments used to measure the characteristics. Ideally, one would like to measure 'the truth' every time these characteristics are measured. Any deviation from this constitutes *measurement error.*

Measurement instruments are usually evaluated for reliability and validity.
- *Reliability* or *precision* refers to the degree of similarity of the results obtained when the measurement is repeated on the same subject or the same group. Is the same value arrived at every time the measurement is taken, or do the values vary a lot on repeated administration?
- *Validity* refers to the extent to which a measurement instrument actually measures what it is meant to measure. The measurement instrument lacks validity if the characteristic in the same individual (or group) is measured repeatedly higher or repeatedly lower than the real value. This systematic error is called *bias*. See Chapter 12 for a full discussion of precision and bias.

These two concepts are illustrated in the bull's-eye diagrams in Figure 9.3a–d. The centre of the bull's-eye represents the 'true value' for the person and deviation from this value will represent poor validity. The small 'shots' represent different measurements for the same person and the star represents the mean value of these repeated measurements. Similar results for repeated measurement are represented by close proximity of the 'shots' to each other (good reliability or high precision). Sometimes, repeated measurements will be similar but their mean will be far from the true value (9.3b). Widely scattered (unreliable or imprecise) results can still produce an unbiased (valid) *mean* (9.3c).

B | Epidemiological research methods and protocol development

(Deviation of a *single* measurement from the true value can therefore be due to unreliability or lack of validity of the instrument or both.)

Figure 9.3 Conceptual representation of reliability and validity, as illustrated by repeated measurement for the same individual

Source: Adapted from Botha & Yach (1986)

Figure 9.3a Neither reliable nor valid measurement instrument

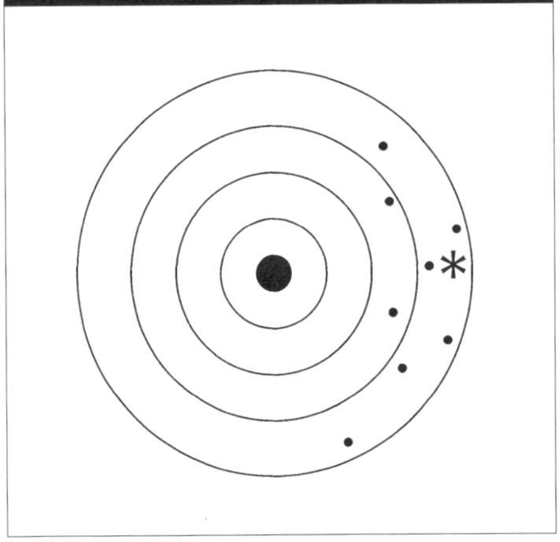

Figure 9.3b Reliable but not valid measurement instrument

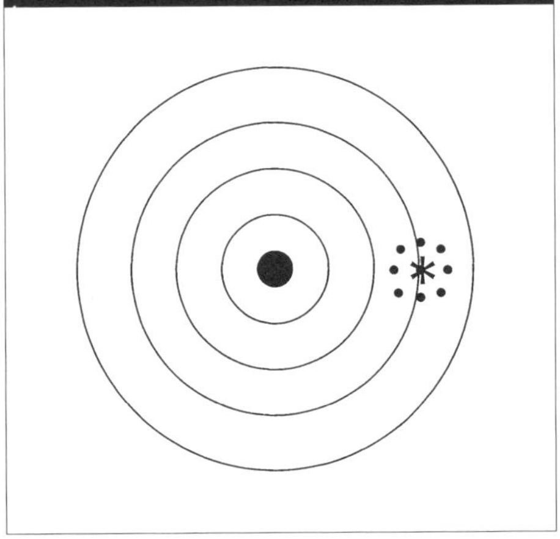

Figure 9.3c Apparently valid but not reliable measurement instrument

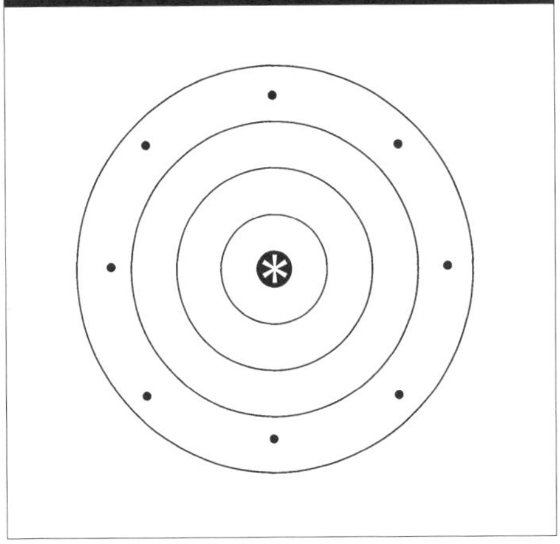

Figure 9.3d Valid and reliable measurement instrument

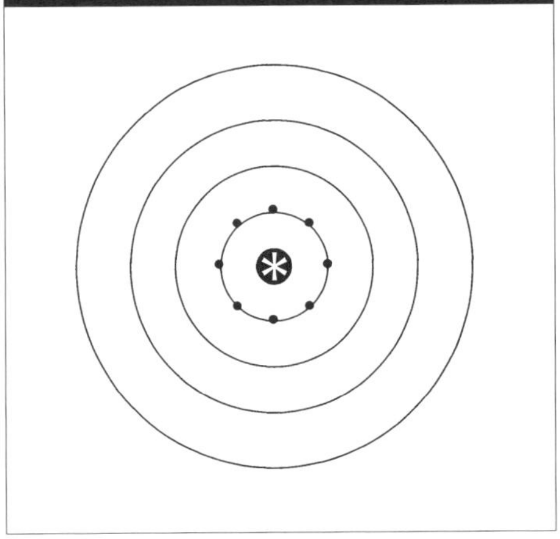

$*$: mean of repeated measurements

Note that the concepts of precision/reliability and validity extend to other research processes as well. For example, we can refer to bias in sampling, method of analysis, and so on. (See Chapter 4 and Chapter 12.)

Data collection and measurement | 9

Sources of error in measurement

The possible sources of error in measurement are:
- the instrument
- the observer
- the subject
- the environment.

Improving and evaluating reliability

Variation between measures (poor reliability) can be decreased by addressing the source of the variation.

- The *instrument variation* (giving different results for the same individuals) can be reduced by standardisation and calibration of the instrument. All measuring instruments have to be calibrated before each measuring session, especially if instruments are handled roughly in the field. So, for example, the weight recorded by a scale should be compared to a standard weight (for example, a 10 litre plastic container filled with water which will weigh 10 kg) which is in the range of weights being measured in the study. When choosing an instrument, one should also take into account the ease with which it can be used.
- *Observer variation* can stem from differences among observers or interviewers (*inter-observer variation*), as well as differences in the same observer or interviewer on separate occasions (*intra-observer variation*).

These variations between measures can be reduced by:
- setting exact ways of measuring (standardisation of measurement or interview)
- appropriate selection of interviewers
- intensive training periods for all observers and interviewers
  For example, during training, each observer and the instructor or supervisor should make repeat measurements on subjects similar to those who will be measured in the study. A simple listing of the different measurements can give an indication of whether there are problems, and whether these are due to carelessness, or show a consistent error.
- supervision and periodic checks on the work of interviewers.
- *Subject variation* may be due to biological variation (for example, blood pressure varies during the day) or inconsistencies of memory. Repeated measures make it possible to assess and adjust for biological variation, for example, by taking the mean value.

Evaluation of variation

Instrument, observer, and subject variation can be evaluated by repeating measures on a subsample of the study sample. In the case of questionnaires, similar questions which should give similar answers could be asked. If their answers are in disagreement, subject variation has been identified.

Statistics used to assess the agreement on repeated application of questions depend on the type of variable, and a biostatistician should be consulted about how to evaluate repeat measures meaningfully. Table 9.2 describes the calculation and interpretation of the Kappa statistic, used to measure the agreement between two observers on a categorical variable with two categories.

Table 9.2 The Kappa statistic

The evaluation by two observers of the same subjects in the form of a categorical variable with only two categories, e.g. condition present or absent, can be depicted as follows:

		Observer 2		
		present	absent	
Observer 1	present	a	b	(a + b)
	absent	c	d	(c + d)
		(a + c)	(b + d)	(a + b + c + d)

The percentage agreement or concordance is (a+d)/(a+b+c+d)*100. However, some agreement will happen by chance. Kappa indicates the agreement, corrected for chance, and is calculated as follows:

$$\frac{2(ad - bc)}{(a + b)(b + d) + (c + d)(a + c)}$$

Kappa can take on values between −1 and 1, with 1 indicating perfect agreement, 0 no agreement other than what would be expected due to chance, and −1 perfect disagreement. Kappa values above 0.8 indicate excellent agreement.

Improving and evaluating validity

Different concepts of validity are used:
- *Face validity* refers to the extent to which the measure or question makes sense to those knowledgeable about the subject or to interviewers familiar with the language and culture of participants.
- *Content validity* requires that the measure accounts for all the elements of the variable or concept being investigated. For example, educational level and occupation may not account for all the elements of the variable 'social class' in a particular setting.
- *Criterion-related validity* (or *criterion validity*) involves evaluating the results of the measurement instrument against the most valid measurement available (the *gold standard*). The gold standard is used as a criterion to see how many values were correctly identified. The *sensitivity* and *specificity* of a measurement instrument can be calculated to assess the criterion-related validity of variables (see Figure 9.4).
- *Predictive validity* requires that the measure, if used, confirms a known or theoretically hypothesised association. For example, higher social class is known to be associated with better school performance. To assess the validity of 'dwelling type' as a measure of social class, the investigator can determine to what extent 'dwelling type' is associated with school performance.
- *Inconsistent validity* refers to a measure which is valid for one group, but may be different in different groups, populations, and environments. So questionnaires or tests designed for a particular population in the northern hemisphere may be invalid for populations in developing communities.

Other issues related to data collection

Ethics

It is important to get permission (informed consent) from potential participants whom researchers want to interview or do measurements on, after the study and methods have been explained to them.

Data collection and measurement 9

> **Figure 9.4 Evaluation of criterion-related validity: sensitivity and specificity**
>
> The true situation as yielded by criterion measure
>
> | | Positive | Negative | |
> |---|---|---|---|
> | **Results yielded by instrument being assessed** Positive | A | B | A+B |
> | Negative | C | D | C+D |
> | | A+C | B+D | A+B+C+D |
>
> **Sensitivity** (true positive rate) = $\frac{A}{(A+C)} \times 100$
> Percentage of positive test results out of all true positives
>
> **Specificity** (true negative rate) = $\frac{D}{(B+D)} \times 100$
> Percentage of negative test results out of all true negatives
>
> Other indices of criterion-related validity (see Chapter 25)
>
> **Positive predictive value** = $\frac{A}{(A+B)} \times 100$
> The percentage of positive test results that are truly positive
>
> **Negative predictive value** = $\frac{D}{(C+D)} \times 100$
> The percentage of negative test results which are truly negative
>
> **Positive likelihood ratio** = $[A/(A+C)]/[B/(B+D)]$ = sensitivity/(1-specificity)
> Probability that the condition is present if the test is positive, divided by the probability that the condition is present if the test is negative
>
> **Negative likelihood ratio** = $[C/(A+C)]/[D/(B+D)]$ = (1-sensitivity)/specificity
> Probability that the condition is absent if the test is positive, divided by the probability that the condition is absent if the test is negative

Ethically, researchers are required to protect the identity of study participants. Ideally information should remain anonymous, that is, names should not be recorded at all on the questionnaire or data capture form. However, often some record of the respondents' names needs to be kept so that follow-up or referral is possible. For example, if the plan is to inform all participants of their personal results (for example, blood results) or the overall study results, names and addresses will be needed. It is then ethically acceptable that information remains confidential, which means that identifying information is available only to the researchers. Ethical issues related to data collection and access to information need to be addressed in the ethics section of the study protocol.

121

Translation

Translation: enhancing communication

Clearly, the best way to obtain information in a project is to address participants in their own language. Translation will be an issue when participants speak a language other than that of the researcher. Interviewers should be fluent in the language of interview. The questionnaire can be drawn up in a language that the researcher understands (for example, English), but fully translated questionnaires need to be used in the interviews. The initial translation should be done by someone fluent in the language, who can judge whether certain phrases are understandable and acceptable. This translation should be proofread by a second person. The next step is for someone else to back-translate the questionnaire into the original language. If the back-translation corresponds well to the original, the translation is considered acceptable. Often health workers who work with people similar to the respondents, rather than linguists, will have a good feel for what can be understood by such respondents. (See Chapter 23 for a further discussion of language.)

Interviewers

Select interviewers carefully (on the basis of, for example, educational level, social skills). Train and supervise them well, and ensure that they are adequately paid. This improves the reliability of information.

One study might employ different types of people to do different tasks in the data collection process. A registered nurse might measure blood pressures, while a high school graduate might be regarded as the best for interviewing. Yet another person, well known in the community and with good interpersonal skills, might inform and motivate people ahead of time of the study.

Training

Training of staff involved in the data collection is fundamental to good quality information. It is well worth spending a few days training interviewers, observers, and motivators so that everyone knows exactly what is expected of them.

During the training period, the nature of and reason for the research, and the objectives of the study, should be carefully explained before the tasks are discussed in detail. Explicitly discuss rules, conditions of employment, and other specific instructions so that the team can work together effectively.

There should be clear lines of accountability, and the nature of the supervision should be explained. For example, the interviewers should know that they will receive instructions from the field co-ordinator or supervisor, who will also check their work for errors and advise on how errors are to be dealt with.

Field supervision

There should be a clear plan of how supervision will be done in the field. Supervision must include site visits, checking of forms, and checking that the data have not been fudged or made up by the interviewer. From time to time, the fieldworkers should meet with the supervisor or co-ordinator to discuss important issues individually or as a group. Field supervision is discussed in further detail in Chapter 14.

Conclusion

Whether data are collected in the community (see Chapter 14), the workplace (see Chapter 21), or the health care setting (see Chapter 25), the measurement tools need to be carefully designed to ensure good quality data. Discussion of results should always include a consideration of the validity and reliability of the measuring instruments.

Useful readings

Bowling, A. 2001. *Measuring disease.* 2nd ed. Buckingham: Open University Press.

Bowling, A. 2005. *Measuring health: a review of quality of life measurement scales.* 3rd ed. Maidenhead, Berks: Open University Press.

McDowell, I & Newell, C. 1996. *Measuring health: a guide to rating scales and questionnaires.* 2nd ed. Oxford: Oxford University Press.

Useful web sites

Department of Health and Ageing, Australia. [Online]. Available: http://www.health.gov.au/internet/wcms/publishing.nsf/. [16 February 2007].

Medical Algorithms Project. [Online]. Available: http://www.medal.org. [25 February 2007].

South East Public Health Observatory. *A review of methods for monitoring and measuring social inequality, deprivation and health.* [Online]. Available: http://www.ihs.ox.ac.uk/sepho/publications/carrhill. [25 February 2007].

World Health Organization. *World health survey.* [Online]. Available: http://www.who.int/healthinfo/survey/. [25 February 2007].

Reference used in this chapter

Botha, JL & Yach, D. 1986. Epidemiological research methods. Part II. Descriptive studies. *South African Medical Journal*, 70:766–72.

Section C

Data presentation, analysis and interpretation

10 Exploring, summarising and presenting data
11 Analysing and interpreting epidemiological data
12 Precision and validity in epidemiological studies: error, bias and confounding

10

Exploring, summarising and presenting data

Gina Joubert

> **OBJECTIVES OF THIS CHAPTER**
>
> The objectives of this chapter are:
> - to provide an (almost) formula-free introduction to the exploration, summarisation and presentation of epidemiological data
> - to characterise different types of variables
> - to emphasise the importance of data checking before analysis
> - to describe ways in which numerical variables should be explored graphically
> - to describe ways in which to summarise information appropriately.

Introduction

As described in Section B, statistics applied to biological and medical problems (*biostatistics*) has a contribution to make in the planning of a project regarding issues such as study design, sample selection and sample size. In Section C we deal with statistical aspects of the presentation, summary and analysis of data. Depending on the complexity of analysis required for the project, a researcher should consult a statistician to discuss the statistical aspects of the research project in the planning phase as well as the analysis and write-up phase. A basic understanding of statistical concepts will enable the researcher to do some initial analyses and ensure that he or she gets the most benefit from interaction with a statistician on the more complex analyses. Such an understanding will also enable a researcher to evaluate published research findings. The statistical techniques used in the literature are not always appropriate. This may be because many statistical textbooks place the emphasis on 'how' a statistical method is applied (the cookbook approach), rather than 'when' and 'why'. In addition, the widespread availability of personal computers (PCs) and statistical software enables a researcher to do complex analyses without having to understand the techniques used or even looking at the data closely. The PC will provide an answer, whether the question asked is appropriate or not. Data analysis cannot be done adequately by simply following a few 'how to' rules.

Many researchers may feel at a disadvantage since they do not have a good mathematical background, and may even fear formulae. Such a background is not necessary to enable one to master the basic statistical concepts. However, researchers should consider upgrading their mathematical skills (by attending courses or working through textbooks) to come fully to grips with statistical methodology. We hope that this section will instil an interest even in those readers who have a fear of numbers and encourage them to develop the necessary skills.

Variables

The characteristics which one measures are referred to as variables (Figure 10.1). Variables are classified according to their *scale of measurement*.

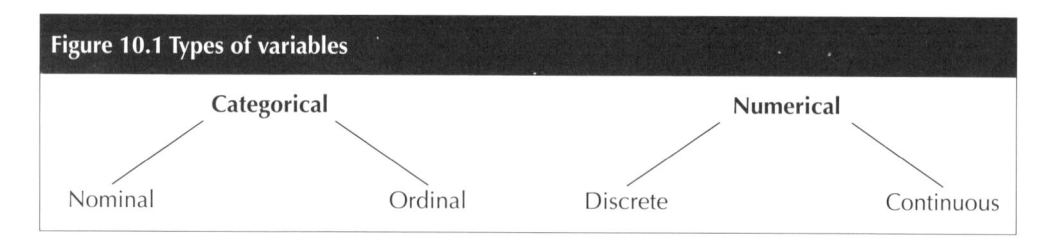

Figure 10.1 Types of variables

```
            Categorical                         Numerical
           /          \                        /         \
      Nominal        Ordinal              Discrete      Continuous
```

Classification of variables

Categorical variables specify into which category an observation falls.

Nominal: Variables are called *nominal* if the categories have no natural order, but are identified only by name, for example, the categories male or female for the variable sex.

Ordinal: If there is some ordering amongst the categories, the variable is called *ordinal*, for example, the variable social class which may be recorded in categories 1 (professional) to 5 (manual), or the severity of a disease (mild, moderate, severe).

Dichotomous or *binary*: A categorical variable which has only two categories is called a *dichotomous* or *binary* variable.

Numerical variables are variables for which the allocated numbers have intrinsic quantitative meaning.

Discrete: Numerical variables are *discrete* if the variable can take on only certain values (for example, the number of children in a family can be 2 but not 2.75 or 2.751). Discrete variables are often counts of events or people, for example, the number of patients seen at a clinic per day.

Continuous: A numerical variable is *continuous* if the variable can assume any numerical value (for example, weight can be measured very precisely on a continuous scale to a number of decimal places).

The scale of measurement determines how the variable is set up in the statistical database. The type of variable also influences sample size calculation and the methods of analysis.

Data checking before analysis

Before any analysis is done, the data set must be carefully checked to identify any strange values and errors which might have occurred in the original source document, during transcription or during data entry.

C Data presentation, analysis and interpretation

Table 10.1 Suggested data-checking procedures

One variable at a time

Categorical variables
- Check any implausible codes e.g. for the variable sex the codes M, F and G appear
- Check missing values

Numerical variables
- Check that the values fall in plausible range. Are the extremes possible?
  e.g. height = 250 cm, height = 5 cm
- Are values of 0 really zero or do they indicate missing values? (If the latter, then 0 must be made missing.)
- Check missing values
- Are missing values really missing or do they indicate 0? For example, a missing value for the number of cigarettes smoked per day may indicate a non-smoker and the missing value should instead be made 0

Cross-checking of variables
- If the same demographic information is asked in more than one question, do the answers disagree: male in one answer, female in another
- In a longitudinal study, are the changes in values between assessments implausible? age at week 1 = 25 years, age at week 52 = 35 years?
- Do related questions give implausible results?
  1. Sex = M, and oral contraceptive usage = Yes
  2. Age = 27 years and age at which started smoking = 33 years
  3. Do you smoke? = No, and How many cigarettes do you smoke? = 10

Such errors can strongly influence and bias the results, and the researcher should therefore detect and correct them before analysing the data (since, as the saying goes, garbage in, garbage out). The data-checking procedures listed in Table 10.1 are done after data entry, but before analysis.

For data-checking procedures, we need a computer listing of the values of all variables, as well as the interrelationship of variables. If any strange values or missing values are found, we should make a list of the subject or questionnaire identifiers of those cases. We should investigate any queries resulting from the data-checking procedure by going back to the raw data (for example, questionnaires), not by guessing. It is therefore important that we keep questionnaires, and that we put them in order according to the questionnaire identifier, so that it is easy to pull out the forms with queries.

Some queries will be easy to resolve, for example, a 1 may be typed as a 7. Others may be difficult to resolve, and if the value in the raw data is completely impossible (for example, sex = Z instead of M or F and the sex cannot be deduced from the name), the value should be classified as *missing*. The aim is to eliminate errors, not 'recreate' the data. Respondents may give conflicting responses; for example, they may express 'contradictory' attitudes where two questions require similar information. These are not data errors and cannot be cleaned.

Stem and branch questions (see Chapter 9) are also frequently incorrectly answered. For example, the respondent marks 'no' to a stem question such as 'does your child have asthma?', but then goes on to answer 'yes' to the branch question 'if yes, has he or she had an attack in the last month?'. The responses to both questions should be coded as missing since it is impossible to know which of the two questions was answered incorrectly. The total number of responses obtained for related questions should also be checked to see whether they add up correctly or whether there are unexpected missing values. Graphical display of the data is described below and is also useful in the data-checking phase.

If data are entered directly onto a PC in the field, the data-entering program (for example, Epi Info) should be set up in such a way that implausible values can be discovered immediately. For example, one should specify a plausible range for a continuous variable such as height. If a value which falls outside this range is typed in, the program alerts the data typist that a strange value has been entered, and must be corrected.

Table 10.2 gives a listing of the information regarding age, sex and certain aspects of smoking history of 10 subjects included in a study of community members aged 20 years and older. How many problems can we identify?

Table 10.2 Listing of 10 observations

Subject	Age (years)	Sex	Current smoker	Ever smoked	Age started smoking (years)
1	45	M	Y	Y	15
2	32	F	Y	N	–
3	35	F	N	Y	31
4	46	M	N	Y	40
5	25	M	Y	Y	28
6	20	M	N	N	–
7	18	M	Y	Y	16
8	20	F	Y	Y	–
9	21	M	Y	Y	18
10	30		N	N	20

Exploratory data analysis

Before any formal statistical analysis is done, we should explore the data (especially numerical variables) through graphical display (also known as exploratory data analysis). Such an exploration helps the researcher to get to know the data. It is possible to detect errors or strange values, and unexpected patterns and relationships in the data. Furthermore, many statistical procedures make assumptions about the data, for example, about the distribution of the data (see below). Through graphical display we can determine whether our data satisfy these assumptions and therefore whether the intended statistical analyses are appropriate. Although these displays are seldom published in final reports or publications owing to space constraints, they should always be done. We can evaluate by formal statistical methods (also called confirmatory data analysis) patterns or relationships detected through, or questions raised by, exploratory data analysis. This exploration of the data is not a fishing exercise to try to pick up any possible associations in the data, but is guided by the objectives of the study.

C | Data presentation, analysis and interpretation

Graphical display of numerical variables

The aim of displaying a numerical variable is to investigate certain characteristics of the data, namely where the central value lies, and what the spread and shape (distribution) of the data are. The distribution shows how many observations have a given value or lie within a certain range of values out of all the possible values. As will be discussed below, the shape of the distribution is important in deciding on appropriate summary statistics and statistical analyses.

The following small data sets will be used to illustrate basic concepts.

- In a hypertension study, diastolic blood pressure was measured on a sample of 16 respondents. Their values, all expressed as mm of mercury (mm Hg), were:
  75, 84, 80, 97, 105, 188, 64, 78, 68, 86, 79, 105, 89, 88, 93, and 92.
- Two groups of children were scored on a psychological test. The scores were (in order):

Group 1 (n = 24)	Group 2 (n = 25)
38 46 46 50 52	41 41 41 41 46
52 55 57 59 62	46 46 48 52 52
63 63 64 65 69	54 54 58 60 60
69 71 71 74 75	61 71 74 76 80
79 81 87 94	84 85 93 104 148

Stem and leaf plot

In a stem and leaf plot, each observation of a numerical variable is plotted. All possible leading values form the stem, and each data value is represented by writing its trailing digit in the appropriate row next to the stem, in this way forming the leaves. Before the plot can be drawn, the data are ordered from small to large.

In the blood pressure example, the ordered data set is:
64, 68, 75, 78, 79, 80, 84, 86, 88, 89, 92, 93, 97, 105, 105, 188

Since the values range from 64 to 188, the leading digits which are to form the stem are 6, 7, 8, 9, 10, 11, 12, 13, 14, 15, 16, 17, 18. The stem and leaf plot is then as follows:

```
18 | 8
17 |
16 |
15 |
14 |
13 |
12 |
11 |
10 | 5 5
 9 | 2 3 7
 8 | 0 4 6 8 9
 7 | 5 8 9
 6 | 4 8
```

Any value which lies far away from the other values (an *outlier*) can be detected easily. The value 188 is suspect and should be checked. It may be a typing error: 88 typed as 188. Apart from the extreme value, the values seem to follow a symmetric distribution. A distribution has a *symmetrical* shape if approximately the same number of observations lie above and below the centre value of the distribution. Figure 10.2 depicts what different data distributions would look like when illustrated by a stem and leaf plot.

If we draw a stem and leaf plot with a very short stem, and many leaves, or a very long stem with very few leaves, the display will not be informative and we should choose our leading digits differently. It is important that the leaves are written neatly in columns; otherwise the shape of the distribution will not be seen clearly.

If groups are to be compared, stem and leaf plots drawn next to one another are useful for detecting distributional differences between groups. The back-to-back stem and leaf plot of psychological data is depicted in Figure 10.3. The value 148 in Group 2 seems to be an outlier and should be checked. From the stem and leaf plot, it is clear that the values in Group 1 follow a

Figure 10.2 Types of data distribution

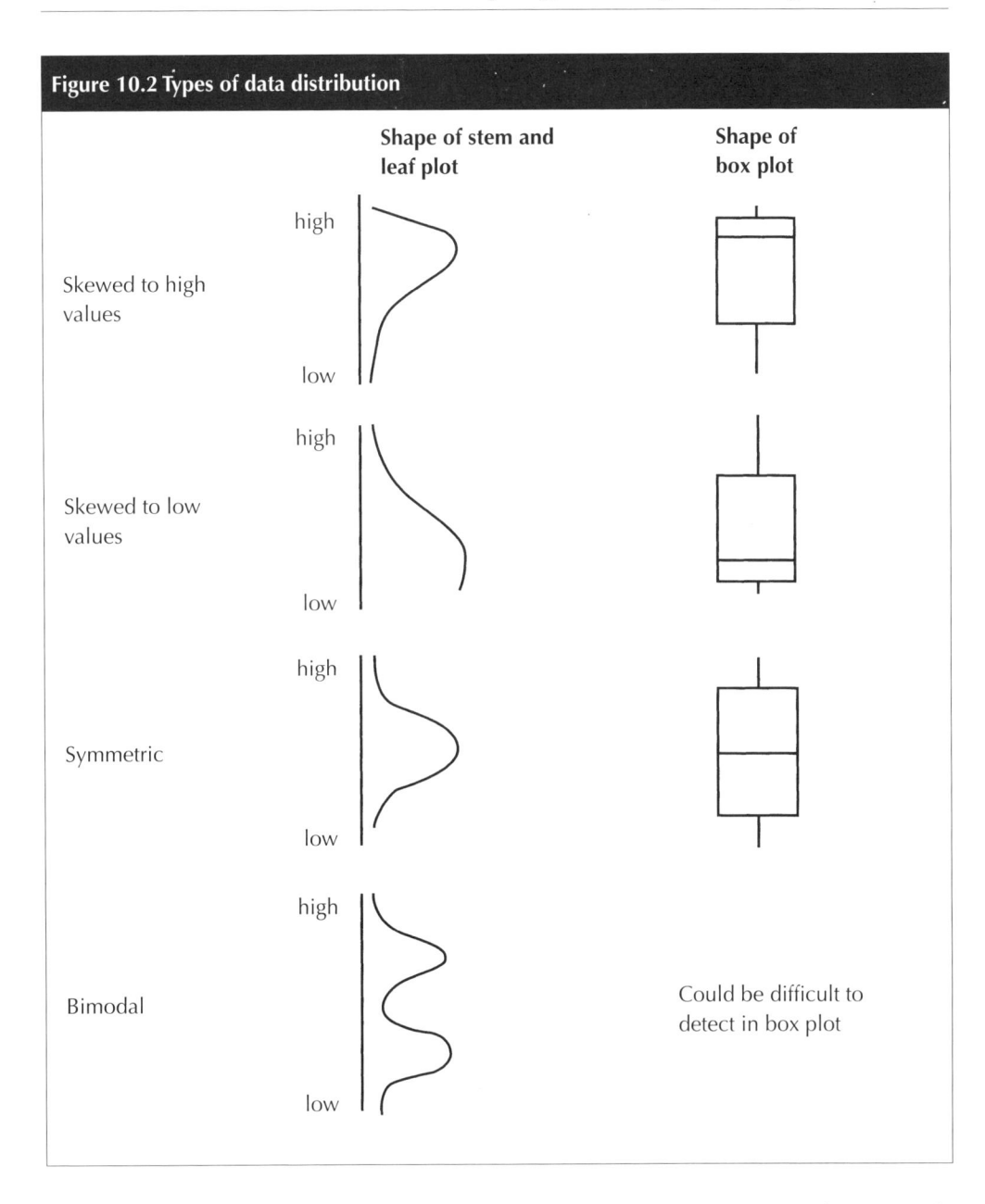

Distribution	Shape of stem and leaf plot	Shape of box plot
Skewed to high values	high to low, peak near low	box with median near bottom
Skewed to low values	high to low, peak near high	box with median near top
Symmetric	high to low, peak in middle	box with median in middle
Bimodal	high to low, two peaks	Could be difficult to detect in box plot

symmetric distribution, but the values in Group 2 are not symmetrical (also called *skewed*), as most of the values are low.

Box plot

A second type of graphical display appropriate for numerical variables is the box plot, which displays the data in summarised form. Not all points are plotted in a box plot, only selected summary values – namely the median, the 25th and 75th percentiles, and the maximum and minimum values.

Median: The median (or *50th percentile*) is that value which divides the sample values, ordered from small to large, in half; that is, half the values lie above the median, the other half below. If the sample size is odd, the middle value in the ordered series

C | Data presentation, analysis and interpretation

Figure 10.3 Stem and leaf plot of children's psychological test scores

```
              GROUP 1                 14 | 8              GROUP 2
              (n = 24)                13 |                (n = 25)
                                      12 |
                                      11 |
                                      10 | 4
                          4            9 | 3
                      7   1            8 | 0  4  5
              9 5 4   1   1            7 | 1  4  6
      9 9 5 4 3   3   2                6 | 0  0  1
        9 7 5 2   2   0                5 | 2  2  4  4  8
                  6   6                4 | 1  1  1  1  6  6  6  8
                      8                3 |
```

is the median. If the sample size is even, the median is the average of the two middle values. Therefore the median of the 16 blood pressure values is the average of the 8th and 9th values, namely the average of 86 and 88, i.e. 87.

Quartiles: These divide the sample values into quarters. The *lower quartile* is also called the *25th percentile*, and the *upper quartile* the *75th percentile*. The distance between the lower and upper quartile is called the *interquartile range*. For the 16 blood pressure values, the lower quartile must lie between the 4th and 5th values in the ordered series (values 78 and 79). The 25th percentile is defined as being a quarter of the way between these two values, namely at 78.25. The upper quartile lies between the 12th and 13th values (values 93 and 97). The 75th percentile is defined as being three-quarters of the way between the two values, namely at 96.

Drawing a box plot

In the box plot, the upper and lower quartiles are displayed by the top and bottom of the rectangle which contains the central 50% of the data. The median is indicated by a horizontal line within the rectangle. The quartiles are connected by lines to the largest and smallest value in the sample. (Some computer packages also indicate extreme values other than the maximum and minimum in the box plot.)

If the distance from the lower quartile to the median is approximately equal to the distance from the upper quartile to the median, the distribution is *symmetrical*. Box plots can therefore be used to detect outlying values, as well as to determine the shape of the distribution of the values. The box plot of the 16 blood pressure values is as follows:

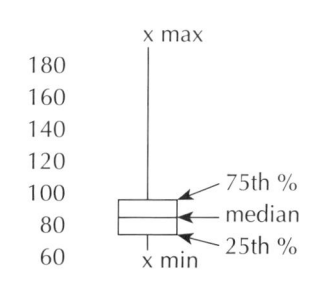

The box plots of the psychological test data are shown in Figure 10.4. The symmetry of Group 1 is clear, since the median lies approximately halfway between the two quartiles. Group 2 is asymmetrical, as can be seen from the fact that the median is much closer to the lower quartile than to the upper quartile. See also Figure 10.2 above, which depicts how different data distributions look when illustrated by a box plot.

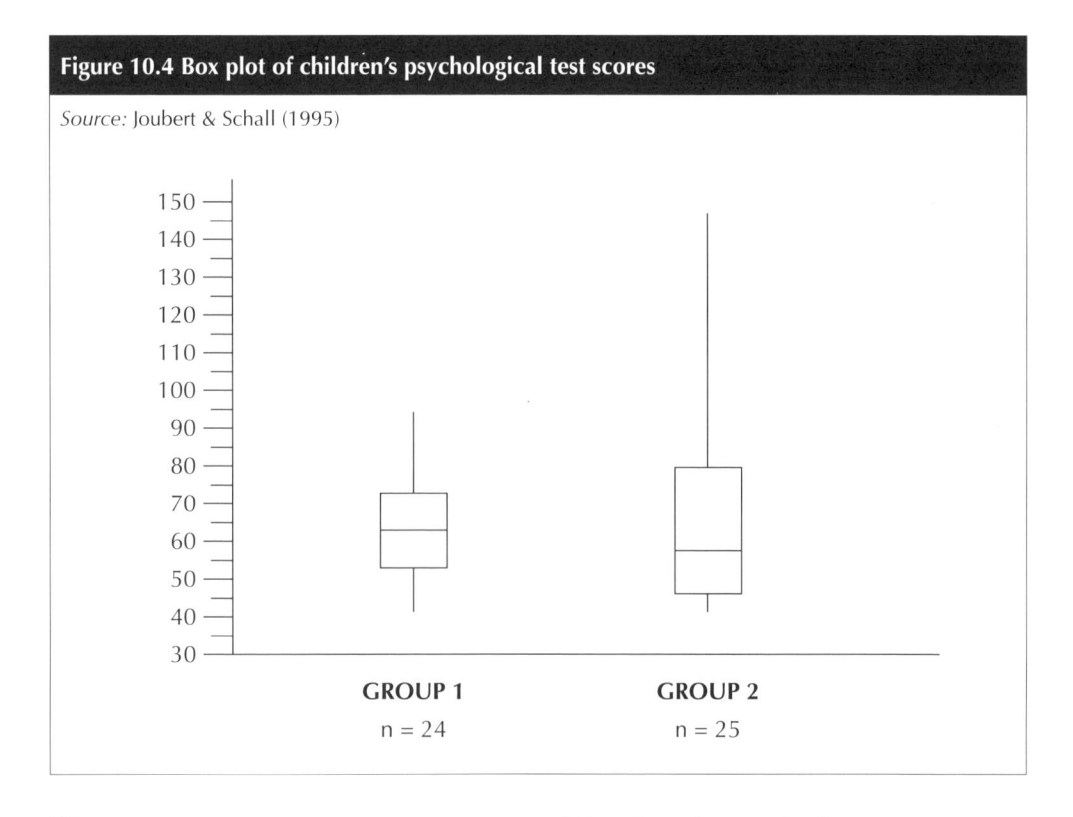

Figure 10.4 Box plot of children's psychological test scores

Source: Joubert & Schall (1995)

Histogram

This graphical display can be used to evaluate the distribution of a numerical variable at the start of the analysis, or to summarise a number of observations in compact form for a presentation or report. A histogram is drawn for a numerical variable which has been grouped into categories. For example, blood pressure can be grouped into 10 mm Hg groups. Each rectangle in the histogram can represent either the number of observations or the percentage of observations that fall in that interval. The population pyramid described in the section on demography in Chapter 2 is a special type of histogram used to depict the age and sex composition of a population.

Bivariate (scatter) plot

Bivariate or scatter plots are used to plot two numerical variables against one another, one variable on the X axis (horizontal); the other on the Y axis (vertical).

These plots are especially helpful when we would like to investigate relationships between variables. We should draw a bivariate or scatter plot before we do a statistical evaluation of a relationship by means of, for example, correlation or regression. Plots of this type can help to identify errors (Figure 10.5) and clarify relationships between variables (Figure 10.6).

C | Data presentation, analysis and interpretation

Figure 10.5 Bivariate plot of height and weight

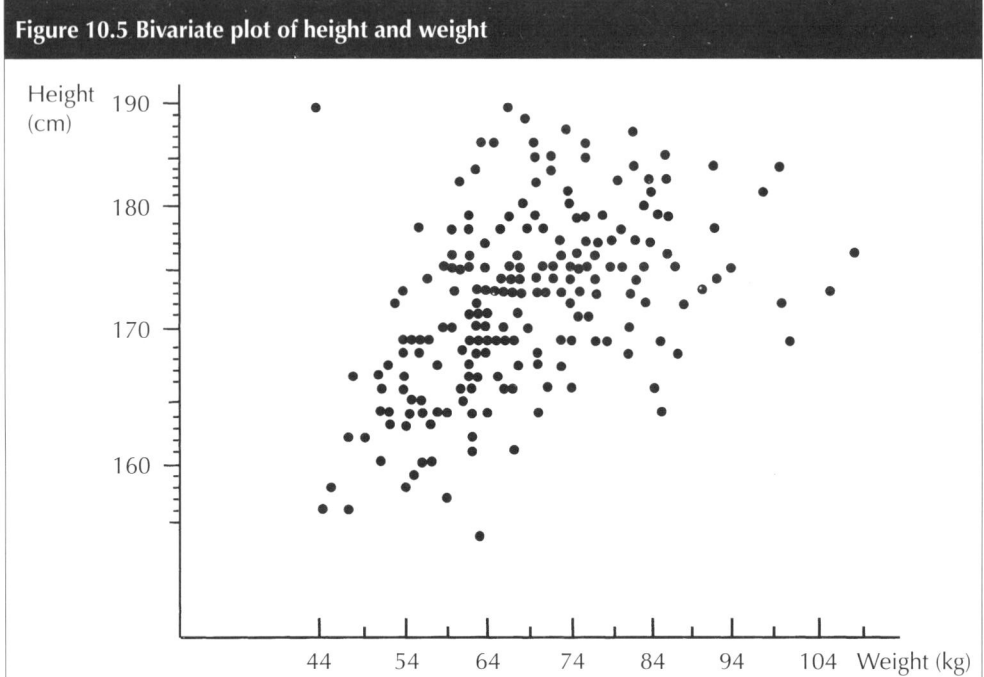

In the bivariate plot of height and weight, the case with height = 189 cm and weight = 44 kg stands out as being questionable. In an investigation of only height or weight, the values for this case would not have seemed strange.

Figure 10.6 Bivariate plot of the relationship between lung function and age

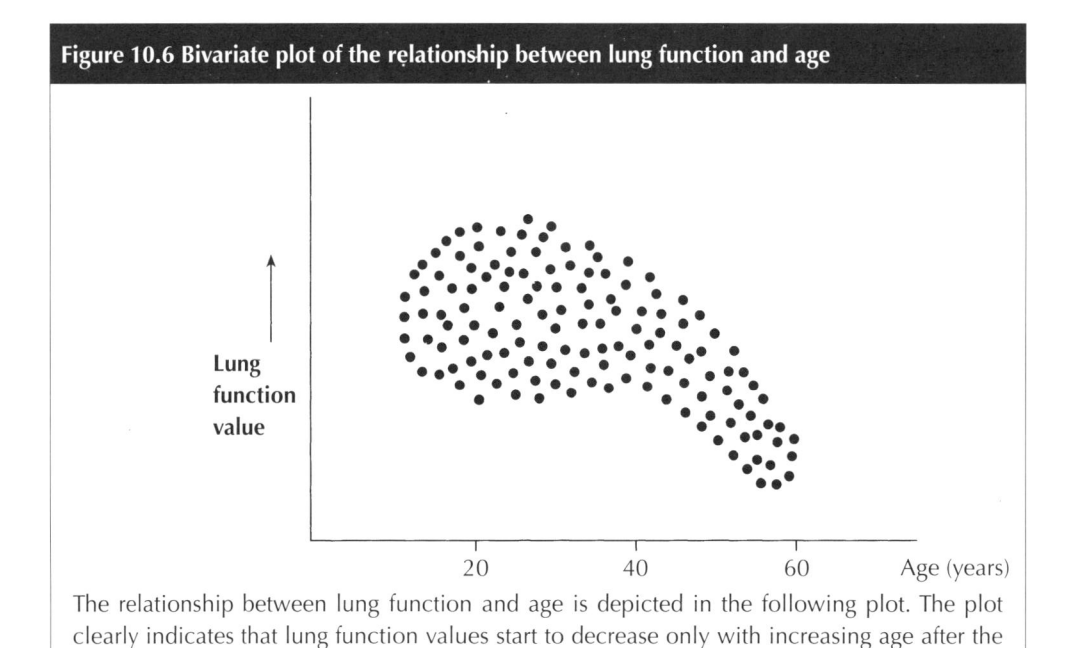

The relationship between lung function and age is depicted in the following plot. The plot clearly indicates that lung function values start to decrease only with increasing age after the age of 40 years.

Graphical display of categorical variables

Whereas the graphical display of numerical variables described above is essential before formal statistical analysis can be done, the methods described here for categorical variables are often used to present the results after the analysis. The choice of method is a matter of personal preference, but it is important that the method used reflects the data correctly. Bar graphs and pie charts can be used to represent categorical variables. The height of the bar in a bar graph (or the size of the slice in a pie chart) can represent either the number of observations in a given category of the variable, or the percentage of all observations that fall in a given category. So, for example, the dust exposure category distribution of factory workers can be represented by a bar graph, as shown in Figure 10.7. It is important that we label the graph clearly, indicating the categories depicted, whether percentages or frequencies are indicated, and the sample size. A bar graph is similar to a histogram, but the bars are drawn with spaces in between.

Figure 10.7 Bar graph showing the dust exposure category distribution of a sample of factory workers (n = 100)

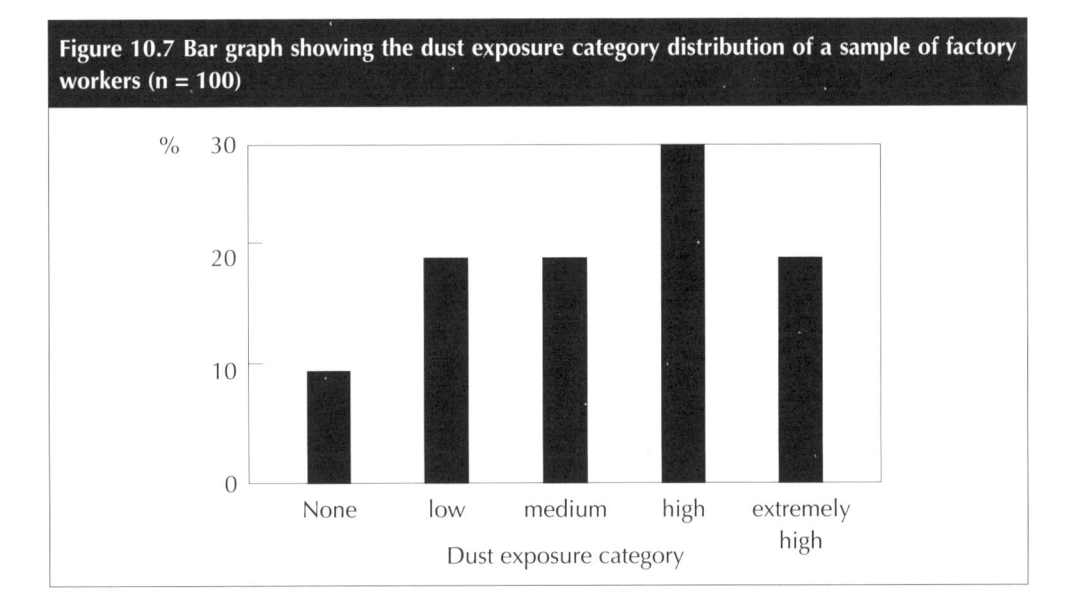

Figure 10.8 is an example of a block chart or three-dimensional bar graph. It displays, for four different age and sex groups, the percentages of respondents who mentioned different categories of Aids prevention strategies (respondents were permitted to choose more than one option). For example, 18.2% of males under the age of 18 years mentioned condoms, whereas only 8.1% of females under 18 years mentioned condoms. From the bar graph it is clear that males tended to mention condoms more often than females did, whereas females mentioned one partner more often than males did.

Summarising the sample data

Summary statistics, also known as descriptive statistics, are used to summarise and describe the data in a concise form. The basic summary of the data is the first step of the statistical analysis, whether we have conducted a descriptive study where the aim is to estimate the level or distribution of a characteristic, or an analytical study where the aim is to

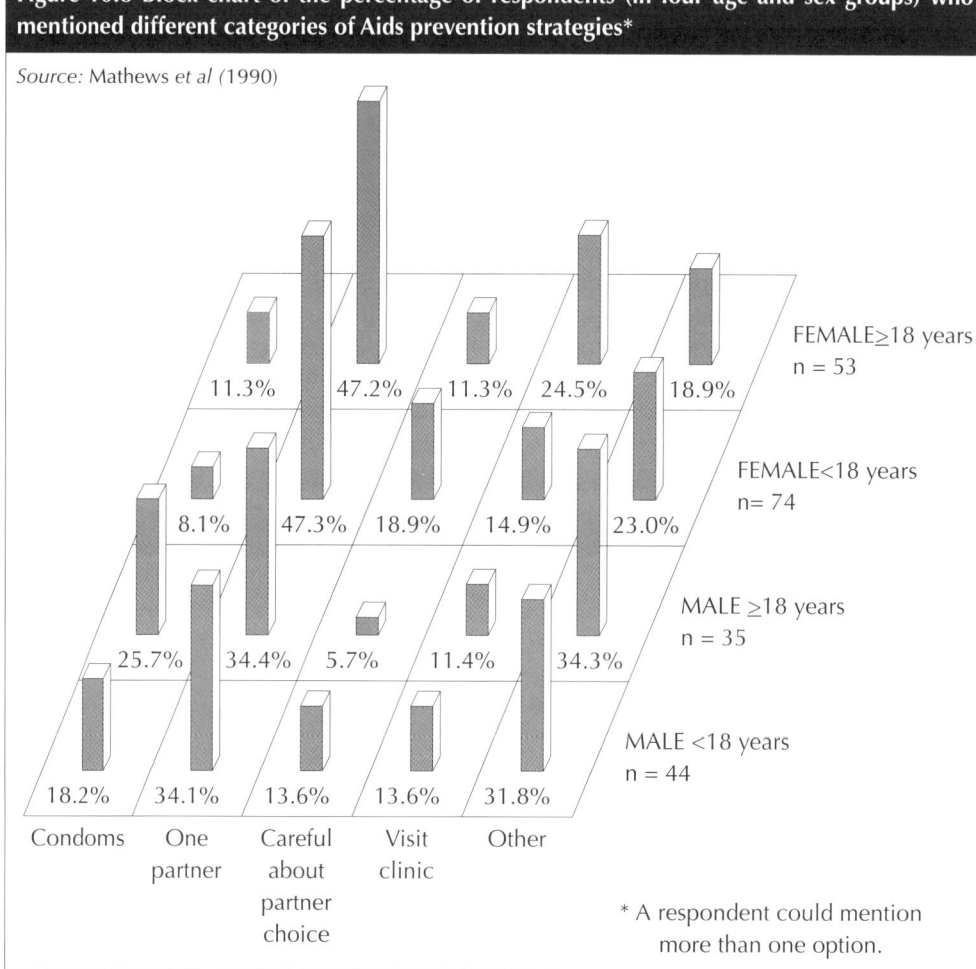

C | Data presentation, analysis and interpretation

Figure 10.8 Block chart of the percentage of respondents (in four age and sex groups) who mentioned different categories of Aids prevention strategies*

Source: Mathews et al (1990)

FEMALE≥18 years n = 53: 11.3%, 47.2%, 11.3%, 24.5%, 18.9%
FEMALE<18 years n= 74: 8.1%, 47.3%, 18.9%, 14.9%, 23.0%
MALE ≥18 years n = 35: 25.7%, 34.4%, 5.7%, 11.4%, 34.3%
MALE <18 years n = 44: 18.2%, 34.1%, 13.6%, 13.6%, 31.8%

Categories: Condoms, One partner, Careful about partner choice, Visit clinic, Other

* A respondent could mention more than one option.

investigate associations between characteristics. By summarising the information as a first step, we can immediately see whether other intended analyses will be meaningful. If, for example, only two individuals out of a sample of 100 have a certain characteristic, there is little point in exploring the association of that characteristic with other factors, because the effective sample is so small.

Categorical variables

Categorical variables can be summarised by the *number* and *percentage* of study subjects which are classified into a given category. For example, a sample of 95 contains 16 males (17%) and 79 females (83%). It is important to state the sample size. The percentage can be rounded to the nearest whole number (especially in small samples), or can be given to one decimal place.

Numerical variables

For numerical variables, on the other hand, one needs to indicate where the central location of the data lies, as well as what the variability of the data is (that is, what the spread of the data is). By examining the graphical display of the data, the researcher determines which measures should be used to summarise the data.

Measures of central location

The most commonly used measure of the central location is the *arithmetic mean* or average (denoted by $\bar{x}$). This is the sum of all individual values (x_i) divided by the number of individuals in the group (n) (where Σ is the sum of all the n observations from 1 to n and x_i indicates the value of the i-th individual):

$$\bar{x} = \frac{\sum_{i=1}^{n} x_i}{n}$$

For the 16 blood pressure values (see page 130) the mean is

(64 + 68 + 75 + 78 + 79 + 80 + 84 + 86 + 88 + 89 + 92 + 93 + 97 + 105 + 105 + 188) / 16 = 91.9

The mean has at most one decimal place more than the original values. The above mean should not be given as 91.9375 since it implies that the original measurements were taken to the fourth decimal place ('spurious accuracy').

Means and medians

The mean is sensitive to *extreme values (outliers)*, especially in small samples. For example, if the sample consists of five values, namely 1, 2, 3, 4 and 5, the mean is 15/5 = 3. However, if the values are 1, 2, 3, 4 and 50, the mean is 60/5 = 12. The high value 50 has a large influence on the mean, pulling it away from the other four values.

If the distribution is asymmetrical or if there are outliers, we should rather use the *median* as the measure of central location (see the part above on the box plot). The median is called a *robust* alternative to the mean, since it is not sensitive to outliers or asymmetry in the distribution of the data. For the values 1, 2, 3, 4, 5, the median is 3. For the values 1, 2, 3, 4, 50, the median is also 3, indicating that the median is not influenced by the extreme value of 50. If the distribution of the data is symmetric, the median and mean will be close together. Since the mean or average is a concept that everyone is familiar with, it would be appropriate to use the mean rather than the median in the latter case.

For the psychological test scores in Group 1, the mean (64.3) is the appropriate measure of central location. For the other group, however, the median has to be used. If we want to compare the two groups, we must, of course, use the same summary statistics for both groups. If the values of one group are asymmetrical or if there is an extreme value, the central locations of both groups should be summarised by medians.

For some variables (especially laboratory determinations), we may encounter *censored* observations. These are observations for which the actual value is not known, but it is known that the value is greater than a certain measured threshold (for example, age greater than 65 years) or smaller than a certain measurable threshold (for example, a laboratory value below the lowest value the instrument can actually measure). In these cases, since the exact extreme values are not known, the median is the appropriate summary measure.

The *mode* is the value which occurs most often. This may be useful in determining whether a measuring instrument has a preference for a certain value (for example, a scale which weighs most respondents as 60 kg), but is of little use as a measure of central location.

In the case of a skewed distribution, a mathematical transformation of each value (for example, the log transformation where the log of each value is calculated) can be used to make the distribution more symmetric. The mean of the transformed values is calculated and then transformed back. In the case of the log transformation, the antilog of the mean of the transformed values is taken. This is known as the *geometric mean*.

Measures of variability (spread)

The variability of a data set is the degree to which observations in the data set vary from each other with respect to a particular characteristic. For example, consider two samples of 10 children each with ages as follows (in years):

Group 1: 2, 4, 6, 7, 8, 10, 11, 12, 14, 16
Group 2: 6, 6, 8, 8, 8, 10, 10, 10, 12, 14

The mean and median ages in both groups are 9 years, but the observations in Group 1 vary much more than those in Group 2. The variability of Group 1 is therefore greater than that of Group 2.

Range: The *range* (the largest value minus the smallest value, or denoted by indicating the largest and smallest values separately) is a measure of variability which we might intuitively consider using. In Group 1, the range is 2 to 16, in Group 2, it is 6 to 14. However, the range is not very useful as a measure of variability, since it can be greatly influenced by one extremely large or extremely small value.

Standard deviation: A commonly used measure of variation is the standard deviation. The standard deviation is defined as:

$$\sqrt{\frac{\sum_{i=1}^{n}(x_i - \bar{x})^2}{n-1}}$$

(See previous page for notation.)
It gives an indication of the average distance from the mean. We seldom have to calculate this without the aid of a calculator or PC, but seeing how it would be done helps to clarify the concept. For example, for each of the 16 blood pressures listed above, we must calculate the difference between the value and the mean. The first difference would be $64 - 91.9 = -27.9$. This difference is then squared (778.4). All 16 squared differences must be added. Divide the total by 15 ($n - 1$) before finding the square root. The *variance* is the standard deviation squared.

Coefficient of variation (CV): The coefficient of variation or CV is often seen in journal articles: it expresses the standard deviation as a percentage of the mean: CV = standard deviation/mean × 100.

Interquartile range: The interquartile range (75th percentile minus 25th percentile, as described earlier) provides a robust alternative to the standard deviation. The standard deviation is used with the mean, the interquartile range with the median. Therefore, if the data are asymmetrical or if there are outliers, the median and interquartile range (or 25th and 75th percentiles) should be used as summary measures.

Conclusion

Graphical display of data is done to let the data reveal their 'truth' to the reader. The way the researcher chooses to depict the data graphically should reflect this truth. Figure 10.9 discusses honesty in graphical display.

Summary statistics should also give a true representation of the data. We should therefore consider the distribution of the numerical data (through some graphical display) in order to decide on appropriate summary statistics. The following types of data are often encountered: grams of alcohol consumed weekly were noted in a heart disease risk factor survey. A total of 76% of respondents did not drink (so grams of alcohol consumed equal zero) and the remainder drank between 20 and 1 000 grams. Is it sensible to summarise the group's alcohol consumption with the overall mean of 78.2 g? In fact, percentiles would be more appropriate (median = 0 and 75th % = 0). Alternatively the researcher could state that 76% did not drink, and then state the mean or the median consumption of the drinkers.

Figure 10.9 Honesty in graphical display

To ensure that the graphical display reveals the truth about the data, one should keep the following in mind.

If bar graphs or pie charts are drawn to reflect percentages in different categories, one should state (in the caption or title of the graphic) the number out of which percentages were calculated. To represent 1 out of 3 as 33.3% without stating that the sample consisted of only 3 individuals is misleading.

When drawing plots, it is important that reasonable scales are used. Reasonable scales are those which do not put too much or too little emphasis on the actual results. Scales should also start at the 0 value if possible. The following plot seems to indicate that there was a big increase in the percentage of mortality owing to cause X between 1985 and 1986. However, close inspection of the scales reveals that the percentage increased from 10.5% in 1985 to 11.0% in 1986, hardly as dramatic an increase as the plot suggests. It would therefore be advisable to include the 0 value in the scales.

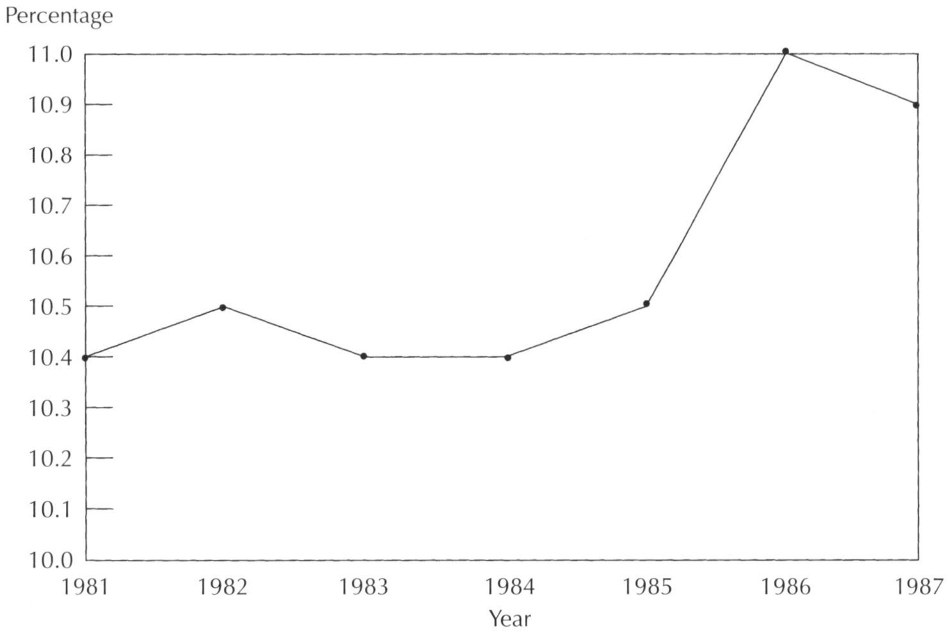

For a given numerical variable, the central value (summarised by the mean or median) may be of little interest. For example, it may be more relevant to the researcher to know what percentage of the sample has high blood pressure than what the mean blood pressure is. We can categorise a numerical variable and then summarise it as a categorical variable. The choice of categories for a numerical variable should make sense clinically. For example, hypertension may be defined as systolic blood pressure of 160 mm Hg and above or diastolic blood pressure of 95 mm Hg and above. The choice of categories can depend on the distribution of the data. For example, we could group all individuals over 65 years of age together in one age group if there are only a few who are between 65 and 74 years, 75 and 84 years, and so on. However, the grouping should not be done in such a way as to influence the results in a given direction.

In conclusion, no matter what the aim of the study was, the basic data should be displayed and described clearly and honestly.

Useful readings

Altman, DG. 1991. *Practical statistics for medical research*. London: Chapman and Hall.

Rosner, B. 2000. *Fundamentals of Biostatistics*. 5th ed. Pacific Grove: Duxbury.

References used in this chapter

Joubert, G & Schall, R. 1995. Some statistical concepts. In Kibel, MA & Wagstaff, L (eds). *Child health for all*. 2nd ed. Cape Town: Oxford University Press.

Mathews, C, Kuhn, L, Metcalf, CA, Joubert, G & Cameron, NA. 1990. Knowledge, attitudes and beliefs about AIDS in township school students in Cape Town. *South African Medical Journal*, 78:511–16.

11

Analysing and interpreting epidemiological data

Gina Joubert

OBJECTIVES OF THIS CHAPTER

The objectives of this chapter are:
- to describe how one uses sample data and probability distributions to make statements about the target population
- to define confidence intervals and describe how they are interpreted
- to describe important aspects of hypothesis testing
- to distinguish statistical significance from clinical or public health significance
- to outline issues which play a role in determining which analysis is appropriate
- to define relative risks, risk differences and odds ratios and discuss their interpretation
- to describe the use of correlation and regression.

Introduction

As outlined in Section B, the objectives of a project determine the research approach and methods to be used. The objectives have the same guiding role regarding the analysis of the data. Depending on the objectives of a study, various sections of this chapter will be of relevance to the specific project.

The STROBE and CONSORT initiatives

The STROBE initiative with the aim of **ST**rengthening the **R**eporting of **OB**servational studies in **E**pidemiology has issued a statement outlining essential items which should be given when reporting on observational studies. Statistical items covered include outlining the statistical methods used, and the reporting of results in terms of participants, descriptive data, outcome data, and main results. The CONSORT statement covers items to report on for clinical trials. (See 'Useful web sites' at the end of this chapter.)

A researcher studies a sample in order to make statements (inference) about the population from which the sample was selected. The summary statistics outlined in Chapter 10 describe the sample data, but what can be said about the population?

From the sample to the population

> **Some useful terminology to start with**
>
> A *parameter* is a characteristic (for example, the mean) of a population. A *statistic* is a characteristic of a sample of the population, and is an estimate of the corresponding parameter in the population (for example, the sample mean estimates the population mean). However, as the simple example in Table 11.1 indicates, different samples of the same size randomly selected from a given population will not necessarily provide the same estimates, nor will they provide estimates which are identical to the population parameters. This is due to random variation in any sample and is known as *sampling error*. If the entire population were studied, the population parameters (for example, population mean) could be calculated exactly. By studying only a sample, the researcher obtains imprecise estimates. It is important, therefore, to calculate the *precision* of a sample estimate (for example, the precision of a mean, mean difference, proportion, or odds ratio). Statistical techniques are needed to enable researchers to make statements based on imprecise estimates.
>
> The precision of an estimate depends on both the variability of the data and the sample size. If all the data values are within a small range, there is small underlying variability in the measurement and the estimate will consequently be more precise. Also, the larger the sample, the more precise the estimate. The *standard error*, which is a measure of the (im)precision of a sample statistic as an estimate of the population parameter, is calculated using the sample size and the variability of the data. For example, the standard error of the sample mean is $\frac{sd}{\sqrt{n}}$ (where sd is the sample standard deviation and n the sample size). The sample estimate remains the best single estimate of the population parameter, as long as the researcher has avoided bias in sample selection and measurement (see Chapter 12).

Before we discuss how the standard error can be used to make a statement about the population parameter, we need to know something about probability distributions.

Probability distributions

A *probability distribution* is a theoretical distribution which provides information on the probability of observing different ranges of values for a given variable. A probability distribution can be thought of as a data distribution based on an infinitely large sample. Such probability distributions exist for categorical as well as numerical variables (see Chapter 10 for scale of measurement). Probability distributions are commonly characterised by their mean and variance. (See Chapter 10 for an explanation of these terms.)

One of the probability distributions used most often is the *Normal (Gaussian) distribution*. Most of the commonly used methods of statistical analysis (for example *t-tests*, *correlation*, and *regression*, which will be described later) are based on the assumption that the numerical variables which are analysed follow a Normal distribution. The Normal distribution is bell-shaped and is symmetrical around its mean (Figure 11.1). Furthermore, the area within one standard deviation on either side of the mean includes 68% of the observations, and the area within 1.96 standard deviations on either side of the mean includes 95% of the observations.

Many numerical biological variables, for example, birth weight, are approximately normally distributed. In small data sets, it may be difficult to validate the assumption of normality adequately, and in small samples with skewed distributions, normality cannot be assumed. In such cases, *non-parametric methods* of analysis need to be

Table 11.1 Estimates yielded by different samples from the same population

The population consists of 50 individuals. Two characteristics are of interest: age and sex

Individual	Age (years)	Sex	Individual	Age (years)	Sex
1	55	F	26	81	M
2	38	M	27	63	F
3	63	M	28	87	M
4	71	F	29	94	M
5	62	M	30	68	M
6	46	F	31	71	F
7	59	F	32	69	M
8	52	F	33	46	M
9	65	M	34	71	F
10	64	M	35	87	M
11	50	F	36	62	F
12	55	M	37	94	M
13	57	M	38	52	M
14	69	M	39	81	M
15	38	F	40	79	F
16	59	M	41	74	M
17	69	F	42	75	M
18	52	M	43	63	F
19	46	F	44	79	M
20	64	M	45	71	F
21	74	M	46	63	F
22	50	F	47	57	M
23	67	M	48	65	M
24	75	F	49	69	M
25	46	F	50	62	M

Two simple random samples of size 10 are selected.

Sample 1: individuals 17, 14, 46, 11, 39, 30, 02, 08, 15, 22
Sample 2: individuals 32, 08, 16, 13, 24, 48, 23, 42, 14, 21

Sample 1 estimates: 4 males out of 10 subjects (40%); mean age 57.8 years

Sample 2 estimates: 8 males out of 10 subjects (80%); mean age 66.2 years

Population parameters: 30 males out of 50 subjects (60%); mean age 64.6 years

---

considered (see the section on parametric versus non-parametric methods below).

Other important probability distributions are the *Binomial distribution* for binary variables (e.g. presence versus absence of disease), the *Poisson distribution* for count data (e.g. number of new cases) and the *Lognormal distribution* for continuous variables which are normally distributed when logarithms are taken. (We will not discuss these distributions further, but for a useful introduction, see Altman (1991) under 'References used in this chapter'.)

Figure 11.1 The Normal distribution

mean − 2sd ... mean − 1sd ... mean ... mean + 1sd ... mean + 2sd

← 68% of area →

← 95% of area →

sd = standard deviation

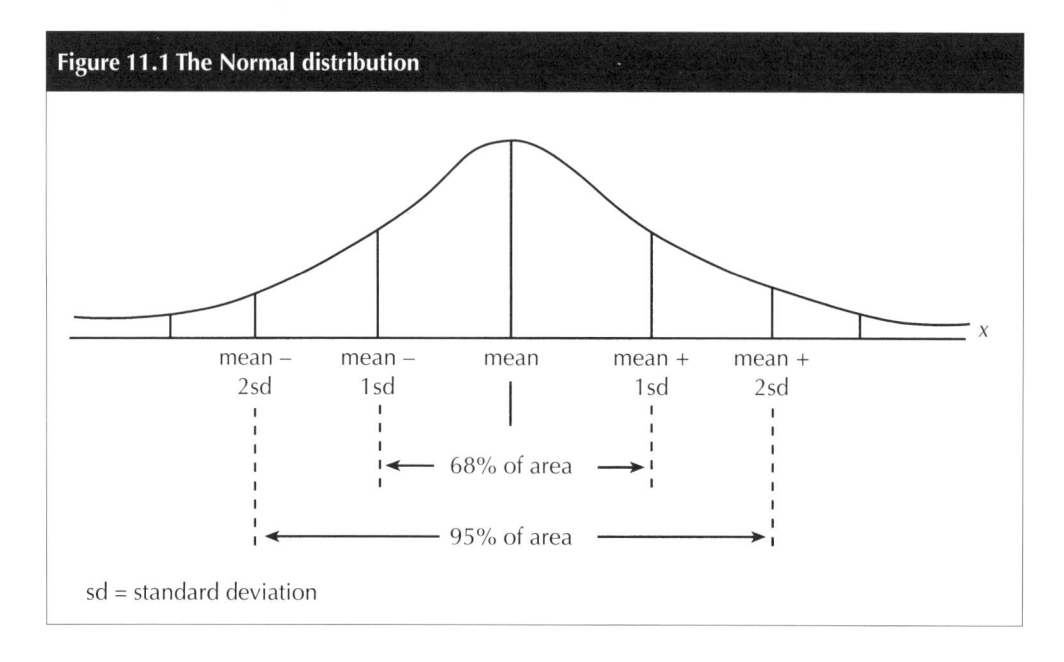

Confidence intervals

As discussed above, if various samples of the same size are drawn from a given target population, a range of different estimates will be obtained. These estimates will follow some theoretical distribution. We use this information to calculate a *confidence interval* for the population parameter.

A confidence interval gives a range of parameter values considered plausible for the population, based on the sample data, and is a useful way of describing the (im)precision of the estimate. We calculate a confidence interval by using the sample estimate, its standard error, the degree of certainty (confidence) we want to associate with the confidence interval (say 95% or 99%), and the cutoff value of the appropriate probability distribution (for example 1.96 in the case of a 95% confidence interval based on the Normal distribution). *If we calculate a 95% confidence interval, we can say that, in a series of identical studies based on different samples from the same population, 95% of the confidence intervals calculated from these studies will include the true population parameter.*

An imprecise estimate (with large standard error as a result of small sample size and/or large variability in the sample data) will therefore lead to a wide confidence interval (that is, a wide range of values which are considered plausible for the population parameter). For example, if in a sample of 10 clinic attenders, four are found to be HIV positive, the percentage positive is 40%, with a 95% confidence interval ranging from 12% to 74% (indicated as (12% ; 74%) or (12%–74%)). The confidence interval is wide since the sample is small. We are therefore highly uncertain as to what the true HIV prevalence is. If, however, the sample consists of 100 attenders and 40 are HIV positive, the percentage positive is still 40%, but the 95% confidence interval now ranges from 30% to 50%, a narrower confidence interval than in the case of the smaller sample. (See Table 11.2 for a further example.) This indicates that the true value is 'less uncertain'.

Methods for calculating confidence intervals for most epidemiological applications (for example, means, differences between means, medians, proportions, relative risks, odds ratios, correlation

Table 11.2 Estimates yielded by increasing sample sizes

The population of 50 individuals is provided in Table 11.1.

Sample 1: Individuals: 17, 14, 46, 11, 39, 30, 02, 08, 15, 22
Sample 2: Individuals: (Sample 1) and 37, 10, 45, 33, 36, 07, 26, 09, 42, 25
Sample 3: Individuals: (Sample 2) and 24, 44, 23, 21, 12, 16, 01, 03, 34, 13

	Sample 1	Sample 2	Sample 3
Sample size	10	20	30
Mean age (years)	57.8	62.1	63.2
Standard deviation	14.4	14.9	13.1
Standard error	4.5	3.3	2.4
95% confidence interval (mean age)	(47.5–68.1)	(55.1–69.0)	(58.3–68.1)
% males	40%	50%	56.7%
95% confidence interval (% males)	(9.6%–70%)	(28.1%–71.9%)	(39%–74.4%)

There are 60% males in the population and the mean age is 64.6 years.

---

coefficients, and survival time) are described, with examples, in *Statistics with Confidence* by Altman *et al* (2000). A computer programme for calculating confidence intervals, Confidence Interval Analysis – CIA – is available with that book (see also http://www.medschool.soton.ac.uk/cia/main.htm).

Hypothesis (significance) testing

If the researcher is interested in determining the level of a characteristic (for example, the prevalence of HIV infection in the Free State), the size of any difference between groups (for example, the mean age difference of mothers with low birthweight babies and mothers with normal birthweight babies), or the strength of an association (for example, the risk of heart disease in hypertensive patients compared to normotensive patients), confidence intervals should be calculated as outlined above. On the other hand, the researcher may wish to test a specific hypothesis: are two factors significantly associated or are two groups significantly different? In this case, the researcher is interested in hypothesis testing.

A *statistical hypothesis* is an assumption made about a parameter of one or more populations (see Chapter 5). To determine whether, for example, two factors are associated, we need to formulate a null hypothesis (H_0) which can then be tested. The *null hypothesis* is the hypothesis of no association or no difference.

We then calculate a test statistic by applying a statistical formula, using the sample data. When the null hypothesis is true (that is, there is no difference or association), this test statistic follows a certain distribution (for example *t*-distribution, chi-squared- (χ^2-) distribution). By comparing the test statistic with this distribution, we can determine how likely it is to obtain the observed sample data if the null hypothesis were true (that is, if there were no association or no difference). This probability is known as the *p*-value associated with the test statistic. The *p*-value is the probability of observing the test statistic or a more extreme result if the null hypothesis is true.

If the *p*-value is large (for example, $p = 0.80$), the data are consistent with the null hypothesis. This implies that the null hypothesis cannot be rejected, using the observed data. However, a large p-value does not imply that the null hypothesis can be accepted. For example, the sample may be too small to detect the difference that really exists. Accepting a null hypothesis that is false is known as a *Type II error*. The *power* of the test (its capability to indicate a difference when there really is a difference) is 1 minus its Type II error, and should preferably be larger than 0.80.

If the p-value is small (for example $p = 0.01$) the data are unlikely to have been as observed if the null hypothesis is true. In other words, there is evidence that there is indeed a significant association or difference, and the null hypothesis is rejected.

An arbitrary cut-off point of the p-value, namely 0.05, is usually chosen. This cut-off value is called the *significance level* of the test, and refers to the probability of rejecting the null hypothesis if it is in fact true (a *Type I error*). P-values are often classified as 'significant' if $p<0.05$ and 'non-significant' (often written in the literature as NS) if $p>0.05$. This over-simplistic use of p-values is now strongly discouraged in most medical literature. If the reader of an article sees that a difference between two groups was found to be 'non-significant', there is no information whether the p-value might have been 0.06 or 0.60. Clearly we should interpret p-values of 0.06 and 0.60 differently and should not simply classify both as 'non-significant'. Exact p-values should be given in papers so that readers can decide for themselves whether they agree with the researcher on the 'significance' of the results. P-values should always be accompanied by the actual values (e.g. the two proportions or means) being compared.

Significance testing can indicate whether there is a statistically significant difference between two groups, or a statistically significant association between two variables, that is beyond chance. As pointed out above, a significance test cannot indicate that there is no difference.

Statistical versus clinical or public health significance

Hypothesis testing determines the statistical significance of an observed effect. If two large samples are compared, the researcher may find small differences between groups to be statistically significant, although such small differences may not be of clinical or public health importance, i.e. of practical value. Similarly, in small samples, large differences may fail to reach statistical significance, although they seem clinically important. (See Table 11.3 below for an example of sample size and statistical significance.) A researcher therefore cannot base decision-making purely on statistical significance, but must consider the clinical or public health significance of the results. This can be done by calculating confidence intervals and interpreting them 'clinically', that is, interpreting the size of the difference or association in terms of its meaning for the patient, disease, or health service.

For example, in a large study of a new blood pressure treatment, assume that a mean change of five units (mm mercury (Hg) pressure) or more is considered to be clinically meaningful. A mean decrease of 3 mm Hg in blood pressure in patients with hypertension could be statistically significant ($p<0.05$). However, a 95% confidence interval of 2 to 4 mm Hg for this mean decrease would be interpreted as not being *clinically* significant, since the entire interval is below the value of 5 mm Hg. A significance test therefore indicates whether there is a difference, but the confidence interval is interpreted to decide whether the difference is clinically important or important from a public health perspective (depending on the subject). A significance test cannot by itself indicate that there is no difference, but a confidence interval can. If, on the other hand, the confidence interval had ranged from 0.5 to 5.5 mm Hg, we would deduce that there is a statistically significant difference (the entire confidence interval is above 0), but we would not be able to draw any clinical conclusion, since the interval includes both values which indicate a clinically meaningful change (> 5 mm Hg) and values which indicate no clinically meaningful change (< 5 mm Hg).

The decision on how large a difference or change is required for it to be clinically meaningful or meaningful from a public health perspective is based on knowledge of the subject matter, the question being asked and the users of the information. In the case of measurements such as blood pressure in a clinical trial, it may be clear what is clinically meaningful, but in other circumstances it may be less clear-cut. For example, if the seroprevalence of HIV infection in one district is 3%, but 5% in another, is that a meaningful difference? The answer may be 'yes' if an epidemiologist is monitoring a rising epidemic in its early stages, but 'no' if a manager is trying to decide in which districts to start HIV treatment services.

Confidence intervals and *p*-values are closely related: if the difference between the means of two groups is significant at the 5% level (that is, $p<0.05$), then the 95% confidence interval for the difference will exclude the value zero (that is, the confidence interval will also indicate that there is a difference). Confidence intervals are consequently sometimes also used for purposes of statistical significance (the result is significant, since the null value is not inside the confidence interval). This is not, however, the purpose of a confidence interval. If the focus is on *estimation*, which is most often the case, the researcher should calculate confidence intervals and interpret the range of the interval to determine whether the findings are clinically important or important from a public health perspective.

Parametric versus non-parametric methods

If we can assume that our data come from an underlying distribution such as the Normal distribution, we can use statistical methods (hypothesis testing or confidence intervals) based on the assumptions of the underlying distribution. These methods are called *parametric*, since the underlying distribution is assumed to come from a parametric family of distributions. *Non-parametric methods* are used if such assumptions cannot be made. For example, the Mann-Whitney U test is the non-parametric equivalent of the two-sample *t*-test. These are called *distribution-free* methods as they make no assumptions about the data distribution. They are often ranking techniques, which focus on the order or ranking of observations, and not on their numerical values.

What to consider when choosing an appropriate analysis

A book of this nature cannot provide a detailed outline of which statistical technique to use under which conditions. Rather, we give some idea of the factors which need to be considered when choosing a statistical analysis.

The type of variable being analysed

Categorical and numerical variables require different statistical techniques. Clearly we would not summarise a categorical variable by a mean (what is the meaning of a 'mean sex of 1.2'?). Similarly, if we wish to compare two groups on a categorical variable, we would not use a *t*-test and a confidence interval for mean differences, but rather a χ^2 *test*, or *Fisher's exact test*, and a confidence interval for the differences in percentages. (For an introduction as to which tests to use when, refer to Altman (1991).)

C | Data presentation, analysis and interpretation

Assumptions necessary for the procedures

As mentioned before, there are many procedures which should be used only if the variables are normally distributed. All distributional assumptions of the intended analysis should be investigated to determine whether they are satisfied by the data. A further assumption one has to consider is whether groups are *independent*. For example, if controls are matched to cases in a case-control study, or repeat measurements are made on the same individuals, the groups (controls and cases, before and after measurements) are not independent, and statistical procedures which take their dependence into account should be used.

The characteristic being tested

Different techniques are appropriate for different characteristics of samples. For example, if normality and independence can be assumed, a two-sample *t*-test would be appropriate to compare the means of two groups, while an *F*-test would be appropriate to compare the variability in the two groups.

Analyses commonly used in epidemiology

Measures of association in a 2 × 2 table

Definitions and interpretation

Many epidemiological studies set out to investigate the association between an exposure (for example, smoking) and a disease (for example, lung cancer). Often we can summarise the information gathered in such studies in a 2 × 2 table (2 rows for levels of exposure; 2 columns for outcomes) as follows:

	Diseased	Not diseased	
Exposed	A	B	A+B
Not exposed	C	D	C+D
	A+C	B+D	A+B+C+D=N

Out of a total of N respondents, there are A who are exposed and diseased, B exposed and not diseased, C not exposed but diseased, and D not exposed and not diseased.

To investigate the association, we could perform a statistical test, namely a χ^2 or *Fisher's exact* test. Such a test would determine whether there is a statistically significant difference between the proportion of exposed who are diseased, and the proportion of unexposed who are diseased. The test result will depend on the sample size. For example, it may be significant in a large sample, but not in a small sample (see Table 11.3). The test result will merely say whether there is a statistically significant difference, and will tell us nothing about how strong the relationship between the exposure and outcome is. Researchers often want an estimate of the degree or strength of the association, for example, that the exposed are twice as likely to develop disease as the unexposed. Such measures of association, also known as *measures of effect*, which have the added advantage of not being dependent on sample size, are outlined below.

Let us first assume that the data have been collected by means of a cohort study in which 100 exposed individuals and 300 non-exposed individuals were followed up.

	Diseased	Not diseased	
Exposed	20	80	100
Not exposed	30	270	300
	50	350	400

Among the exposed (A + B) we can say that the *risk* of disease is A/(A + B) (in the example 20/100 = 0.2 or 20%). Similarly, among the non-exposed (C + D) the risk of disease is C/(C + D) (in the example 30/300 = 0.1 or 10%). One measure of association between exposure and disease is the ratio of the risk among the exposed to the risk among the non-exposed. This is called the *relative risk* (or *risk ratio*) and is given by the following formula:

148

Table 11.3 Statistical significance, strength of association and sample size

A study is done on 50 subjects to investigate the association between exposure A and disease B. The following results are obtained.

	B present	absent	
A: present	15 (75%)	5 (25%)	20 (100%)
absent	20 (67%)	10 (33%)	30 (100%)
	35	15	50

Null hypothesis: the two factors are not associated.

A test statistic which follows the χ^2 distribution is calculated to evaluate the association between the two categorical variables A and B, and the p-value equals 0.53. One would thus conclude that the two factors are not associated. If, however, the study was done on 500 subjects and exactly the same configuration of results obtained, namely:

	B present	absent	
A: present	150 (75%)	50 (25%)	200 (100%)
absent	200 (67%)	100 (33%)	300 (100%)
	350	150	500

the test statistic results in a p-value of 0.05; therefore there seems to be evidence of an association.

The statistical test measures the significance of the association (which depends on the sample size), but not the degree of association. The odds ratio, on the other hand, measures the degree or strength of the association, independent of sample size.

The odds ratio in the 50 subjects is 1.50 with a 95% confidence interval of 0.36 to 6.42. For the 500 subjects, the odds ratio is also 1.50, but the narrower confidence interval of 0.99 to 2.28 reflects the better precision of the odds ratio estimate from the bigger sample.

$$\frac{A/(A + B)}{C/(C + D)}$$

In this example, it is 20%/10% = 2.

Since risks are probabilities or proportions which lie between 0 and 1 (or percentages which lie between 0% and 100%), the relative risk is always a positive number. A relative risk of 1 indicates that the risk of disease in the exposed group is the same as in the unexposed group. The exposure and disease are therefore not associated. A relative risk larger than 1 (as in our example) indicates that the exposure is a risk factor, whereas a relative risk less than 1 indicates that the exposure is protective. The sample relative risk (and the risk difference, odds ratio, and attributable risk which are outlined below) is an estimate and should therefore be reported and interpreted with a 95% confidence interval to indicate the precision of the estimate.

A *risk difference*, that is, the difference between the risk among exposed and non-exposed, can also be calculated: $A/(A + B) - C/(C + D)$. In our example, the risk difference is 20% − 10% = 10% (or 0.10 in proportions). The risk difference lies between −100% and 100% (or −1 and 1 if the risks are expressed as proportions) with a difference of 0 indicating no association.

In the instances outlined above, the denominators are counts. If the denominators are person-time (see Chapter 2), one can calculate a *rate ratio* (the ratio of two rates) or a *rate difference* (the difference between two rates).

A third measure of association is the *odds ratio*. In a cohort study the chances of disease can be measured by the *odds*, where the *odds of disease* among the exposed is A/B (20/80 = 0.25 in our example) and among the non-exposed C/D (30/270 = 0.11 in our example). The odds ratio in this case equals:

$$\frac{(A/B)}{(C/D)} = \frac{AD}{BC}$$

In our example the odds ratio is therefore 0.25/0.11 = 2.25.

In a case-control study typically a target or predetermined number of cases (diseased) and controls (not diseased) are selected. Their numbers may not reflect the true proportions of diseased and non-diseased in the population. It is therefore not usually possible to estimate the risk of disease directly among the exposed and unexposed, and the relative risk and risk difference cannot be calculated. A case-control study does, however, provide information on the *odds of exposure* among the cases (A/C) and controls (B/D), which can be used to calculate an odds ratio:

$$\frac{A/C}{B/D} = \frac{AD}{BC}$$

Note that the odds ratio has the useful property of reducing to the same formula under both study designs, despite the different derivation.

The interpretation of the odds ratio is similar to that of the relative risk. Under certain circumstances, for example, if the disease is rare (that is, if A is very small relative to A + B, and C is very small relative to C + D), the odds ratio approximates the relative risk.

If we are analysing data from a cross-sectional study (in which n individuals have been sampled and cross-classified as to exposure and disease status), a *prevalence ratio* can be calculated which is analogous to the risk ratio in the cohort study. A *prevalence odds ratio* is calculated in a similar way to the odds ratio in a cohort study.

The type of study thus determines which measure of association can be estimated.

The value of a relative risk

The odds ratio and relative risk are dimensionless and have been criticised because of this feature. Say, for example, the rate among the exposed is 5 per *million* and 1 per million among the unexposed, then the relative risk is 5 and the risk difference 4 per million. If the rate among the exposed is 5 per *thousand* and among the unexposed 1 per thousand, the relative risk is also 5 but the risk difference is now 4 per thousand, indicating a more serious increase attributable to exposure than in the first case, although the relative risks are the same. It has therefore been said that the risk difference is the appropriate measure of the practical magnitude with regard to public health importance of an association. However, if one risk factor has a higher relative risk than another, the first risk factor is interpreted as being more important in the causation of the disease.

If we can assume that the association is causal, the risk difference is also called the *attributable risk in the exposed*, which is the excess risk due to exposure. The *attributable proportion* (or attributable fraction) *in the exposed* is defined as (RR-1)/RR where RR is the relative risk.

The *population attributable proportion* (or fraction) indicates the proportion by which the rate of disease would be reduced if the exposure were eliminated, assuming the association is causal. It takes into account the relative risk, as well as how common the risk factor is in the population being studied. The population attributable proportion is calculated as follows:

$$\frac{P(RR-1)}{1 + P(RR-1)}$$

where P is the proportion of the population who are affected by the factor and RR is the relative risk. As an example, if factor A has a relative risk of 2 and 10% (that is P = 0.1) of the population is exposed to the risk factor, the population attributable proportion would be $(0.1 \times 1)/(1 + 0.1 \times 1)$ = 0.09. If factor B has a relative risk of 3 but only 2% (P = 0.02) of the population is exposed to that risk factor, the population attributable proportion would be $(0.02 \times 2)/(1 + (0.02 \times 2)) = 0.04$. So factor A may have a lower relative risk than risk factor B, but because more people are exposed to risk factor A, the population-attributable fraction indicates that factor A is more important to the health of the community. The proportion by which the rate of disease would be reduced if the exposure were eliminated is higher for factor A. The population-attributable fraction is therefore of great importance in health services planning, namely in deciding which risk factors to target for prevention and intervention.

More than two levels of exposure

If an exposure has more than two levels, an $r \times 2$ table can be set up (where r is the number of levels of exposure). For example, daily cigarette smoking can be classified as 0, 1–2, 3–4, 5–9, 10 cigarettes and more. If the association between the level of smoking and the presence of lung disease is to be studied, a 5×2 table can be formed. To calculate relative risks or odds ratios, one level of exposure is chosen as the *reference level* (generally the level with the least risk of disease is taken as the reference, in this case, the level of 0 cigarettes) and each of the other levels is compared to the reference level in turn (effectively forming four 2×2 tables and calculating four relative risks or odds ratios).

Stratification

Factors such as sex or age may complicate the estimation of the measure of association between exposure and disease. By using a stratified analysis, the researcher attempts to adjust for, or remove the effect of, an extraneous factor (*confounder*) which is related to both the exposure and the disease (see Chapter 12 for a discussion of confounding). Rather than using only one (crude) measure of association, one would calculate measures of association for each of the strata of the extraneous factor and possibly compute an adjusted (common) measure. See Table 12.6 in Chapter 12 for a detailed example.

Correlation

Measures of association between two dichotomous variables have been outlined above. If, however, the researcher wants to describe the relationship between two numerical variables, he or she could calculate a *correlation coefficient*. (The term correlation is often used loosely to apply to an association between categorical variables when in fact it should be reserved for numerical variables.)

Two variables are positively correlated if an increase in one variable is associated with an increase in the other (for example, an increase in height is usually associated with an increase in weight). If a decrease in one variable is associated with an increase in the other, the two variables are negatively correlated (for example, lung function decreases as age increases). If a decrease or increase in one variable is not associated with any change in the other variable, the variables are not correlated (for example, birthweight and hour of birth). The correlation coefficient can range from −1 (perfect negative correlation) to 1 (perfect positive correlation), with 0 indicating no correlation. The sample correlation coefficient is an estimate and should be reported and interpreted with a confidence interval.

If the variables are normally distributed, the *Pearson correlation coefficient* is calculated. If either or both of the variables have a skewed distribution or have outlying values, we can calculate a non-parametric correlation coefficient based on the ranks of the observations. This is called the *Spearman rank correlation coefficient*.

A high correlation does not imply cause and effect. Furthermore, the correlation between two variables may be spurious owing to the influence of a third variable, that is, a confounder. The effect of a third variable can be removed by calculating a *partial correlation coefficient*.

Correlation measures the linear (straight line) relationship between two variables. A strong correlation coefficient therefore implies a strong linear relationship. It is important to draw a scatter plot (see 'Exploratory data analysis' in Chapter 10) to see whether the relationship is indeed linear, before calculating a correlation coefficient. Figure 11.2 shows the relationship between two variables. The correlation between the two equals zero, but from the scatter plot it is clear that there is in fact a very distinct relationship between the two variables. This relationship is not linear, however: where x is less than 100, the two variables are negatively correlated, whereas for x above 100, the correlation is positive.

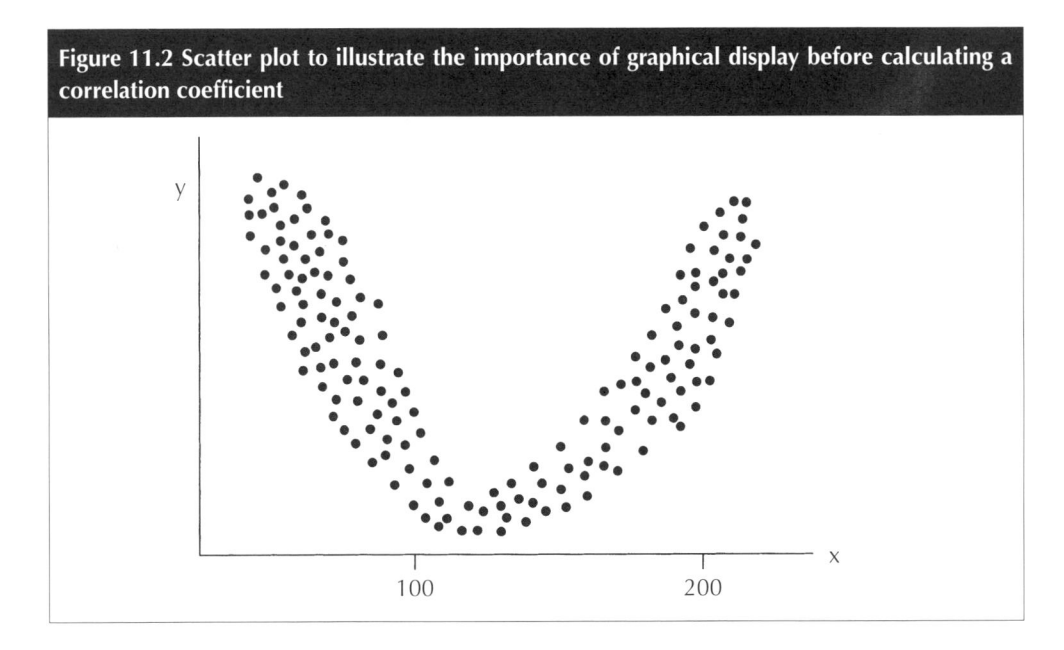

Figure 11.2 Scatter plot to illustrate the importance of graphical display before calculating a correlation coefficient

Measuring agreement

Correlation should not be used to measure inter-observer agreement (i.e. precision or reliability – see Chapter 9). If, for example, two examiners have to do blood pressure readings, and they both evaluate the same 20 patients to determine how well their measurements agree, it is not appropriate to calculate the correlation coefficient as the measure of agreement. As Figure 11.3

indicates, there can be a strong linear relationship (that is, a strong correlation) even if one examiner consistently notes a higher reading than the other. Correlation measures whether the readings 'go in the same direction' (that is, whether if one examiner notes a high reading, the other does as well), not whether they actually get exactly the same readings. Altman (1991) describes the appropriate methods of analysis to measure agreement between numerical variables.

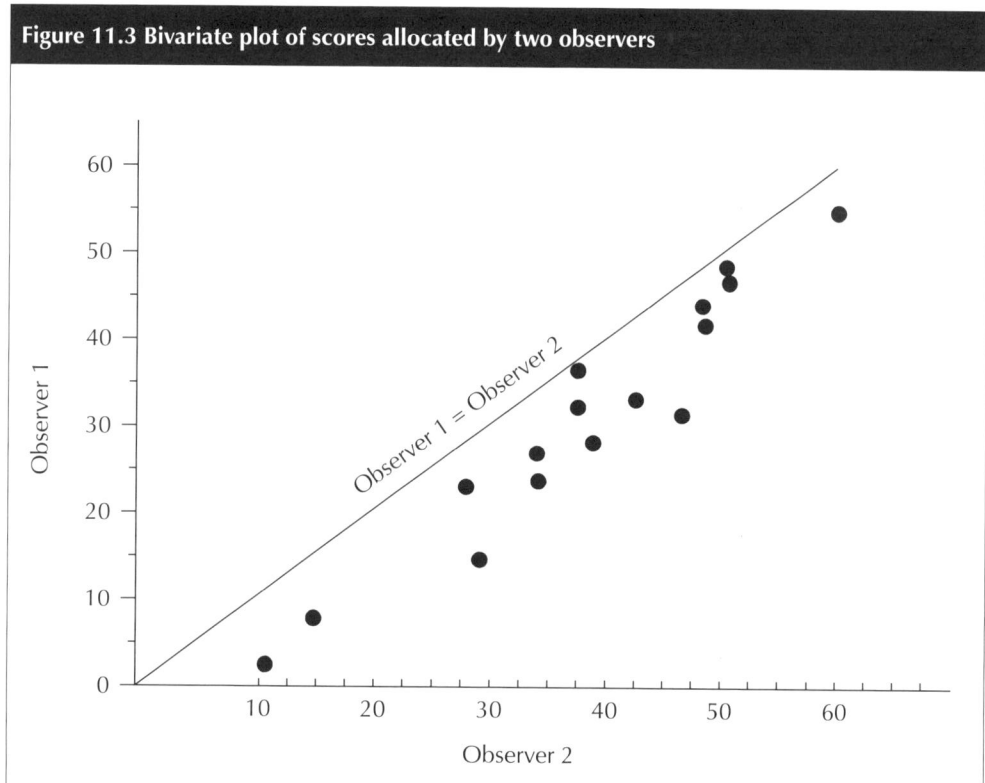

Figure 11.3 Bivariate plot of scores allocated by two observers

Two observers were asked to score 16 individuals. A strong positive correlation was found when calculating a correlation coefficient. The graphical display is more informative, however, indicating that observer 2 consistently gave higher scores than observer 1.

Correlation is closely related to the statistical technique known as simple linear regression. In *simple linear regression*, the actual values of one numerical variable (the dependent variable) are predicted by the values of the other variable (the independent variable) and an equation is determined. For example, lung function can be predicted using age. In this way the relationship between two variables can be described.

Multivariate analysis

Multivariate analysis encompasses a range of statistical techniques which, on the basis of mathematical models, can evaluate the inter-relationship of more than two variables, for example more than one outcome (dependent) variable and/or more than one predictor (independent) variable. A mathematical model is one which describes the relationship between variables in mathematical form. Whereas simple linear regression is used to predict a dependent variable (*y* variable or outcome variable) from one independent variable (*x* variable), *multiple linear regression* is a multivariate technique which predicts a dependent variable from two or more independent variables, assuming a linear relationship. So, for example, a person's lung function (such as forced vital capacity expressed in litres) can be predicted from their age, height and weight.

Multiple linear regression can be used only if the dependent variable is numerical, for example, a person's lung function. However, often the dependent variable is dichotomous, for example, died/survived or recovered/not recovered. In such cases, *multiple logistic regression* is the appropriate method of analysis. The *proportional hazards model*, which is used to investigate the role of independent variables on survival time in a cohort, is a further example of a multivariate technique.

Multivariate techniques can use data very efficiently and enable the researcher to identify which variables from a large set of independent variables are related to the dependent variable, after adjusting for other important independent variables (confounders). However, these techniques are complicated and ideally we should not perform them without some understanding of the mathematical models and assumptions underlying them. This understanding is also required for an accurate interpretation of the computer output of such analyses. One should consult a statistician for assistance with such analyses.

Multivariate techniques also place a barrier between the researcher and the data. Other methods of analysis (e.g. stratification) can bring about a closer understanding of the data, for example, by presenting them in 2 × 2 tables. It is therefore important to do the simpler analyses first, in order to get to know the data and their irregularities, before an appropriate multivariate analysis is considered. (See Chapter 10 for exploratory data analysis.)

Conclusion

This chapter has provided an introduction to statistical concepts, and we encourage readers to refer to the recommended reading for further details. Not every researcher needs to become a statistician to be a good epidemiologist. Rather, researchers should make a point of working closely with statisticians on more complex research projects. However, an understanding of the terminology and principles used by statisticians will make the collaboration with statisticians more fruitful and enjoyable, and will enable researchers to handle many analyses themselves.

Useful readings

Fleiss, JL, Levin, B & Paik, MC. 2003. *Statistical methods for rates and proportions*. 3rd ed. New York: Wiley.

Rosner, B. 2000. *Fundamentals of biostatistics*. 5th ed. Pacific Grove: Duxbury.

Rothman, KJ & Greenland S. 1998. *Modern epidemiology*. Philadelphia, PA, USA: Lippincott Williams & Wilkins.

Useful web sites

Confidence Interval Analysis – CIA. [Online]. Available: http://www.medschool.soton.ac.uk/cia. [25 February 2007].

CONSORT statement. [Online]. Available: http://www.consort-statement.org. [25 February 2007].

STROBE statement. [Online]. Available: http://www.strobe-statement.org. [25 February 2007].

References used in this chapter

Altman, DG. 1991. *Practical statistics for medical research*. London: Chapman and Hall.

Altman, DG, Machin, D, Bryant, TN & Gardner, MJ. 2000. *Statistics with confidence*. 2nd ed. London: BMJ Publishing.

12

Precision and validity in epidemiological studies: error, bias and confounding

Landon Myer   Salim Abdool Karim

> **OBJECTIVES OF THIS CHAPTER**
>
> The objectives of this chapter are:
> - to describe the concepts of precision and validity and their relationship in epidemiological studies
> - to describe the most common sources of random error (leading to imprecision) in epidemiological research, and how different kinds of random error can influence study findings
> - to describe the most common sources of systematic error (leading to bias or lack of validity) in epidemiological research, and how different kinds of bias can influence study findings
> - to describe the way in which confounding can influence study findings, and how confounding variables can be identified and dealt with in epidemiological research.

Introduction

In the process of selecting individuals from a population to participate in a study, taking measures on those participants, and analysing these measurements to produce study findings, we are seeking to make statements that are as close to the truth as possible. Typically, this concerns the size of the problem or the difference between two groups.

Different kinds of *error*, or undesired variation, can enter the process of selecting participants and measuring study variables. Different sources of error in research, and how these may influence the *validity* and *precision* of a study, are cross-cutting concerns that are relevant to epidemiological and clinical studies.

Reliability versus validity

As described in Chapter 9, precision refers to the repeatability or reproducibility of a measurement or study finding: whether the same result would be found if the measurement were taken (or study conducted) over and over again. The term *reliability* is also used for this characteristic, particularly in regard to a measurement or construct, e.g. a diagnosis, derived from a questionnaire.

On the other hand, validity refers to how close a measurement or study finding comes to the truth. The term *accuracy* is sometimes used to refer to the same concept, particularly in relation to a single measurement using a clinical or laboratory instrument.

The relationship between precision and validity can be understood through the example of an archer shooting at a target, aiming to hit its centre (see Figure 9.3 in Chapter 9). If the archer hits the same spot on the target regularly, we would describe the result as having high precision (or as highly repeatable) regardless of its proximity to the centre of the target. If the archer hits the centre of the target, we would describe the result as having high validity (or accuracy).

Precision and validity are commonly confused by students at all levels, but it is important to understand that they are distinct concepts (Table 12.1).

Table 12.1 The relationship between precision and validity

It is important to emphasise that validity and precision (or their inverse, bias and imprecision) are different phenomena that need to be considered separately. It is common for students and even some researchers to see a very precise study result, usually indicated by a narrow confidence interval or a low *p*-value, and infer that this precision means that the study finding is valid. This is a mistaken inference.

For example:
- A large study may find a very strong association between two variables, and the measure of association may be highly statistically significant, as reflected by a very narrow confidence interval or small *p*-value (eg, $p<0.0001$). However, if this association is due to bias (confounding, information bias, or selection bias), the results are invalid regardless of the precision of the measure of association.
- Conversely, the results of a small study may be somewhat imprecise (as indicated by a wide confidence interval or $p\text{-value} > 0.05$) but still be valid, in that the estimated measure of occurrence or association is unbiased.

This is an important lesson, that *the validity of a study result should be considered separately from its precision*. Related to this, increasing the number of participants in a study does not as a rule increase its validity. Increasing the sample size may be important in increasing the precision of the study results, but ensuring that the sample selected or groups compared (regardless of size) are unbiased is necessary to ensure the validity of the study results.

It is important to keep in mind that different kinds of error, leading to imprecision and lack of validity, can affect every kind of study design regardless of whether the study is descriptive or analytical. The exact sources of imprecision and lack of validity vary with the specific details of a study, including how participants are sampled, how measurements are taken on participants and what type of variables are defined. However, the basic concepts regarding error discussed here are of concern in every research setting.

There are two general classes of error that affect studies. First, there is error that occurs at random, which introduces imprecision into study results. Second, there is error that occurs systematically (i.e. more in one direction than the other), that leads to invalidity in study results. *Bias* is a term that is commonly used for sources of invalidity in epidemiological studies. Common sources of invalidity are *selection bias*, *information bias*, and *confounding bias* (or simply *confounding*). Table 12.2 provides a guide to the terminology commonly used to describe these concepts.

Table 12.2 Terminology used in describing sources of variation which influence epidemiological study results

Factor	Also known as*	Threats in study design/conduct	Also known as
Precision	Reliability or repeatability	Random sampling error	
		Random measurement error	
Validity	Accuracy	Selection bias Information bias Confounding bias	Systematic sampling error Systematic measurement error Confounding

* Exact equivalence depends on context (see text).

Factors that influence precision of study results: random error

There are two major sources of random error in epidemiological and clinical research: random *sampling* error and random *measurement* error.

Random sampling error

The most common source of random error that influences epidemiological studies is *random sampling error*. If we have used a random sampling technique (see Chapter 8) to obtain the study data, any deviation of the estimate (e.g. prevalence) from the true population value can be thought of as being due to chance. Different samples drawn from the larger population will produce different estimates. The degree of imprecision or *uncertainty* in how the study results relate to the true population value is reflected in the size of the confidence interval around the estimated mean or proportion or around some measure of association such as risk ratio.

As outlined in Chapter 11, increasing the sample size of a study has an important influence on the precision of study results by reducing random sampling error. Large studies therefore produce more precise findings with narrower confidence intervals than small studies. In the extreme, if all members of a population are studied, random sampling error disappears and the calculation of confidence intervals is not necessary.

Random measurement error

A second major source of random error in epidemiological studies is random measurement error. Random error in the measurement of a variable means that the variation from the true population value occurs in an unpredictable way (i.e. the random error is not more likely to be in one direction than another). It also occurs independently of the values of other variables in the study. This form of error can be thought of as arising as a result of 'chance' (even if the source of the error is known).

In an analytical study comparing two groups, error is random if it occurs equally in both comparison groups; i.e. it does not influence one group of participants (exposed or unexposed, diseased or non-diseased) more than the other group.

There are different ways of quantifying measurement error in *categorical* variables. These include *sensitivity* and *specificity* for situations when a 'gold standard' measure exists, i.e. criterion validity (see Chapter 9). For situations when there is no gold standard, measures of agreement such as the kappa statistic are used (see Table 9.2). When working with *continuous* variables, different types of correlation coefficients or limits of agreement can be used to assess measurement error (although simple correlation coefficients should be avoided). For further discussion of kappa and measures of agreement for continuous variables, the reader is advised to see Szklo and Nieto (2000) or other more advanced epidemiology texts.

Random measurement error

It is important to note that random measurement error can affect any type of measurement in a study, including biological measures such as laboratory assays, or behavioural variables such as participants' responses to a questionnaire. The key feature of random error (which distinguishes it from systematic measurement error or information bias, discussed below) is that the error does not occur in a patterned or predictable way within a study. For example, a particular assay used to measure CD4 cell count (in cells/µl) may be imprecise, with a 'margin of error' for a single measurement of ± 25 cells/µl. If this error potentially affects all participants in the study and is as likely to overestimate as underestimate the true CD4 cell count in a particular specimen, it can be thought of as a source of random measurement error.

What is the influence of random measurement error on study results? The impact depends on how we analyse the variables with measurement error. If the variable in question is being used in a descriptive manner (such as in a mean, prevalence or incidence), random measurement error will increase the standard error of the variable and will be reflected in wider confidence intervals. The greater width of these confidence intervals reflects the increased imprecision (greater uncertainty) of the estimated mean or proportion.

If the variable in question is being used to produce a measure of association, then random measurement error will usually work to *reduce* the measure of association closer to the null value. The null value equals 1.0 for relative measures of association (such as relative risk) and 0 for absolute measures of association (such as risk difference). For example, if there is a true positive association between exposure and outcome, the relative measure of association (such as relative risk) will be greater than 1.0; the influence of measurement error will be to move the observed association closer to 1.0 (Table 12.3). Conversely, if there is a true negative (inverse) association between exposure and outcome, the relative measure of association will be less than 1.0; the influence of measurement error will be to move the observed association closer to 1.0.

When dealing with categorical variables, this kind of measurement error is sometimes referred to as *non-differential misclassification*, which can also be regarded as a form of information bias (discussed below). Note that while we have used categorical variables in the above example, the same concept holds for continuous variables – if there is random measurement error in one of the variables, the resulting measures of association will be moved closer to the null value of no association.

The best way to reduce random measurement error in research is to use measurements

Table 12.3 Example of the effect of random measurement error in a case-control study

These are 2 × 2 tables from a hypothetical case-control study of the association between maternal smoking in pregnancy and risk of stillbirth. The true association (without measurement error in mothers' reporting of whether they smoked or not) is shown in Situation A. Using the language of Figure 9.4 in Chapter 9, smoking is measured with 100% sensitivity and 100% specificity in both cases and controls with respect to the truth.

Situation A *Hypothetical association with no random measurement error*

Self-reported history of smoking during pregnancy	Mothers with stillbirths (cases)	Mothers without stillbirths (controls)
Smoked	60	40
Did not smoke	140	160
Total	200	200

Odds ratio with no measurement error = (60/140)/(40/160) = 1.71 (95% confidence interval (CI) 1.06–2.79)

In Situation B, the exposure is measured imperfectly (with 70% sensitivity and 95% specificity in both cases and controls). To complete the 2 × 2 table with measurement error, 30% (i.e. 100%–70%) of the exposed individuals in the 'true' table were reclassified as unexposed, while 5% (i.e. 100%–95%) of the unexposed individuals were reclassified as exposed. Cell values have been rounded as necessary. Note that the error is *random* because it affects cases and controls equally. This is an example of non-differential misclassification of exposure.

The result is a weakening of the association (odds ratio in Situation A) towards a smaller association observed in the measured study data (odds ratio in Situation B).

Situation B *Observed association with measurement error: exposure measured with 70% sensitivity and 95% specificity in both cases and controls*

Self-reported history of smoking during pregnancy	Mothers with stillbirths (cases)	Mothers without stillbirths (controls)
Smoked	49	36
Did not smoke	151	164
Total	200	200

Observed odds ratio with measurement error = (49/151)/(36/164) = 1.48 (95% CI 0.89–2.48)

that are known to be precise. For this reason, researchers usually prefer measurement instruments that have been used, tested and standardised. Researchers should always test the quality of their measurements in small preliminary or pilot studies (e.g. 'test-retest' studies or split-sample measurements for laboratory tests). These studies are used to measure the precision (as well as validity if possible) of a measurement

Factors that influence validity of study results: bias

Concerns about the validity of study results are separate from issues of precision. *Bias* is the term commonly used to refer to problems in the design or conduct of epidemiological studies that lead the study results to be invalid. A biased study finding is one that does not represent the truth. (Note that this does not imply that the researchers are necessarily 'biased'.) Biased study results are generally attributable to one or more of (a) systematic error in the selection of participants into a study (*selection bias*), (b) systematic error in the collection of data on participants within a study (*information bias*), or (c) the intercorrelation of risk factors in the study population of interest that can lead to the appearance of false results (*confounding bias*, or simply *confounding*).

Selection bias

Selection bias occurs when there are systematic or directional errors in how participants are sampled into a study, which leads the study sample to be systematically different from the population that is of interest to the researchers. As a result of selection bias in a study, measures of occurrence (incidence or prevalence) and association (risk ratios, rate ratios, odds ratios) will lack validity.

Selection bias can take different forms in different study designs. In cross-sectional descriptive surveys, selection bias is often referred to as *sampling bias* (see Chapter 8). For example, in a descriptive cross-sectional study to assess vaccination coverage in Durban, a random sample of houses from the municipal register of electricity consumers was chosen to participate. Randomly selected households were visited to obtain information on vaccination coverage of children in the household. This study found a vaccination coverage level which was higher than all previous estimates. This was probably due to selection bias resulting from the exclusion of houses without electricity (for example, shacks in informal settlements), where vaccination coverage is likely to be lower. Sampling bias that systematically excludes the poorest individuals is a common problem in cross-sectional studies that attempt to sample the entire population.

Another example of selection bias is the *healthy worker effect*, in which only healthy employees are present at work (because the ill workers are taking sick leave or have stopped working), which may bias the results of occupational epidemiological research (see Chapter 21).

Volunteer bias

A further example of selection bias is *volunteer bias*. Individuals who volunteer to participate in epidemiological or clinical research studies may be very different from the population at large, to such a degree that the information collected on volunteers may not be representative of the broader population. One example of this is the use of volunteers to measure the prevalence of a particular disease or health behaviour. A volunteer sample is likely to be healthier than the general population, consequently underestimating the prevalence of the condition of interest. Similarly, if a study offers significant incentives to participants, individuals who choose to participate may be of lower average socioeconomic status than the population at large. It is for this reason that observational epidemiological studies which are based on random sampling are generally preferable to studies that employ non-random sampling methods, such as recruiting volunteers.

Selection bias can take other forms in analytical studies. In a case-control study, the most common form of selection bias is the selection of an inappropriate control group. As discussed in Chapter 7, controls in a case-control study should be representative of the population which gave rise to the cases. If the controls do not represent this group, then the resulting measure of association (the odds ratio) will be biased. For example, in a case-control study of the association between hormonal contraceptive use and cervical cancer in Cape Town, cases were patients living anywhere in Cape Town with cervical cancer. If controls had been drawn from only one neighbourhood (for example, around a major hospital), a biased study result would have been likely (Shapiro *et al*, 2003).

> **Loss to follow-up**
>
> In a cohort study, loss to follow-up through time can be a major source of selection bias. If individuals who are lost to follow-up (and drop out of the study) have a different pattern of exposure and disease from those retained in the cohort, the resulting measure of association (e.g. risk ratio or rate ratio) will be biased. Table 12.4 shows an example of how loss to follow-up can introduce bias into a cohort study. It is critical to note that it is not actually the *amount* of loss to follow-up that introduces bias, but rather *how* the loss to follow-up is distributed with respect to exposure and outcome status. If loss to follow-up occurs *evenly* in all groups under comparison (Situation A), the study results will be unbiased. If the loss to follow-up occurs in a way that differs according to exposure and outcome status, then selection bias will occur (Situation B). (This example is for illustration. Since we would not know the outcome status of participants who are lost to follow-up in a real life cohort study, the true association would be unknown.)

In these examples of analytical studies the presence of selection bias has acted to increase the apparent association between exposure and outcome. However, it is important to note that selection bias can have a varying impact on study results depending on the situation. Usually, we are most concerned with selection biases that create an association between exposure and outcome when there is truly no association. In other situations, it is possible that a true association may be masked by the presence of selection bias.

The best method of preventing selection bias depends on the study design, but as a general rule researchers want to ensure that the participants sampled by their study are representative of the target population of interest (which is not necessarily the 'general' population).

- In a *cross-sectional* study, this means ensuring that the sample is a random selection of the target population.
- In a *case-control* study, this means selecting an appropriate control group to compare to the cases.
- In a *cohort* study, this means maintaining low levels of loss to follow-up, so that the participants analysed at the end of the study are similar to those who entered the study originally.

Note that random sampling is important mainly in descriptive cross-sectional studies where the interest is typically in prevalence. Random sampling is usually less important when selecting cases or controls (in case-control studies) or exposed or unexposed subjects (in cohort studies). Regardless of the specific study design, it is important to note that the time to prevent selection bias is during the design and conduct of

C Data presentation, analysis and interpretation

Table 12.4 Example of loss to follow-up as a source of selection bias in a cohort study

The following illustrates a hypothetical cohort study in which there is no association between exposure and disease in the cohort, as the proportion of participants developing the outcome is the same in the exposed and unexposed groups (risk ratio = 1.0; 95% CI 0.86-1.16).

The cohort with 20% loss to follow-up is shown in Situation A. Here, the result is unbiased: despite the loss to follow-up, there is still no association between exposure and outcome (risk ratio = 1.0). This is because the proportion of participants lost to follow-up did not differ according to exposure and outcome status; that is, every category of exposure and disease suffered 20% loss to follow-up, so that 80% of each group was retained in the study. Note however that the loss of participants had a slight impact on the precision of the risk ratio, as reflected by slightly wider 95% confidence intervals (0.84 to 1.18).

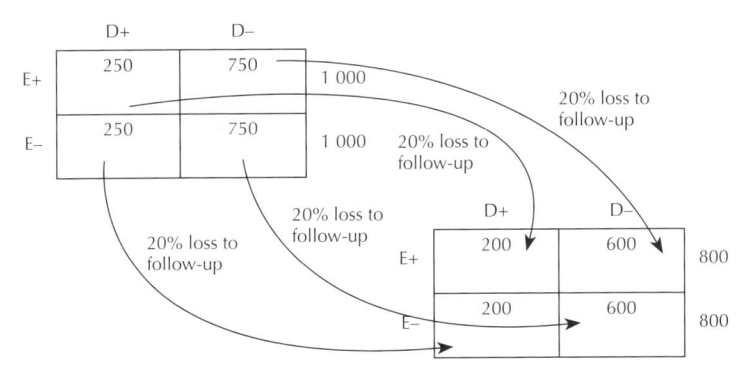

Situation A

	D+	D−	
E+	250	750	1 000
E−	250	750	1 000

20% loss to follow-up (applied to each cell)

	D+	D−	
E+	200	600	800
E−	200	600	800

The cohort with loss to follow-up that occurs differently for exposure and disease categories is shown in Situation B. Note that the proportion of participants lost to follow-up now varies according to the exposure and outcome status. Here, the result is biased. The risk ratio observed in the cohort that is retained (not lost to follow-up) is greater (1.21; 95 % CI 1.02–1.44) than the true risk ratio (1.0). This is because there is greater loss to follow-up among individuals who are both unexposed (E−) and have the disease (D+), leading to an overestimate of the true risk ratio among those participants who are retained.

Situation B

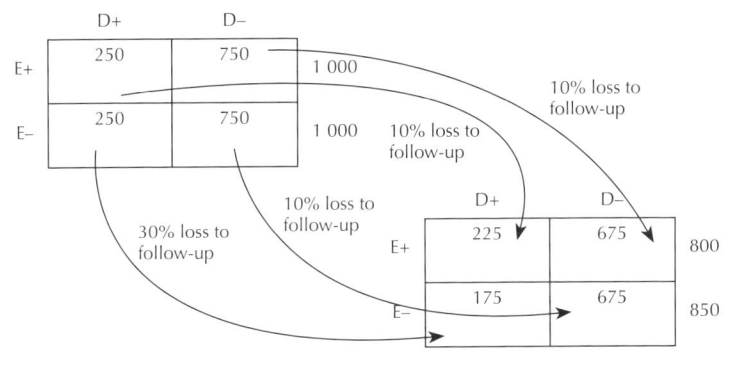

	D+	D−	
E+	250	750	1 000
E−	250	750	1 000

Losses to follow-up: E+/D+ 10%, E+/D− 10%, E−/D+ 30%, E−/D− 10%

	D+	D−	
E+	225	675	800
E−	175	675	850

Note that in Situation A (in which the risk ratio is unbiased), the total proportion of participants who are lost to follow-up (20%) is higher than the total proportion of participants lost to follow-up in Situation B (12.5%, i.e. 250 out of 2000). This is an important demonstration of the concept that it is not the absolute amount of loss to follow-up but the distribution of loss to follow-up that introduces selection bias into a cohort study.

the study. After a study is complete, it is not generally possible to remove selection biases during data analysis (although one could try to estimate the effect of bias).

Information bias

Information bias occurs when there is systematic or directional error in how measurements are taken on participants within a study. This error in measurement can affect any kind of variable, including a clinical measure (owing to diagnostic error) or a behavioural measure (owing to error in self-reporting). As a result of systematic measurement error, the measures of occurrence (incidence or prevalence) and/or association (e.g. risk ratio, rate ratio or odds ratio) will lack validity.

In descriptive studies, information bias can lead to an overestimate or underestimate of the variables being described. For example, in a cross-sectional study of self-reported substance abuse among school-going adolescents in Cape Town, it is likely that some adolescents will systematically under-report their use of alcohol and drugs. If this is the case, then the prevalence of substance abuse will be underestimated (Flisher et al, 2003). A similar phenomenon is commonplace in the reporting of sexual risk behaviours, in which study participants often under-report their sexual activity or high risk sexual practices. These are examples of *social desirability bias*, in which participants respond to particular questions with the answers that they consider to be most socially desirable (or least stigmatising), rather than answering with complete honesty.

In analytical studies, information biases that lead to incorrect estimates in the measures of association are often referred to as *misclassification*, particularly in the case of categorical variables. With *differential misclassification*, the measurement error (misclassification) is systematically different in the groups being compared in a study. As a rule, differential misclassification leads to a bias in the measure of association being estimated, *either* towards *or* away from the null result of no effect. This is distinct from *non-differential misclassification* (discussed earlier), which is random measurement error in categorical variables. This type of error causes the observed measure of association to shift closer to the null value, i.e. the direction of bias is towards finding no effect.

The types of information bias that are most common vary between study designs. In prospective studies (cohort studies or randomised controlled trials), a common form of systematic measurement error is *diagnostic* or *detection bias*. Here researchers assessing the outcome are systematically more (or less) likely to detect the outcome because of their knowledge of the participant's exposure status. For example, in a cohort study of hormone replacement therapy (HRT) and breast cancer, doctors who are aware of participants' HRT use may be more likely to conduct a thorough examination for and to detect breast cancer. If this is the case, then this detection bias will lead to an overestimate of the association between HRT use and the incidence of breast cancer (Grodstein et al, 1996).

In a case-control study, *recall bias* in the assessment of exposure is a common form of information bias. In the most common form of recall bias, cases are more likely to have thought about and to remember past exposures owing to concern about their condition (Table 12.5).

The first step in preventing information bias or non-differential misclassification in epidemiological research is to ensure that variables are measured in the same way on all participants. In situations where a variable is measured in different ways for participants in a study (for example, in a cohort study where outcomes are measured by laboratory assay for the exposed participants and by self-report for the unexposed participants), information bias is very likely.

C | Data presentation, analysis and interpretation

Table 12.5 Example of information bias: recall bias in a case-control study

These data are from another hypothetical case-control study of maternal smoking during pregnancy and risk of stillbirth. In the unbiased situation, maternal smoking is measured perfectly (100% sensitivity and specificity) for cases and controls, and there is no association between smoking and risk of stillbirth (Situation A).

Situation A *Hypothetical situation with no recall bias*

Self-reported history of smoking during pregnancy	Mothers with stillbirths (cases)	Mothers without stillbirths (controls)
Smoked	50	200
Did not smoke	150	600
Total	200	800

Odds ratio with no recall bias = 1.0 (95% CI 0.68-1.45)

In Situation B, mothers without a stillbirth (controls) were more likely to forget or under-report their smoking during pregnancy than were cases (sensitivity 80% for controls but 100% for cases; specificity remains 100% for both). Note that the sensitivity is different for cases and controls. This is an example of differential misclassification of exposure. Smoking now appears less frequent among the controls, and thus the odds ratio reflects a positive association between smoking during pregnancy and stillbirth.

Situation B *Observed association with recall bias: exposure measured with 80% sensitivity in controls*

Self-reported history of smoking during pregnancy	Mothers with stillbirths (cases)	Mothers without stillbirths (controls)
Smoked	50	160
Did not smoke	150	640
Total	200	800

Observed odds ratio with recall bias = 1.33 (95% CI 0.91-1.94)

Another way to prevent information bias in epidemiological research is through the process of *blinding* or *masking*, that is, making sure that study personnel involved in taking measurements on participants know as little as possible about the participants. In the conduct of a case-control study it may be beneficial (assuming it is feasible) to blind interviewers who are assessing the exposure status of all participants from knowing whether the participant in question is a case or a control. In a case-control study, this may also require refraining from telling study participants what the exact exposure of interest is, in order to prevent them from focusing their recall on that specific exposure and not on others. In a cohort study, blinding usually means preventing the personnel assessing outcomes from knowing the exposure status of the participants. This is most commonly practised in a randomised controlled trial, in which blinding of study personnel is commonplace, but we can apply the principles of blinding in taking measurements during cohort and case-control studies as well.

Confounding

Confounding bias, or simply confounding, is the third major source of invalidity in epidemiological and clinical research. Confounding occurs when a 'third variable' (other than the exposure or outcome) results in an apparent association between an exposure and outcome which is not the true association.

Confounding is a common problem in observational studies that seek to analyse an association between exposure and outcome, and can appear in cohort, case-control or cross-sectional studies alike. Confounding is not of concern in purely descriptive studies that do not examine the associations between variables.

Confounding can operate either to increase or to decrease the association observed between the exposure and the outcome. A confounder can create the appearance of a positive exposure-disease association when in fact the true association is at the null (e.g. a risk ratio = 1.0). In other situations, a confounder can make the association between exposure and outcome appear smaller than it truly is.

Figure 12.1 provides a graphical portrayal of confounding. Three criteria are generally necessary in order for a variable to act as a confounder:

- the confounder must be an independent risk factor for the outcome
- the confounder must be associated with the exposure; and
- the confounder cannot be caused by the exposure.

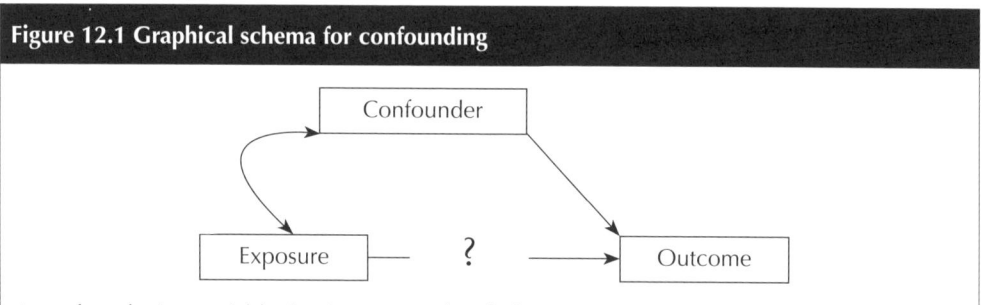

Figure 12.1 Graphical schema for confounding

A confounder is a variable that is associated with the exposure of interest (but not caused by the exposure of interest) and that is an independent risk factor for the outcome. The presence of the confounder obscures the true exposure-disease association, making the observed association larger or smaller than it truly is (denoted by the question mark).

Confounding occurs because risk factors for health outcomes are strongly associated with each other in many situations. For example, inadequate nutritional intake (owing to low socioeconomic status) is a common independent risk factor for tuberculosis (and many other diseases). Inadequate nutrition is also often associated with many behavioural risk factors for tuberculosis, such as smoking and alcohol consumption. It may therefore be difficult to determine which factor is truly causal for tuberculosis and which a confounder. This association of risk factors in the source population is the essential problem of confounding in observational research.

> C | Data presentation, analysis and interpretation

Identifying confounding in data can be difficult. The simplest approach, evaluating the exposure-diseases association separately for each level of the confounder ('stratified analysis') is described in Table 12.6.

Table 12.6 Recognising confounding: the role of stratified analysis

The most common way to evaluate the potential for a variable to confound the association between exposure and outcome is through stratified analyses (where a stratum refers to one level of the confounding variable, e.g. non-smoker versus smoker). The exposure-disease association is then evaluated separately for participants within each stratum, i.e. who have the same value of the confounding variable. If the results of each stratum specific analysis are similar to each other but different from the original (or "crude") analysis (containing all participants), confounding is said to be present.

For example, in a study examining the association between women's use of hormonal contraception (the exposure) and incident HIV infection (the outcome), sexual behaviours are a likely confounder. Women who use hormonal contraception are more sexually active generally speaking, and sexual activity is associated with increased risk of HIV. That is, the confounder in this case is associated with, but not caused by, the exposure, and the confounder is a risk factor for the outcome.

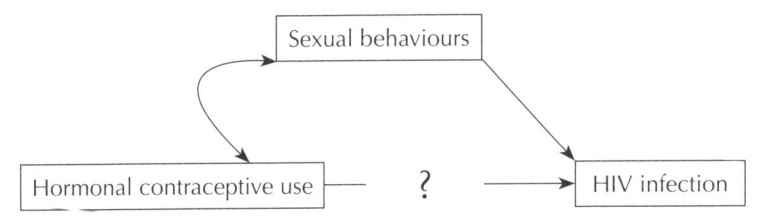

The overall results of a hypothetical cohort study of 2 000 women are shown in Table 12.6a below. They suggest an association between hormonal contraceptive use and HIV risk (unadjusted risk ratio, 2.18).

Table 12.6a Unadjusted association among all women

	HIV-infected	HIV-uninfected	Total
Use of hormonal contraceptives	120	1 880	2 000
No use of hormonal contraceptives	55	1 945	2 000

Unadjusted risk ratio
= (120 × 2 000)/(55 × 2 000) = 2.18; 95% CI 1.60–2.98

However, we have said that sexual behaviours are a possible source of confounding bias. In order to examine the potential confounding role of sexual behaviours, participants are divided into two strata: those reporting high-risk sexual practices, and those reporting low-risk sexual practices, during the study. The results are shown in Tables 12.6b and 12.6c, respectively. Note that the total number of women in the study has not changed. Similarly, the total numbers of women who do or do not use hormonal contraception, and who do or do not become infected with HIV during the study, have not changed. We have simply divided the total study population into two subgroups (strata).

Table 12.6b Association among women with high risk sexual behaviours

	HIV-infected	HIV-uninfected	Total
Use of hormonal contraceptives	101	945	1 046
No use of hormonal contraceptives	20	190	210

Stratum-specific risk ratio for women with high-risk sexual behaviours
= (101/1046)/(20/210) = 1.01; 95% CI 0.64–1.60

Table 12.6c Association among women with low risk sexual behaviours

	HIV-infected	HIV-uninfected	Total
Use of hormonal contraceptives	19	935	954
No use of hormonal contraceptives	35	1 755	1 790

Stratum-specific risk ratio for women with low-risk sexual behaviours
= (19/954)/(35/1 790) = 1.02; 95% CI 0.59–1.77

Note that the stratum-specific risk ratios for women reporting high-risk and low-risk sexual behaviours both show that there is no association between hormonal contraceptive use and HIV infection (the risk ratios are both very close to 1.0). These similar null associations suggest that there is no true association between the exposure and the outcome. The apparent association shown in Table 12.6a was confounded by sexual behaviours; when sexual behaviours were accounted for through stratified analyses, the association disappeared.

In this example, the confounder falsely created the appearance of an association where in truth there was no association. However, it is important to remember that in other instances confounding can hide a true association. The role that confounding might play in an exposure-disease association requires careful consideration on a study-by-study basis.

There are a number of different ways of dealing with confounding in epidemiological studies. These may take place during study design (such as matching and then stratifying in the analysis, or by randomisation) or in data analysis (such as stratified analysis or statistical modelling). Each of these options has different strengths and limitations. However, it is important to emphasise that potential confounding variables must be identified before a study starts in order to measure and account for them adequately. If we do not measure a possible confounder before the study begins, we cannot deal with it with later in data analysis. For a fuller description of confounding, see Rothman & Greenland (1998) or other more advanced epidemiology texts.

Note that distinguishing information bias, selection bias, and confounding can be difficult. Table 12.7 summarises the difference between them.

Mediation and effect modification

We have referred above to confounders as a kind of 'third variable' in a study, other than the exposure and outcome. It is useful for the introductory reader to be aware

> **Table 12.7 The difference between selection bias, information bias, and confounding**
>
> Because they can each cause invalidity in an analytical study, the relationship between selection bias, information bias and confounding can be confusing. One simple way to distinguish these is to ask: *Is the source of the invalidity part of the study, or does it exist outside the study?*
> - Confounding is the result of the correlation in the underlying population between risk factors for a particular outcome, and this correlation exists regardless of whether or not a study is undertaken.
> - Selection and information biases are the direct result of study procedures, either in the selection of participants into the study (selection bias) or in taking measurement on participants (information bias).

that there are other kinds of 'third variables' in epidemiological data that may be confused with confounding variables. These include *mediators* (sometimes called *intermediate variables*) which are part of the causal pathway linking exposure and outcome. One example would be the association between multiple sexual partners and increased risk of cervical cancer among women. Here, the presence of human papilloma virus (HPV, which is sexually transmitted and the 'necessary' cause of cervical cancer) would act as a mediator: an increased number of sexual partners is associated with an increased risk of HPV infection, which in turn increases the risk of cervical cancer.

Another category of 'third variable' is *effect modifiers*. These variables produce a phenomenon called *interaction*, in which the magnitude and/or direction of the exposure-disease association is dependent on the value of the effect modifier. For example, in a cohort study of South African gold miners, silicosis (an occupational lung disease that is common among gold miners) increased the risk of developing tuberculosis disease by approximately 3-fold among HIV-negative men, but more than 5-fold among individuals who were HIV positive. So we say the effect of silicosis on tuberculosis is *modified* by the presence or absence of HIV infection, or alternatively, that there is interaction between silicosis and HIV infection in their influence on tuberculosis.

Conclusion

The issues described here regarding precision and validity frequently present problems in epidemiological and clinical research. Concerns about random error, bias and confounding are widespread, and it is commonplace to hear a dismissive critique of a study such as 'that association is confounded' or 'this study is biased'. This chapter highlights the fact that the consideration of measurement error, bias and confounding is considerably more complex than such remarks suggest. The sources of imprecision and invalidity in epidemiological research, and their impact on study findings, will depend on the specific details of the research question, the study design, and variable measurement. When designing and carrying out studies, investigators need to consider how best to prevent random error, bias and confounding from affecting the precision and validity of the study results. In evaluating the quality of studies, or in interpreting their own data, students and researchers alike need to think carefully about how different types of random error, bias and confounding could have affected the study findings.

Useful readings

Rothman, KJ & Greenland, S. 1998. *Modern epidemiology*. Philadelphia, PA, USA: Lippincott Williams & Wilkins.

Susser, E, Schwartz, S, Morabia, A & Bromet, EJ. 2006. *Psychiatric epidemiology*. NY: Oxford University Press.

Szklo, M & Nieto, FJ. 2000. *Epidemiology: beyond the basics*. Gaithersburg, MD: Aspen Publications.

References used in this chapter

Flisher, AJ, Parry, CD, Evans, J, Muller, M & Lombard, C. 2003. Substance use by adolescents in Cape Town: prevalence and correlates. *Journal of Adolescent Health*, 32(1):58–65.

Grodstein, F, Stampfer, MJ, Manson, JE, Colditz, GA, Willett, WC, Rosner, B, Speizer, FE & Hennekens, CH. 1996. Postmenopausal estrogen and progestin use and the risk of cardiovascular disease. *New England Journal of Medicine*, 335(7):453–61.

Shapiro, S, Rosenberg, L, Hoffman, M, Kelly, JP, Cooper, DD, Carrara, H, Denny, LE, du Toit, G, Allan, BR, Stander, IA & Williamson, AL. 2003. Risk of invasive cancer of the cervix in relation to the use of injectable progestogen contraceptives and combined estrogen/progestogen oral contraceptives. *Cancer Causes & Control*, 14(5):485–95.

Section D

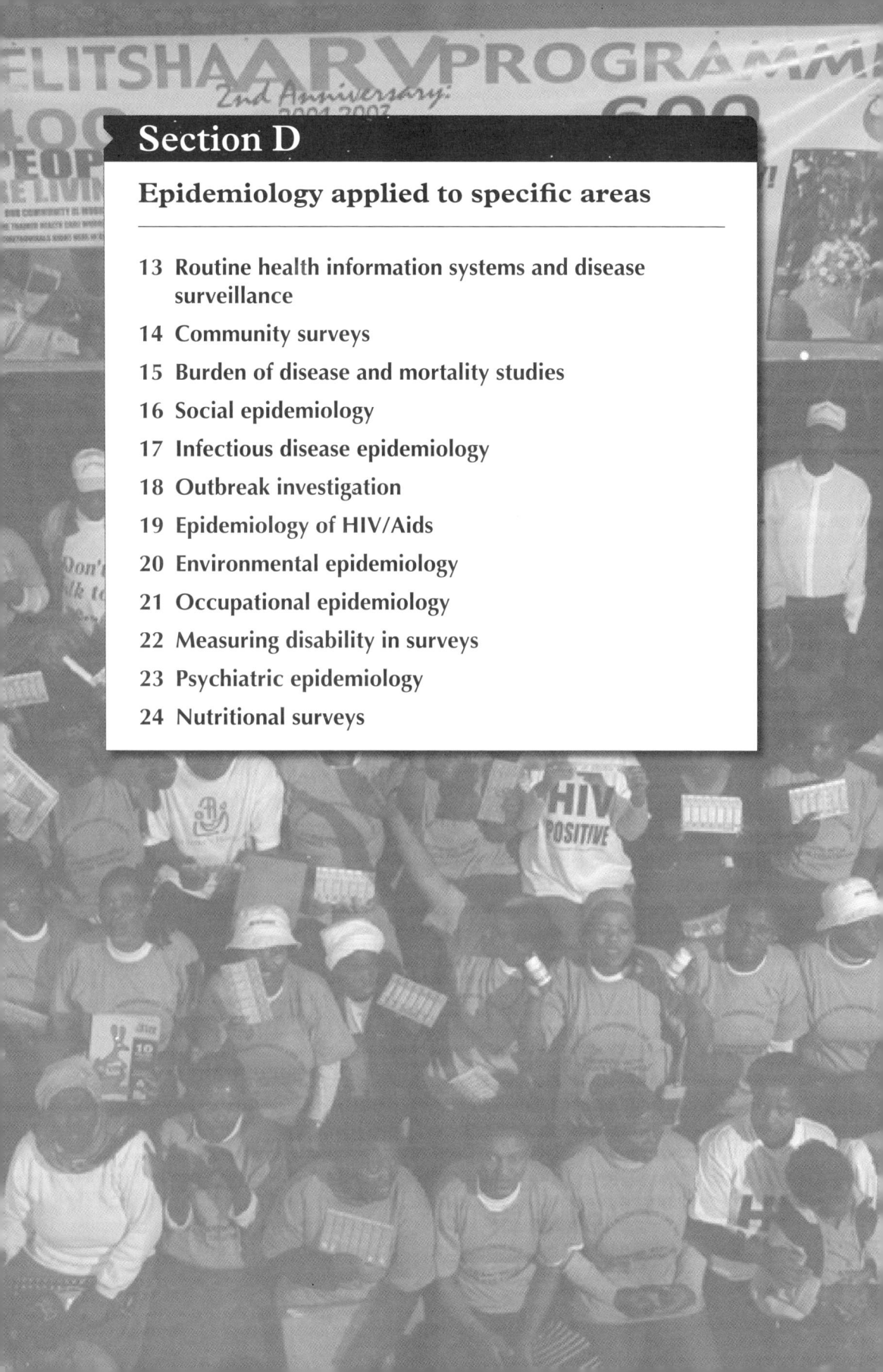

Epidemiology applied to specific areas

13 Routine health information systems and disease surveillance
14 Community surveys
15 Burden of disease and mortality studies
16 Social epidemiology
17 Infectious disease epidemiology
18 Outbreak investigation
19 Epidemiology of HIV/Aids
20 Environmental epidemiology
21 Occupational epidemiology
22 Measuring disability in surveys
23 Psychiatric epidemiology
24 Nutritional surveys

13

Routine health information systems and disease surveillance

Hassan Mahomed

OBJECTIVES OF THIS CHAPTER

The objectives of this chapter are:
- to define routine health information systems and outline the main sources of routine information available in South Africa
- to define disease surveillance, describe its uses and set out some ways of presenting and interpreting surveillance data
- to provide examples of disease surveillance systems in South Africa
- to define health indicators and their uses
- to outline the limitations of routine health information systems.

Introduction: what is a routine health information system?

In a country with significant health problems and limited resources, we need to know what diseases are responsible for the main burden on health care services and how well health services are running so that we may use our resources effectively and efficiently. Routine health information systems play a central role in providing such data.

A routine health information system collects and processes data on particular health related events in an ongoing way (hence the term 'routine data'). For example, government departments, health programmes and health institutions usually define a set of data needed to guide operational decision making and programme management. National and international goals and policies also influence what data are collected. Both manual and computerised collection systems may be used.

Internationally, the Health Metric Network (HMN) of the World Health Organization has developed a framework for country level routine health information systems whose target is expressed as follows: '... by 2011, the HMN comprehensive Framework will be the universally accepted standard for guiding the collection, reporting and use of health information by all developing countries and global agencies'. (See 'Useful web sites' at the end of this chapter.)

What are the main routine health information systems in South Africa?

A number of the routine health information systems in South Africa are set out in Table 13.1. Specific sources of data are discussed in more detail thereafter.

Table 13.1 Types, sources and limitations of routinely available data

Type	Source	Limitations	Aggregate or individual
Mortality			
National	Statistics South Africa	Usually not current (several years out of date)	Aggregate
	Department of Home Affairs	Summary data by office without cause of death information	Aggregate
Local	Municipalities, provincial health authorities	A few selected areas only	Individual
Diseases, health services			
Notifiable conditions (mainly infectious)	National Department of Health Municipal Health Departments	Usually incomplete; degree of incompleteness varies by condition	Aggregate or individual depending on source
Tuberculosis	Electronic and paper-based tuberculosis register: available at clinic, municipal, provincial and national level	Incomplete reporting in certain areas Incomplete records Data capture errors	Aggregate or individual depending on source
Cancer	South African National Cancer Registry (Department of Health, the Cancer Association of South Africa, the National Health Laboratory Service and the University of Witwatersrand)	Histology-based but also incomplete owing to inconsistent reporting	Individual and aggregate
Infectious diseases	National Institute for Communicable Diseases	Microbiologically confirmed cases only	Individual and aggregate
Primary care data on nutrition, immunisation, chronic diseases, trauma and workload	District Health Information System at clinic, sub-district, district, provincial and national levels	Type of data collected may vary in different parts of the country Data may be incomplete or incorrectly captured	Aggregate (individual records available through record review)

Hospital (including disease information)	Hospital, provincial and national annual reports Hospital information systems	Type and quality of data collected may vary by hospital Data may be incomplete or incorrectly captured	Aggregate or individual depending on source (additional data on individuals available through record review)
HIV/Aids	There are a number of registers at health facilities reflecting data on voluntary counselling and testing, prevention of mother-to-child transmission programmes and antiretroviral treatment programmes Summary data usually available from provincial and national levels	Data may be incomplete Access to this kind of data may be difficult	Aggregate (individual records available through record review)

Population

National	Statistics South Africa provides data from the five-yearly Census Estimates and population projections for the period between censuses	Under-counting, particularly for specific age or gender groups	Aggregate
Local	Municipalities often provide population estimates for their areas	Estimates may be influenced by political considerations	Aggregate

Births

National	Statistics South Africa provides estimates of births	Dependent on assumptions May be based on Census data (with limitations as above)	Aggregate
Local	Local municipalities, provincial health authorities and individual health facilities	Incomplete data common	Aggregate or individual depending on source

Occupational injuries and diseases

National	Compensation Commissioner (general) Medical Bureau for Occupational Diseases (mining lung disease)	Data incomplete owing to under-reporting	Aggregate

The tuberculosis register system

All new cases of tuberculosis (TB) are required to be recorded in a register once diagnosed, usually at primary care level. Data on case finding (at baseline), smear conversion (after 2–3 months of treatment), and treatment outcome are recorded in these registers. In most provinces these registers have tear-out sheets which are sent to the sub-district level where the data are captured into an electronic tuberculosis register.

Routine primary care facility data

Primary health care facilities usually have a monthly report form which is a compilation of data such as patient head-counts, immunisations given, curative care patients seen (including specific chronic disease visits), and family planning methods issued. These data are usually collected manually on tick sheets or extracted from registers and the monthly aggregates are captured into a computerised programme called the District Health Information System (DHIS).

Hospital data

Hospitals collect data on the number of admissions, length of stay and reasons for admission. Discharge summaries provide a profile of final diagnoses, procedures performed and hospital mortality rates. Many hospitals have computerised systems from which the data are extracted.

Birth and death data

These can be obtained from different sources such as the Department of Home Affairs, Statistics SA, municipalities, provincial health departments and health facilities.

HIV/Aids information systems

Data on programmes such as Prevention of Mother-to-Child Transmission (PMTCT), Voluntary Counselling and Testing (VCT) and antiretroviral treatment (ART) are being collected by the relevant health services. Ease of access by researchers to such information will depend on the type of data required and the existing uses of these data by programme researchers.

The National Institute for Communicable Diseases (NICD)

The newly established National Institute for Communicable Diseases (NICD) (http://www.nicd.ac.za/about.html) aims to be an important source of data on communicable diseases in South Africa. Specifically, its role is to be 'the national organ for South Africa for public health surveillance of communicable diseases'.

The statutory notification system

In terms of the previous Health Act, 1977, and its regulations, there is a statutory list of conditions which are required to be reported by health practitioners at the time of diagnosis to the local, provincial and national health departments (Table 13.2). The new National Health Act 61 of 2003 makes provision for this surveillance function, but until new regulations have been put in place the old regulations still apply.

Specified forms are in place for the reporting of cases and deaths caused by the listed conditions. This system represents primarily the traditional type of surveillance system focused on communicable diseases where the main response is outbreak investigation and control. The list has changed over time but there are only two non-communicable diseases listed (pesticide poisoning and lead poisoning). Up-to-date statistics on these notifiable conditions are available on the Department of National Health website (www.doh.gov.za/facts/notify/index.html).

Table 13.2 Notifiable diseases in South Africa

Source: Department of Health (http://www.doh.gov.za/docs/nds.html/)

Acute flaccid paralysis	Tetanus
Anthrax	*Tetanus neonatorum*
Brucellosis	Trachoma
Cholera	Tuberculosis, primary
Congenital syphilis	Tuberculosis, pulmonary
Crimean-Congo haemorrhagic fever, other haemorrhagic fevers of Africa	Tuberculosis (other respiratory organs)
	Tuberculosis of meninges
Diphtheria	Tuberculosis of intestine, peritoneum
Food poisoning	Tuberculosis of bones and joints
Haemophilus influenzae type B	Tuberculosis of genito-urinary system
Lead poisoning	Tuberculosis of other organs
Legionellosis	Tuberculosis, miliary
Leprosy	Typhoid fever
Malaria	Typhus fever (lice-borne)
Measles	Typhus fever (ratflea-borne)
Meningococcal infection	Viral hepatitis type A
Paratyphoid fever	Viral hepatitis type B
Plague	Viral hepatitis non-A non-B
Poisoning: agricultural stock remedies	Viral hepatitis, unspecified
Poliomyelitis	Whooping cough
Rabies, human	Yellow fever
Rheumatic fever	

Disease surveillance as part of routine health information systems

Disease surveillance is an important part of such routine systems. This chapter will focus on disease surveillance as a component of routine information systems because of the central role of surveillance in epidemiology, but many of the quality issues raised are of relevance to all uses of routine information systems.

Formal disease surveillance in South Africa started in the late 19th century with a focus on a few highly prevalent infectious diseases, primarily smallpox. However, the system has evolved over the last 120 years to include surveillance of a much wider range of infectious diseases as well as chronic diseases, mortality and injuries. Also, there is increasing emphasis on risk factor or aetiological factor surveillance such as for smoking and sexual practices.

In the modern world, disease surveillance is an integral part of the function of local, national and international health agencies. The proliferation of surveillance systems has led the World Health Organization (WHO) to propose the implementation of 'integrated disease surveillance programmes' (http://www.who.int/csr/labepidemiology/projects/surveillance) at country level to achieve synergy and sharing of resources.

What is disease surveillance?

The World Health Organization (WHO) defines 'surveillance' as: 'the process of systematic collection, collation and analysis of data with prompt dissemination to those who need to know, for relevant action to be taken' (WHO, 2001). The application of this process to diseases is known as

disease surveillance. The key elements of a disease surveillance system are that:
- it is an ongoing activity and is therefore routine
- it is systematic, even legislated, i.e. it happens in a standardised and organised way
- data are disseminated in a timely way, i.e. to those who need such data in time for action to be taken
- it should lead to prevention and control actions.

Disease surveillance can therefore also be described as 'a state of watchfulness to detect trends or changes in disease patterns which require a public health action or response' (WHO, 2001). The actions required may be rapid as for acute infectious disease outbreaks or more measured as in monitoring established diseases such as tuberculosis and HIV/Aids.

How is surveillance different from monitoring? Surveillance and monitoring are similar and the terms are often used interchangeably, but the term surveillance implies a more active state of 'watchfulness' for diseases which require an active public health response.

Over time, specific systems for certain diseases have been put in place. Besides the statutory notifiable diseases system, there are special surveillance systems for maternal deaths and for certain childhood diseases covered by the Expanded Programme on Immunisation, such as acute flaccid paralysis (polio) and measles. These are covered in more detail later in the chapter. Historically, but still very relevant today, one of the key purposes of surveillance has been to detect infectious disease outbreaks. This is dealt with in Chapter 18.

Traditionally, surveillance has been divided into active and passive surveillance. WHO defines active surveillance as 'public health officers seek(ing) reports from participants in the surveillance system on a regular basis, rather than waiting for the reports' (WHO, 2001). Passive surveillance refers to the situation where 'reports are awaited and no attempts are made to seek reports actively from participants in the system' (WHO, 2001). The distinction may be blurred in practice. However, it is important to keep in mind that the degree of effort put into detecting diseases may vary and this will influence the quality of the data obtained. Regularly repeated surveys can also form the basis of a surveillance system.

Why is disease surveillance necessary?

The functions of disease surveillance according to the Centers for Disease Control, Atlanta, USA (CDC), are listed in Table 13.3 and discussed with examples below.

Table 13.3 Functions of disease surveillance

Source: Centers for Disease Control, Atlanta (http://www.cdc.gov/idsr/)

1. Estimate the magnitude of a problem
2. Determine the geographic distribution of illness
3. Portray the natural history of disease
4. Detect epidemics/define a problem
5. Generate hypotheses, stimulate research
6. Evaluate control measures
7. Monitor changes in infectious agents
8. Detect changes in health practices
9. Facilitate planning

D | Epidemiology applied to specific areas

Estimating the magnitude of a problem

Table 13.4 sets out the top five reported notifiable diseases for 2004 in South Africa. This is an example of how surveillance can show the relative magnitude of infectious diseases. If we assume that the data are reasonably accurate, it is clear what the relative burden of each of these diseases is. One can take this a step further and calculate incidence rates based on the population at risk. (The potential problems with these data will be discussed later in this chapter.) Diseases such as HIV/Aids and diarrhoea are not reflected because they are not notifiable.

Table 13.4 Top five notifiable diseases in South Africa, 2004

Source: Department of Health (http://www.doh.gov.za)

Disease	Numbers
Tuberculosis	48 061
Malaria	13 263
Cholera	2 760
Measles	786
Viral hepatitis	325

Determining the geographic distribution of illness

Table 13.5 shows a higher percentage of stillbirths in the sub-district of Nyanga, which is consistent over three years. Data of this kind focus attention on where the problem is greatest.

Portraying the natural history of disease

Disease surveillance can show what the outcomes are for various diseases in the form of mortality, long-term sequelae or recovery, depending on the amount of data collected. We can also observe long-term trends such as cyclical patterns in incidence of diseases or outbreaks.

Detecting epidemics or defining a problem

An increase in reported cases of typhoid fever from Delmas, Mpumalanga, in 2005 heralded the onset of an outbreak or epidemic in that area (see Chapter 18).

Table 13.5 Stillbirths as a percentage of total births in Cape Town and four sub-districts

Source: City of Cape Town Municipality: City Health Directorate, unpublished data

	Cape Town (overall)	Athlone	Central	Mitchells Plain	Nyanga
1997–1998	1.8	1.8	1.4	1.5	2.6
1998–1999	2.0	1.9	1.4	1.7	3.1
1999–2000	3.0	1.3	1.4	2	2.9

Generating hypotheses or stimulating research

The high rate of tuberculous meningitis in 1988-1990 of 19/100 000 in children in the Western Cape led to an investigation of the tool used for percutaneous BCG vaccination against tuberculosis (Kibel et al, 1995). The finding was that BCG vaccination was inadequate with this tool.

Evaluating control measures

The Expanded Programme on Immunisation is meant to ensure high coverage with certain vaccines. Two national surveys, one in 1994 and the other in 1998, showed levels of coverage and changes over time (Table 13.6). The drop between 1994 and 1998 of coverage for all vaccines was of great concern.

Table 13.6 Vaccination coverage (%) of children aged 12–23 months in South Africa, by card or maternal history, 1994 and 1998

Sources: (1994 figures) Labadarios & van Middelkoop (1995); (1998 figures) Department of Health et al (2001)

Vaccine	1994 (n = 2 166)	1998 (n = 973)
BCG	95.2	96.8
DTP 3	80.6	76.4
OPV 3	78.5	72.1
Measles 1	84.5	82.2
All vaccines	74.4	63.4

Explanation of terms:

> DTP 3: 3rd diphtheria, tetanus, pertussis vaccination
> OPV 3: 3rd oral polio vaccination
> Measles 1: 1st measles vaccination

Monitoring changes in infectious agents

The monitoring of antibiotic resistance patterns is an example of this function. A second example would be collection of microbial strain profiles. Figure 13.1 below sets out the serogroup ('subspecies') pattern for meningococcal disease in South Africa. These are measured over time and changes in the patterns may have implications for disease control measures; e.g. certain serogroups have proven vaccines while others do not.

Detecting changes in health practices

Periodic surveys, for example, of smoking practices, can help to determine if anti-smoking legislation or cigarette taxes have had any impact.

Facilitating health systems planning

Data on the magnitude of disease trends over time and their geographic distribution are necessary in planning disease control programmes and resource allocation.

The epidemiology of disease surveillance

Routine data require interpretation. Epidemiological techniques and understanding are needed to take quality issues into account and to maximise the informational value of such data.

D | Epidemiology applied to specific areas

Figure 13.1 National serogroup patterns for meningococcal disease cases

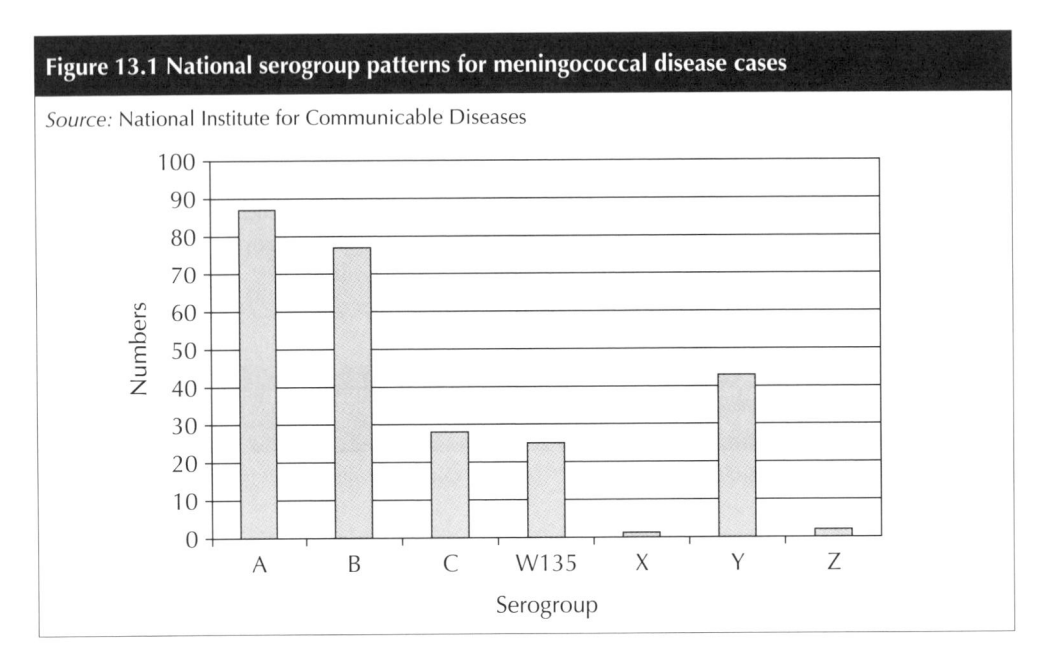

Source: National Institute for Communicable Diseases

Simple *counts* may be used as a first step in the epidemiological evaluation of disease trends (as in Table 13.4 above). However, one should try to go beyond count data to incidence and prevalence data in order to monitor trends. Tuberculosis notification is an example of *incidence* data surveillance. There were 22 999 new cases of tuberculosis reported in 2003 in Cape Town (Table 13.7). Since the total population is at risk for tuberculosis and the population of Cape Town was estimated to be 3 392 183 in 2003 (mid-year estimate), the incidence rate of tuberculosis (represented by the case detection rate) was calculated at 678/100 000 population per year for 2003.

Table 13.7 Incidence (case-detection) rate of tuberculosis, City of Cape Town, 1997–2003

Source: City Health Directorate, City of Cape Town, and Department of Health, Provincial Government of the Western Cape (2004)

Year	All TB	Case-detection rate/ 100 000 population: all TB	New smear-positive cases	Case-detection rate/ 100 000 population: new smear-positive TB
1997	13 870	521	–	–
1998	14 970	520	6 089	212
1999	15 769	530	6 639	223
2000	17 244	562	7 262	237
2001	18 361	581	7 761	247
2002	20 950	638	8 769	266
2003	22 999	678	8 853	261

As an example of *prevalence* data surveillance, National HIV and syphilis antenatal seroprevalence surveys are conducted annually in South Africa in October. In 2004, 16 061 pregnant women attending public antenatal clinics were tested for HIV, of whom 4 738 were found to be HIV positive, giving a prevalence of 29.5%. The trends in HIV prevalence for South Africa and the Western Cape Province for 1990 to 2004 are shown in Figure 13.2.

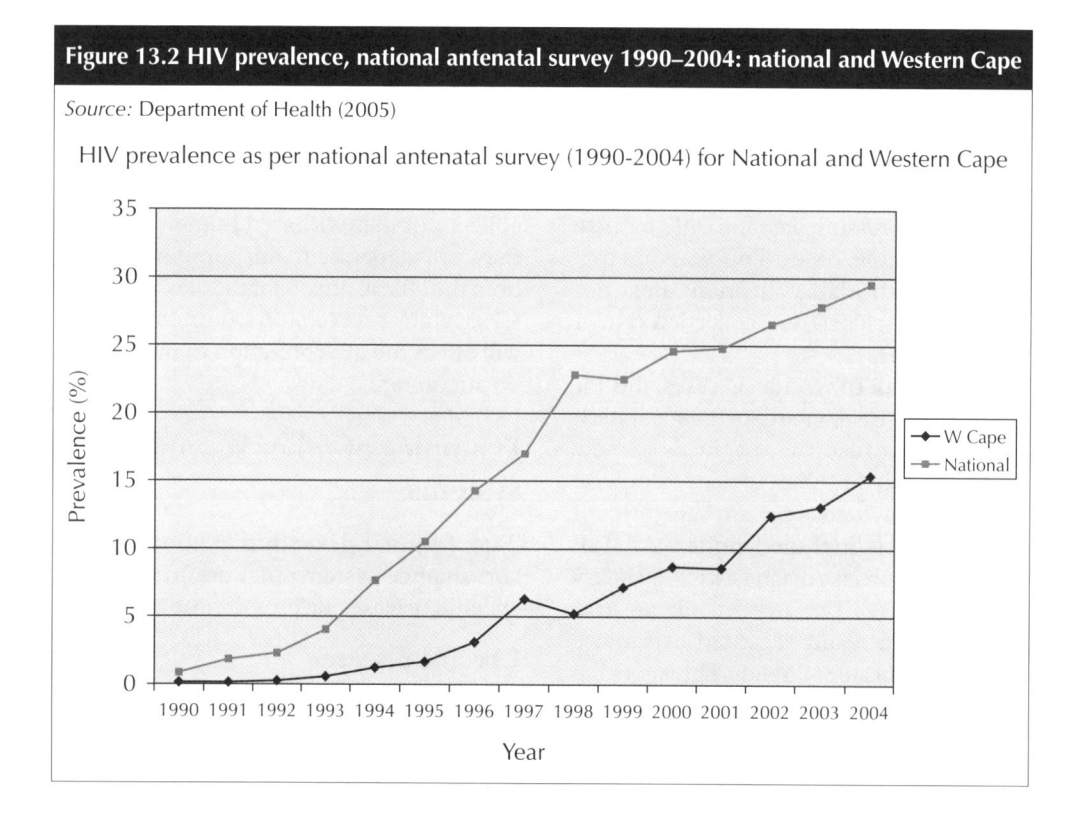

Figure 13.2 HIV prevalence, national antenatal survey 1990–2004: national and Western Cape

Source: Department of Health (2005)

HIV prevalence as per national antenatal survey (1990-2004) for National and Western Cape

Interpreting trends

Interpreting trends in disease surveillance includes evaluating the statistical significance of trends, possible biases, and in some cases causation. This is where the role of the epidemiologist is crucial. Surveillance data are often collected without the kind of controls and rigour present in research projects. Several studies have shown disease notification data to be incomplete, leading to reporting bias. Routine data therefore have the advantage of large numbers of people covered but the disadvantage of poor quality data. We need to take the problems of routine data into account when interpreting such data (see below under 'Limitations of routine health information systems').

Statistical testing is useful in comparing different geographic areas or trends over time. However, since different communities have different age structures, we should use age standardisation (see Appendix I) in comparing rates between different communities. Where the number of cases is small, statistically non-significant trends may still be important in public health terms.

Table 13.7 can be used to illustrate some of the interpretation issues which need to be considered when dealing with routine surveillance data.

- There is a clear upward trend over the period 1997 to 2003 in cases and rates.
- The term *case-detection rate* is used interchangeably with incidence rate. The point the authors of the table are making is that as not all tuberculosis cases were detected, the case detection rate was used as a surrogate for true (total) incidence rate.
- There are missing data for 1997 for new smear positive cases. This was due to a change in the data collection categories of the tuberculosis data collection system at that time.
- Rates for all tuberculosis cases and for new smear cases are reported separately. This is because the diagnosis of new smear-positive tuberculosis is a precise diagnosis, whereas certain categories of tuberculosis included under 'All TB' have a less precise diagnosis, e.g. 'primary tuberculosis'. The new smear positive rate is as a result regarded as a more reliable indicator of trends. This approach is, however, becoming problematic because of HIV co-infection, where smear negative but culture positive tuberculosis as well as extra-pulmonary forms of tuberculosis are becoming more common.

While surveillance data may have a range of problems, the question is often whether the data are 'good enough' for those working in the health services to take necessary action. Surveillance data may also be a rich source of research questions, which may vary from 'Are the observed trends valid?' to 'Why do similar services and communities have such differing trends?' Routine surveillance data provide only a limited set of data attached to each reported case and further research is usually needed for investigation of associations between the disease and possible causal factors. Research can also help to improve surveillance systems, e.g. by paying greater attention to accurate data collection, clear data definitions and by defining and answering specific research questions.

Denominator data

Because surveillance systems generally collect population-based numerator data, they are dependent on population data from the official census for the denominators. Clearly, any problems in denominator data will affect the interpretation of rates based on surveillance data.

Examples of other surveillance systems

The following section elaborates on surveillance systems that are in place for specific diseases or programme areas.

Chronic diseases

Chronic diseases such as hypertension, heart disease, cancer and stroke have not traditionally been part of surveillance efforts in developing countries. However, with the increasing recognition that such diseases cause a significant burden of disease in poor communities, this is changing. While such diseases are not reported as part of the notification system, health services usually collect some routine data on such conditions. There are layers of surveillance for chronic diseases – the actual outcomes themselves, the risk factors, risk factors for risk factors, and so on. Mortality trends are an important source of data on chronic diseases (see Chapter 15).

The South African National Cancer Registry (NCR)

The South African National Cancer Registry (NCR) is a co-operative venture of the Department of Health, the Cancer Association of South Africa, the National Health Laboratory Service and the University of Witwatersrand. The NCR reports cancers diagnosed by histology, haematology and cytology laboratories in South Africa. The NCR is a voluntary cancer notification system and receives copies of pathology reports from both public and private laboratories nationally. In a year, about 80 000 cancer cases are reported and of these approximately 55 000 are new cases. Cancer incidence is reported in annual incidence reports, which are available from the National Cancer Registry (Department of Health, 2003). Information can be obtained from: http://www.nhls.ac.za.

Injury surveillance

The National Injury Mortality Surveillance System (NIMSS), hosted by the South African Medical Research Council and University of South Africa, 'produces and disseminates descriptive and epidemiological information on deaths due to non-natural causes that in terms of the Inquests Act 58 of 1959 are subject to medico-legal investigation' (see web site address below). This started as a research project focused on data mainly from urban centres but the 'ultimate goal is to establish a permanent system that will register all such deaths that occur annually in South Africa'.

A *sentinel surveillance* system is one in which data are collected at carefully selected sites which are then used to get a more general picture of disease patterns. The NIMMS is an example of a sentinel surveillance system in which data are collected from selected urban and rural mortuaries which give some idea of broader trends on non-natural deaths in South Africa. Information is available from: http://www.sahealthinfo.org/violence/nimss.htm.

Maternal death notification system

Any maternal death is a source of particular concern as most of these deaths are preventable. To this end the Department of Health established a National Committee for the Confidential Enquiry into Maternal Deaths which started its work in October 1997 to investigate maternal deaths. This reporting system is special in that each death is evaluated thoroughly by an expert in the field with a view to determining if the death could have been prevented. The data from these deaths are collated annually and reported to the government, and provide both insight into what factors play a role in maternal deaths and recommendations on how these factors must be corrected.

Expanded Programme on Immunisation (EPI) surveillance

All EPI diseases are part of the normal notification process. These include measles, polio, tetanus, diphtheria, whooping cough, hepatitis B and *Haemophilus influenzae* type b. However, polio and measles are targeted for eradication and therefore have particular reporting needs. In order to monitor progress towards polio eradication, there is a requirement that all cases of acute flaccid paralysis (AFP), the manifestation of polio, are reported and adequately investigated. WHO has set a target of two AFP cases per 100 000 per year that need to be detected to indicate adequate surveillance, because this is approximately the expected rate of acute flaccid paralysis cases which are not due to polio.

Similarly, because measles can be confused with other conditions such as rubella, South Africa is required to investigate each case of suspected measles serologically. Specific surveillance systems have been set up for these two conditions, although linked to the general surveillance system. Data not just on disease occurrence but on surveillance programme activities are collected. For example, for polio, adequacy of stool collection for each case of AFP is reported as well. This is another example of how the traditional simple reporting system has been expanded.

Health indicators

A health indicator is a quantitative measure used to evaluate progress towards a goal or target. It usually but not always has a numerator and denominator and is therefore a calculated measurement. International agencies, governments, programmes and local level organisations often set broad goals with a set of specific targets arising out of these goals. Indicators then follow from these as measures of progress towards these goals and targets. For example, the World Health Organization in the context of a goal of controlling tuberculosis worldwide has set a target of an 85% cure rate for newly diagnosed smear-positive pulmonary tuberculosis cases. The numerator for this indicator is the number of new smear-positive pulmonary tuberculosis cases who were cured and the denominator is the number who started treatment.

Health indicators are used in the planning cycle in situation analyses, in the setting of targets and in assessing progress towards targets. Routine data are usually the source of health indicators but regular surveys are used from time to time.

Epidemiological measures such as incidence and prevalence are sometimes used as indicators. Since routine data are used to calculate indicators, possible biases in such data should be taken into account when interpreting trends. Assessing whether changes are significant might require statistical analyses and evaluating causation

Table 13.8 Selected indicators from the 'Revised National Essential Data Set for Primary Health Care'*

Source: Department of Health (2003)

*As approved by the National Health Information System for South Africa Committee in principle on 16 August 2002

Indicator	Numerator (routine data elements)	Denominator
Incidence of severe malnutrition under 5 years	Severe malnutrition under 5 years – new	Population under 5 years
Incidence of diarrhoea under 5 years with dehydration	Diarrhoea with dehydration under 5 years – new	Population under 5 years
Incidence of pneumonia under 5 years	Pneumonia under 5 years – new	Population under 5 years
Incidence of hypertension	Hypertension cases put on treatment – new	Target population
Male urethral discharge incidence	Male urethral discharge – new	Male target population 15 years and older

may be an important part of the process. Health indicators often have specific definitions and these should be considered when interpreting the data. Selected national indicators are set out in Table 13.8 on the previous page.

Limitations of routine health information systems

A summary of the problems which may be encountered in routine data collection systems is set out in Table 13.9 below.

Table 13.9 Summary of problems in routine data collection systems

- Missing data
- Incomplete data
- Duplicate data
- Differential reporting owing to resource differences
- Data recording problems, e.g. errors on tick sheets, in registers or in patient notes
- Data capture errors, e.g. incorrect capture of data records into computer databases
- Small numbers which may not be statistically significant but may be of public health significance, e.g. disease outbreaks
- Inaccurate denominator data for rates
- A lack of depth in the data (few data items collected per case)

The main problem with routine data is that they are incomplete. This has been demonstrated in a number of studies worldwide. Nevertheless, trends may be of value provided that reporting systems do not change significantly from one year to the next.

A second major limitation is duplication of data. While modern information technology can assist in minimising this problem, there will always be limits to solving it completely, for example, owing to misspelling of names. This is a particular problem in South Africa, with its historically low level of literacy and the need to convert names phonetically into single written spellings. We are not yet at the point where unique identifiers such as ID numbers can be used for information systems.

Data are often obtained from different sources which may vary in their quality of reporting. Under-resourced services dealing with very poor communities often have poorer data. As limited information is collected on each reported case, there is often a lack of depth in the data, making further investigation and collection of more data necessary to answer questions. There may also be data recording and data capture errors, which computer systems can limit to a certain extent. However, differences in ability to procure and maintain information technology equipment and systems remain a major obstacle to equalising data quality across facilities and regions.

D | Epidemiology applied to specific areas

> **EXAMPLE 13.1**
>
> **A profile of fatal injuries in South Africa: a platform for safety promotion**
>
> The National Injury Mortality Surveillance System (NIMSS) has been described above. In a report on the pattern of fatal injuries in South Africa for 2002, data were obtained from 36 mortuaries in six provinces representing between 35% and 40% of all non-natural deaths but mainly from urban areas. Their main findings were as follows: homicide was the most significant contributor of non-natural mortality (45% of non-natural deaths); 54% of homicides were perpetrated with firearms and 30% with sharp objects. Unintentional injuries accounted for 37% and suicide for 10% of non-natural deaths. In 8%, the manner of death was undetermined. Males were the victims in 81% of non-natural deaths giving a ratio of 4:1 with females, with homicide being the main manner of death in males. Mainly young adults were affected, with 73% being between 15 and 44 years of age. Drowning and burns were the main cause of death in children less than 2 years of age and motor vehicle pedestrian collision was the main cause in children 3 to 14 years of age. Alcohol was a significant factor in both homicide and transport related deaths.
>
> The authors recommended a range of public health interventions that have been established in other countries to deal with injury related mortality. They emphasised that 'there are numerous advantages to effective permanent data collection systems'. These will be 'used to prioritise and drive public health programmes on an ongoing basis'.
>
> *Reference:*
>
> Matzopoulos, R, Seedat, M, Marais, S & Van Niekerk, A. *South African Medical Research Council policy brief*. [Online]. Available: http://www.mrc.ac.za/policybriefs/fatalinjuries.pdf. [25 February 2007].

> **EXAMPLE 13.2**
>
> **Notification of pesticide poisoning in the Western Cape**
>
> This study compared official notification data and hospital record data and found that in 1991, 78% of cases had not been notified, a very high level of incompleteness.
>
> Further findings were that the majority of notifications that did take place were from rural areas and that farmers, farmworkers and their families were most often affected by these poisoning events. Direct occupational contamination made up 11% of cases while 35% were due to self-inflicted injury and 44% of events occurred outside of workplace activities. Farm pesticide stores were the most common source of pesticides. The mortality rate was higher among those with self-inflicted injury.
>
> Based on their findings, the authors called for improved notification of pesticide poisoning given its public health importance. While this study showed up the incompleteness of the data, useful information was nevertheless gleaned from the data which provided a basis for further research.
>
> *Reference:*
>
> London, L, Ehrlich, RI, Rafudien, S, Krige, F & Vurgarellis, P. 1994. Notification of pesticide poisoning in the Western Cape, 1987–1991. *South African Medical Journal*, 84:269–72.

Useful readings

Abdool Karim, SS & Abdool Karim, Q. 1991. Under-reporting in hepatitis B notifications. *South African Medical Journal*, 79:242–4.

Nsubuga, P, Eseko, N, Wuhib, T, Ndayimirije, N, Chungoing, S & McNabb, S. 2002. Structure and performance of infectious disease surveillance and response, United Republic of Tanzania, 1998. *Bulletin of the World Health Organization*, 80:196–203.

Useful web sites

Health Metrics Network, World Health Organization. [Online]. Available: http://www.who.int/healthmetrics/tools/en/. [25 February 2007].

Health Systems Trust: *Health status review reports.* [Online]. Available: http://www.hst.org.za. [25 February 2007].

World Health Organization. [Online]. Available: http://www.who.int/mediacentre/factsheets/fs200. [25 February 2007].

References used in this chapter

Cape Town TB Control. 2004. *Progress report 1997 to 2003.* City Health Directorate, City of Cape Town, and Department of Health, Provincial Government of the Western Cape. [Online]. Available: http://www.hst.org.za/uploads/files/tb_ct.pdf. [25 February 2007].

Centers for Disease Control, Atlanta, USA. [Online]. Available: http://www.cdc.gov/idsr. [25 February 2007].

Department of Health: *Data on notifiable diseases in South Africa.* [Online]. Available: http://www.doh.gov.za/facts/notify. [25 February 2007].

Department of Health, Medical Research Council & ORC Macro. 2001. *South African demographic and health survey, 1998.* Full report. Pretoria: Department of Health. [Online]. Available: http://www.mrc.ac.za/bod/dhsfinl.pdf. [24 May 2007].

Department of Health. 2003. Research update: *National Department of Health: health systems research, research co-ordination and epidemiology,* 5(4). [Online]. Available: http://www.doh.gov.za/docs/research/vol5-4cancer.html. [9 April 2007].

Department of Health. 2005. *National HIV and syphilis antenatal sero-prevalence survey in South Africa 2004.* Pretoria: Department of Health.

Kibel, MA, Hussey, GD, Marco, C & van der Wal, L. 1995. An evaluation of the 'Japanese tool' for percutaneous vaccination with BCG in neonates. *South African Medical Journal*, 85:988–91.

Labadarios, D & van Middelkoop, A. 1995. *Children aged 6 to 71 months in South Africa, 1994: their anthropometric, vitamin A, iron and immunisation coverage status.* Technical report, University of Stellenbosch. [Online]. Available: http://www.sahealthinfo.org/nutrition/vitamina.htm. [29 March 2007].

National Institute for Communicable Diseases. 2004. *Communicable Diseases Surveillance Bulletin.* Johannesburg: National Institute for Communicable Diseases of the National Health Laboratory Service. [Online]. Available: http://www.nicd.ac.za/. [10 May 2007].

South Africa. 1959. *Inquests Act 58 of 1959.* Pretoria: Government Printer.

South Africa. 1977. *Health Act 63 of 1977.* Pretoria: Government Printer.

South Africa. 2004. *National Health Act 61 of 2003.* Pretoria: Government Printer.

World Health Organization (WHO). *Integrated disease surveillance programme.* [Online]. Available: http://www.who.int/csr/labepidemiology/projects/surveillance/en/index.htm. [25 February 2007].

World Health Organization. 2001. *Protocol for the assessment of national communicable disease surveillance and response systems.* WHO/CDS/ISR/2001.2. Geneva: World Health Organization.

14

Community surveys

Zaid Kimmie Aislinn Delany Bongani Khumalo

> **OBJECTIVES OF THIS CHAPTER**
>
> The objectives of this chapter are:
> - to characterise the role of community surveys, including knowledge, attitude, belief and practice (KABP) studies, in epidemiology
> - to outline the main steps in setting up a community survey, including defining the study population and the respondent, sampling and selecting respondents
> - to describe the stages and pitfalls involved in fieldwork planning, logistics and execution of community surveys.

What are community surveys?

Community surveys are studies that try to estimate health-related events in a population by interviewing a random sample of that population. Although the data for these studies are usually collected by interviewing respondents in their homes, the interviews could also be conducted at central locations such as schools or clinics. Community surveys are typically cross-sectional studies, but they may form part of other study designs such as intervention studies.

The key difference between community surveys and other types of study is that the respondents are randomly selected from some general population, often geographically defined. Surveys aim to make inferences about health-related events in this population. Community surveys therefore generally avoid the forms of selection bias that may accompany studies which draw their respondents from a restricted population such as, for example, those attending a health facility (who may be less healthy or have better access to health services than the community at large), or a school (which would exclude children who do not attend school or who are off sick).

We can conduct community surveys to measure the prevalence of health states such as diabetes or a history of injury, or the frequency of use of local health services by residents. We may also use them to assess the impact of an intervention (see Example 14.1 at the end of this chapter).

> **Knowledge, attitude, belief and practice (KABP) surveys**
>
> Common applications of community-based studies are surveys of knowledge, attitudes, belief and practice (KABP) within a community. The KABP approach is based on the theory that an individual's health-related behaviour ('practice') is influenced by their knowledge of a disease

and the necessary health-promoting actions associated with it, and by their attitudes and beliefs (positive or negative) regarding the disease and its prevention. For example, KABP surveys are widely used to evaluate programmes and campaigns that aim to change health-related behaviour so as to prevent the spread of HIV infection.

The difficulty of accurately measuring behaviour change is one of a number of problems in KABP studies. KABP surveys measure reports of behaviour rather than behaviour itself. These reports can be influenced by recall and perceptions of social desirability. For example, youth may report that they always use condoms because they know that this is what they should do rather than because this is actually the case. Another criticism levelled at KABP studies is that knowledge, attitudes and beliefs are poor predictors of behaviour. Young people may be knowledgeable about HIV infection and appear to have positive attitudes towards health-promoting behaviours such as practising safe sex, but this does not necessarily mean that they do not engage in risky behaviour.

Conducting a community survey

Defining the study population and the respondent

The first step in conducting a community survey is to define both the study population and the respondent. It is worth noting that the study population and the respondents may not necessarily be the same. For example, a study that wishes to collect information on infant access to the health system will have the set of infants as the study population and would use the primary caregiver of the infant as the respondent. In contrast, in the South African Medical Research Council (MRC) study on the link between substance abuse and sexual behaviour (see Example 14.2), the study population was the set of adolescents living in the Cape Town and Durban municipalities and the respondents were the adolescents themselves.

With respect to the selection of the respondent we can distinguish between studies which have as their main focus the household, the individual, or some combination of the two.
- *Household:* These are studies in which the bulk of the information required will be household level information (the level of household income, or household access to the health system or basic services). The definition of 'household' will vary with the nature of the study. For most studies the household is defined as a group of people who live together for at least four nights a week and share the same pot. However, studies that also aim to examine the economic linkages of the household may include members of the household living in other locations.

In these cases one respondent from within the household is usually chosen to provide this information on behalf of the household. This respondent may be chosen *purposively* (e.g. the senior female, the senior male or the head of the household) or may be *randomly* selected from a list of qualifying household members (e.g. all adult members of the household). The manner in which the respondent is chosen will depend on the nature of the information required – randomly choosing a respondent may eliminate any bias that may be associated with the purposive selection of a respondent, but such a respondent may not be able to provide accurate information about the entire household. Specifying the head of the household as respondent may also introduce gender bias into the study (Budlender, 1997).

- *Individual:* These studies require the bulk of their information about an individual selected from the household, such as in the abovementioned MRC adolescent study. In such cases the respondent is usually selected from a list of eligible respondents in the household using a random selection procedure.
- *Combining household and individual data:* In some studies it is necessary to collect information about both the household and about a number of individuals from within the household. An example of such a study is the 1998 *South African Demographic and Health Survey* (Department of Health et al, 2001). In this study a household questionnaire was administered within each selected household. In addition all women between the ages of 15 and 49 years were identified and interviewed with a women's questionnaire. In half of the selected households all adults over 15 years of age were also identified and interviewed with an adult health questionnaire.

The choice of respondent depends on the nature of the study as well as time and budgetary constraints. Although the option of combining household and individual level data may be the most appropriate, the additional costs and personnel time associated with collecting multiple questionnaires in each household may not make this feasible.

Securing access to the community

The logistics of securing access to a community form an important part of implementing a community survey. In rural areas, for example, access to the community may have to be negotiated with the traditional leadership structure. Ignoring these structures may result in a lack of co-operation from the community since they may be suspicious of or offended by fieldworkers operating without the permission of the local chief. Similar conditions may exist in urban areas – entry to a hostel, a block of flats or a housing complex may have to be negotiated with the management or appropriate controlling structure.

Sampling

An important component of the sampling process is determining an appropriate sample size. For details on calculating sample size, see Appendix IV.

Most large community studies will use a *multi-stage stratified random sampling* design. This is usually the most efficient design since it does not require the complete enumeration of the study population (i.e. a list of all members of the population such as residents in an area), a step which is generally neither feasible nor affordable. However, if it is possible within budgetary and time limitations to enumerate the entire study population, then the selection can take place directly from such a list. This is possible, for example, in school- and workplace-based studies as well as studies of registered professionals such as nurses.

A national study (such as the evaluation of the Khomanani Campaign – see Example 14.1) would use the latest available census data to divide the country into a large number of Primary Sampling Units (PSUs). These are usually the Census Enumerator Areas (EAs), consisting of approximately 200 households each. (The 2001 census contained approximately 90 000 EAs.) The researchers then stratify the sample by at least province and type of area (urban or non-urban) and randomly select a specified number of PSUs from within each stratum. They conduct a number of interviews within each PSU (the number of interviews per PSU is usually fixed, but may vary with the size of the PSU). A similar approach would be followed if the study area is reasonably large, such as in the study of adolescent behaviour in greater Durban or greater Cape Town.

Community surveys

A smaller area-specific study (e.g. a study based in a particular town or suburb) could also use census information as a basis for sampling but will usually update this information, for example by visiting the area and verifying the accuracy of the sampling information. Local authorities may have additional information on their areas, including informal settlements. The households to be visited in this study can then be randomly selected from this list, subject to whatever stratification is imposed.

Selecting visiting points

Visiting points (i.e. the points at which the interview will be conducted) are usually 'stands', i.e. plots of land that may contain more than one structure and may consist of multiple households.

It is advisable to obtain a complete listing of all the possible visiting points in the selected area – this can be in the form of a street map showing individual stands (e.g. Figure 14.1), an aerial photograph or a hand-drawn map. In each case the information should be updated by a member of the fieldwork team to reflect recent changes in the area.

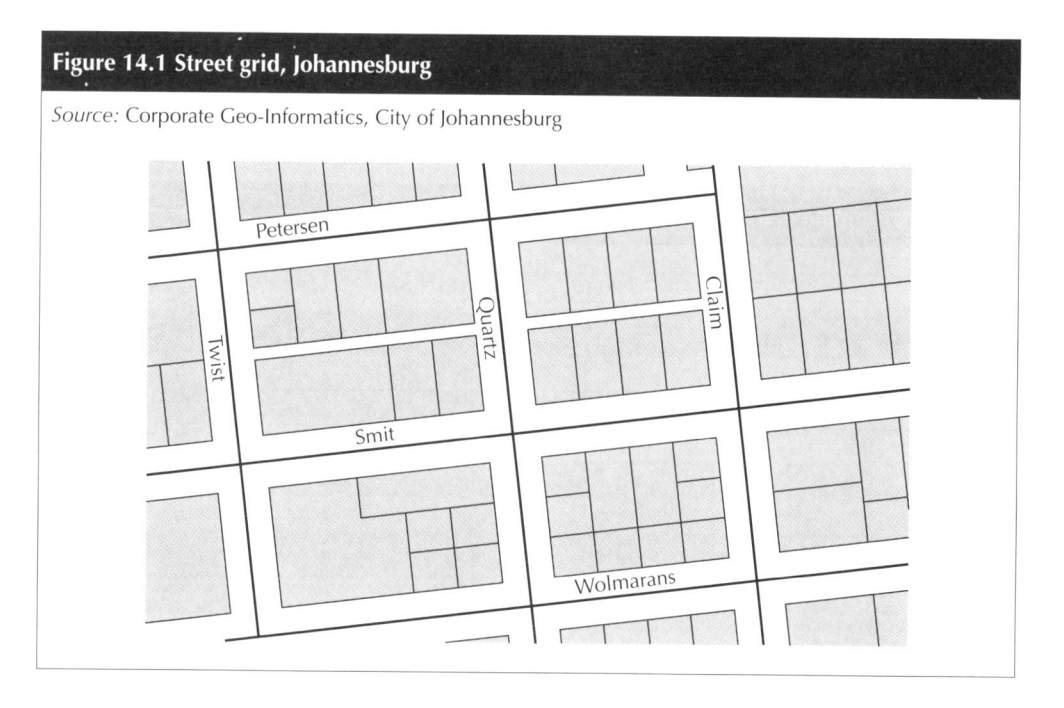

Figure 14.1 Street grid, Johannesburg

Source: Corporate Geo-Informatics, City of Johannesburg

The visiting points can either be chosen randomly (usually by numbering all the visiting points in the area and then using a random number table (see Appendix II) or a random number generator (see below)) to pick the sites to be visited.

An alternative is to choose a starting point for the interviewer and prescribe a rule to be followed to pick visiting points (e.g. to move in a specified direction and to conduct an interview at every 5th or 10th stand, i.e. by systematic sampling – see Chapter 8). Particular attention has to be paid to the difficulties that different types of areas may present for each of these approaches – in densely-populated areas apartment blocks may be difficult to enumerate from maps or aerial photographs, while in sparsely-populated rural areas selecting every nth visiting point may involve excessive amounts of travelling. In either case the selection rule should be strictly applied – allowing interviewers to choose their own visiting points will bias the results of the study.

Selecting households and respondents

Once a visiting point has been selected it is sometimes necessary to choose among different households living on the same stand. There are several possibilities for the distribution of the households – there could be several structures on the stand, each housing a separate household, or there could be multiple households sharing one or more structures.

Generating random numbers

Most spreadsheets are able to generate random numbers – in Excel you can type = ROUNDDOWN(RAND()*6 + 1.0) to generate a random whole number between 1 and 6, for example.

In order to construct the grid below in a spreadsheet we would enter the formula = **rounddown(rand()*2+1.0)** in the column where the size of sample = 2 (generating a random number between 1 and 2) and the formula = **rounddown(rand()*3+1.0)** in the next column (where the size of the sample = 3). We can continue this process until the grid is complete.

Figure 14.2 Example of a random number grid

Qu. No	Size of sample								
	2	3	4	5	6	7	8	9	10
01	1	3	1	3	2	7	3	4	6
02	1	1	1	2	3	2	2	7	10
03	2	2	2	5	1	5	3	6	7
04	1	3	2	1	1	7	4	7	4
05	1	1	4	3	5	1	3	4	5
06	2	1	3	5	1	7	3	1	8
07	1	2	1	4	1	7	7	7	2
08	1	3	3	1	6	5	4	2	9
09	1	2	1	2	2	2	5	5	5
10	2	2	4	1	4	1	5	2	8

To use the random number grid, proceed as follows:
1. Find the last two digits of the identifying number of the questionnaire (usually each questionnaire has a unique number) in the first column of the grid.
2. Find the size of the population (in this case, the total number of households) in the top row.
3. The intersection of the selected row and column will give us the number of the selected household. For example, if the questionnaire to be used was no. 07 and we had to select one household randomly from five on a stand, we would choose the fourth (numbered) household.

One way of formalising this selection process is to ask the fieldworker to list the households starting with the main household and then the remaining households in a fixed (e.g. clockwise) order. Supply the fieldworker with a random number grid (Figure 14.2) for each questionnaire, which will specify which household is selected. This method has the advantage that the selection process can be checked on subsequent visits.

If it is necessary to select a respondent randomly in the selected household, the fieldworker will have to list all the qualifying members of the household (e.g. all adolescents or all adults) even if they are not present at the time of the first visit, and then randomly select a subject for an interview (using one of the methods described above). Fieldworkers may have to return to interview a person who is not present at the time of the initial visit.

It is important to collect accurate information on the selection process itself, in particular the number of households at the visiting point and the number of qualifying respondents in the selected household, since this information may be used to weight the data. Information on the number of respondents who decline or who cannot be contacted should also be meticulously recorded, as this is needed to calculate response rates.

Fieldwork planning and logistics

The following sections outline the key steps to be followed in preparing for and conducting a community survey.

Steps in a community survey

Community surveys present a number of challenges and sufficient planning and preparation are necessary in order to successfully complete the data collection. The planning needs to be realistic and anticipate the problems that may affect data collection. In the *South African Stress and Health Study* (Williams, 2004) the researchers expected that a 4-hour questionnaire could be completed in one session. Instead most interviews were completed over two or three sessions, resulting in an extended data collection period. The logistical steps in executing a community-based survey are:
- the recruitment of fieldworkers
- the training of fieldworkers
- the piloting of the data collection instruments
- quality control measures
- compiling a fieldwork report.

Recruiting fieldworkers

Among the factors we need to consider when recruiting fieldworkers are the following.

Number of fieldworkers required

The number of interviewers required depends on the time allocated to data collection, the estimated number of interviews a fieldworker can complete per day, and the geographic distribution of the areas selected in the study (particularly with respect to the distances between areas and the predominant languages in these areas). The number of interviews a fieldworker can complete is clearly dependent on the length, complexity and content of the questionnaire. In particular, fieldworkers working on studies that include questions covering trauma and abuse may require regular debriefing or counselling sessions. Some studies may also require multiple visits to complete an interview – for example, in the MRC adolescent study, the initial visit dealt only with selection and ethical clearance issues, and the interview was conducted during a second visit.

In addition to fieldworkers, the data collection phase will need *fieldwork supervisors* in order to ensure the quality of the data collected. The number of fieldwork supervisors required depends on the composition of the fieldwork teams – a combination of one supervisor for every four interviewers is commonly used. However, in smaller studies the research team will usually take on the task of fieldwork supervision.

Demographic characteristics

Depending on the sensitivity of the topic under investigation and the areas in which the study is being conducted, it may be necessary to match interviewers and respondents in respect of age, gender and population group. One possible scenario where gender- and age-matching may be necessary is if the instrument contains questions about the respondent's sexual history. Another difficulty may arise where men may be reluctant to allow male interviewers to interview their female partners in confidence.

Qualifications

Different types of studies may require differing skill levels among interviewers. For example, a study that includes measurement of lung function will require a higher skill level than a study which collects simple demographic information. In general fieldworkers will need a basic level of proficiency in English (since training sessions are often conducted in English) and in the language in which they will conduct the interview.

Areas

It is preferable to recruit fieldworkers from within the communities being studied. Such fieldworkers have a number of advantages. Communities may be suspicious of strangers or people from outside their areas resulting in a high refusal rate. Local fieldworkers are also more likely to understand and be sensitive to local cultural and language issues. However, there may be circumstances in which the use of local fieldworkers is not possible or not advisable – the skills needed to conduct the interview may not be available within the community or the subject matter being investigated may be sensitive, with the result that the use of local interviewers could lead to a high refusal rate.

Training

The training sessions for fieldwork staff are crucial in ensuring the accuracy of the data collected and the correct implementation of data collection procedures. The duration of the training session will usually be determined by the complexity and length of the survey instruments and selection procedures. Normally training sessions last between two and five days and have the objective of ensuring that all fieldworkers:

- have a common understanding of the purpose and content of the study, as fieldworkers who understand the study will be better at conducting interviews and answering queries from potential respondents in the field
- are proficient at implementing the selection procedures, e.g. enumeration of areas and the use of random number grids
- are able to administer the instrument in the language of the respondents
- are able to administer the instrument accurately, e.g. implementing questionnaire instructions such as prompts and skip patterns, and coding responses.

Other areas covered in the training session are general interviewing skills (interviewers will generally read out the questions and record the responses on an interview schedule) and appropriate dress. Contractual issues such as payment (e.g. whether there is a rate per questionnaire or a rate per day), and compensation for travel and telephone costs should also be covered.

Methods used in training interviewers

Some of the more common methods used at training sessions include:
- *Role-plays:* The trainers play the role of interviewer and interviewee and conduct a complete interview. The responses which the interviewee gives should highlight possible misunderstandings in the questionnaire with respect to skip patterns, refusals and unclear responses.
- *Mock interviews:* The fieldworkers conduct mock interviews among themselves, playing the role of interviewer and interviewee respectively. This component should be supervised by the trainers to ensure that the instrument is being correctly applied. Fieldworkers should also conduct at least two mock interviews with their family or friends in order to familiarise themselves with the instrument.
- *Tests or quizzes:* Regular tests or quizzes during training will allow the trainers to evaluate the effectiveness of the training session. One of the most common pitfalls during fieldworker training is the assumption by trainers that there is a common understanding of even the most basic procedures – it is worth verifying these assumptions before the data are collected.

Piloting the questionnaire or data collection instrument

The process of testing the data collection instruments is necessary to determine whether the instruments are free of errors and will provide the information required when implemented in the field. Chapter 9 details how questionnaires should be designed and how the reliability and validity of measuring instruments should be evaluated and improved. Chapters 9 and 23 describe in detail issues relating to translation, which are important if the interviews are to be conducted in different languages.

Quality control

The purpose of quality control procedures is to verify that:
- the correct sampling procedures have been followed
- every interview has taken place; and
- the information collected during the interview has been correctly recorded.

The quality control takes place at several levels. The first involves the fieldwork supervisor, whose main task is to ensure that the interviews have been conducted correctly. There are a number of steps that the fieldwork supervisor will follow in this process.

Steps in quality control of field interviews

- Review the selection procedures and the administration of the questionnaire for at least the first two interviews conducted by each interviewer under their supervision. Where possible the supervisor should be physically present at these first two interviews so that errors can be rectified immediately.
- Review every completed questionnaire, ensuring that all the questions have been asked and all the questionnaire instructions have been followed. If necessary questionnaires that are incomplete or incorrectly completed should be given back to the interviewer and the appropriate sections re-administered.

- For a random sample of approximately ten percent of the interviews the supervisor should find the visiting point, check the selection procedure and re-administer a sub-section of the questionnaire to the respondent (usually the sections dealing with factual demographic information). This also serves as a check that the interview has actually been conducted as interviewer fraud does occur.

The second level of quality control is the tracking and checking of all questionnaires by members of the research team. The researchers should construct a database (Excel is a useful tool for this purpose) listing each of the questionnaires by questionnaire number, the name of the interviewer responsible for the questionnaire, the name of the supervisor, the area in which the interview took place (e.g. the PSU number), the date of the interview, whether a check-back was performed by the supervisor, and whether a check-back was performed by a member of the research team.

The final stage of quality control happens after the data have been captured electronically – an analysis of inter- and intra-interviewer patterns may reveal problems in the data collection process and may lead to questionnaires being omitted from the analysis. For example, the results of one interviewer may be very different from those obtained by all the others. One then needs to make a judgement as to whether that interviewer ended up with a sub-sample that was truly different, or whether there was a problem with his or her interviewing process.

Fieldwork report

The fieldwork report is an important component of the study, detailing the procedures used and the difficulties experienced during data collection. Each of the fieldwork supervisors has to write a short report on the data collection in their area, paying particular attention to problems experienced with the selection procedures, with the instrument, with fieldworkers and with refusals on the part of respondents. The project team member with overall responsibility for data collection will write a detailed fieldwork report combining the individual supervisor reports. The fieldwork report is an important supplement to the report on the findings of the study since it provides other researchers with information on the quality of the data.

EXAMPLE 14.1

Quantitative evaluation of the Khomanani Campaign

An example of a large household or community study is the national evaluation of the Khomanani Campaign. The evaluation was part of a series of qualitative and quantitative studies to assess the impact of the Khomanani Campaign, a government sponsored mass media and communication campaign that aimed to prevent HIV infection and increase care and support for those infected and affected.

The Khomanani Campaign used a combination of print, radio and television and consisted of three major campaigns, namely a Youth Campaign, a Positive Living Campaign and a Circles of Support Campaign, all of which promoted the care and support of vulnerable children. The aim of the study was to assess changes in knowledge, attitudes, beliefs and practices (KABP) amongst the general public with respect to the key messages of each campaign.

Two large national household surveys were conducted approximately 18 months apart. The first was a baseline survey conducted prior to the airing of the campaigns in March and April 2002. The second survey was carried out in August and September 2003, after the major campaigns had been on air for approximately a year. A random sample of 2 500 respondents (aged 15 to 65 years) was drawn from 284 enumerator areas (EAs) in each survey, using the 1996 National Census conducted by Statistics South Africa. The samples were stratified by province, race and area. The data were collected by a fieldwork team consisting of 98 fieldworkers and 15 supervisors.

The 'pre-test, post-test' design allowed the research team to compare KABP responses over time. Respondents in the follow-up survey were also asked questions about their level of exposure to the campaigns, so that the responses of those who had been exposed to the campaigns and those who had not could be compared. Where differences were found, the effect of potential confounding factors such as media consumption patterns and other factors were explored.

The table below provides an example of how the analysis was conducted. One of the key objectives of the Youth Campaign was to reduce acceptance of inter-generational sex amongst youth. To measure this attitude or belief, youth in both surveys were asked how much they agree with the statement, 'It is okay for a girl younger than 18 years to have a relationship with a man five or more years older than her.'

Table 14.1 Proportion of 15 to 19 year olds who disapprove of intergenerational sex, by exposure to Khomanani Campaign

Exposure		'Disapprove of intergenerational sex' %	n
Baseline		60%	493
One year follow-up	Not exposed	59%	161
	Exposed	69%	317

The table above indicates that exposure to the Youth Campaign had a positive impact on young people's attitudes towards intergenerational sex (p = 0.028). This effect was evident even when differences in education, race, sex and patterns of media consumption between the exposed and unexposed groups were taken into account.

Reference:

Community Agency for Social Enquiry. 2004. *Khomanani national evaluation survey.* Johannesburg: Community Agency for Social Enquiry.

> **EXAMPLE 14.2**

A community study of adolescents

Researchers from the Medical Research Council conducted a study among adolescents in selected suburbs of Cape Town and Durban to determine the prevalence of alcohol, tobacco and drug use and risky sexual behaviours. The research team decided to interview the adolescents (aged 12 to 17 years) in their homes rather than schools to ensure that parental consent for the interview could be obtained. The decision to collect the information using a community- or household-based methodology resulted in a number of hurdles for the researchers to overcome.

There were initial logistical problems in identifying households with adolescents falling within the specified age range. Enumerator areas were randomly selected to ensure a representative sample, but as some areas were more likely to be inhabited by families and adolescents than others, it was difficult to meet the required number of interviews in each EA. Interviewers also received contradictory information on whether or not an adolescent lived in the selected household. This was particularly the case when the original contact was not available on follow-up visits.

Once a qualifying household had been identified, both the parent and the adolescent had to sign the informed consent forms before the interview could continue. In many instances the interviewers found that either the parent or the adolescent was not present at the time of the first visit, and therefore the interviewer had to return at a later date when both would be available. This meant that interviewers often had to make several visits to households before an interview could be conducted, which delayed the data collection. The interviewers and adolescents also had to be 'matched' by age, gender and ethnicity, again causing numerous delays.

Other obstacles to conducting the interviews included the parents' suspicion of having to sign a legal document, and a high rate of refusal because parents objected to the interviewer discussing topics such as drug use and sexual behaviour with their children. Another obstacle was the stipulation that the interviews should be conducted in private so that the child would not be inhibited by the presence of others. In many poorer households this is not possible owing to limited space. In addition, a number of parents wanted the interview to take place in their presence.

In most community surveys, the interviewer reads out questions from a structured questionnaire and records the respondent's verbal answers in the spaces provided. In an attempt to obtain honest answers to particularly sensitive questions, the interviewers in this study were required to ask the adolescent to fill in some sections (such as sections on sexual behaviour) by themselves. The interviewer had a master copy and would ask and explain a question, after which the adolescent was asked to record his or her response on a second questionnaire. When the interview was completed, the questionnaire that the respondent had filled in was sealed in a separate envelope and the interviewer signed a confidentiality pledge stating that only the researchers doing the analysis would view the questionnaire. However, this meant that the interviewers could not check whether all the questions had been answered or understood correctly, and this affected the quality of the data received.

Reference:

Morojele, N, Brook, J, & Moshia, M. 2003. Adolescent risk behaviour study: update. *SACENDU: proceedings of report back meetings, April 2003*. Cape Town: Medical Research Council – Alcohol and Drug Abuse Research Group.

Useful reading

Terre Blanche, M, Durrheim, K & Painter, D (eds). 2006. *Research in practice: applied methods for the social sciences.* 2nd ed. Cape Town: University of Cape Town Press.

Useful web site

Household sample surveys in developing and transition countries. [Online]. Available: http://unstats.un.org/unsd/hhsurveys/. [25 February 2007].

References used in this chapter

Budlender, D. 1997. *The debate about household headship.* Pretoria: Central Statistical Services.

Corporate Geo-Informatics, City of Johannesburg. [Online]. Available: http://www.eservices.joburg.org.za/joburg/eservices. [25 May 2007].

Department of Health, Medical Research Council & ORC Macro. 2001. *South African demographic and health survey, 1998.* Full report. Pretoria: Department of Health. [Online]. Available: http:/www.doh.gov.za/facts/1998/sadhs98/. [25 May 2007].

Williams, DR, Herman, A, Kessler, RC, Sonnega, J, Seedat, S, Stein, DJ, Moomal, H & Wilson, CM. 2004. The South African stress and health study: rationale and design. *Metabolic Brain Disorders*, 19(1-2):135–47.

15

Burden of disease and mortality studies

Debbie Bradshaw

> **OBJECTIVES OF THIS CHAPTER**
>
> The objectives of this chapter are:
> - to explain the concept of burden of disease
> - to describe methods to calculate and standardise mortality rates
> - to introduce summary measures of burden of disease and mortality
> - to outline methods to analyse geographic and time trends in mortality data
> - to describe how cause of death statistics are collected in South Africa.

Introduction

Information about the disease profile of the population is essential for identifying strategies for improving lifespan and quality of life. In the last few years there has been considerable development in the area of summary measures of population health and ill-health. *Burden of disease* is the comprehensive assessment of the ill-health and causes of death in a population combining fatal outcomes (mortality) and non-fatal outcomes (morbidity and disability). Mortality is often considered the foundation measure of the burden of disease and selected mortality rates are used as key indicators of the health status of the population. The routine collection and analysis of mortality data therefore form the cornerstone of the health information system to monitor population health. (See also Chapter 13.)

A range of epidemiological studies involving mortality or burden of disease data can be undertaken using data from a variety of sources, including routinely collected data and data from surveys or follow-up studies. In the most basic type of study, the level of mortality is assessed for a particular population or study group. In more sophisticated analyses, geographic variations, trends over time, seasonal or occupational variations, or other factors related to the burden of disease are investigated to gain an understanding of the risk factors associated with ill-health.

Burden of disease studies

A burden of disease study is a particular type of study that aims to estimate the overall burden of disease and its causes. This requires substantial amounts of data including cause of death statistics, incidence of conditions and the duration and severity of the diseases or disability. Most countries, including South Africa, do not have all the requisite data for such a study. However, they do have several data sets that can be used together with mathematical models of disease dynamics and

Mortality rates

In order to measure the level of mortality, we need to calculate a *rate* by taking the number of deaths relative to the population over a defined period of time. We can calculate mortality rates only if the death data as well as the population figures are reliable. (The terms 'death rates' and 'mortality rates' are used interchangeably in this text.)

Mortality levels vary considerably with age. Rates typically follow a 'bath-tub' shape, with high infant and child mortality, low adolescent and young adult mortality, and increasing rates with increasing age. With the substantial decline in maternal mortality rates since the middle of the last century, male mortality rates at adult ages are typically higher than those for females. This pattern can be seen in Figure 15.1, which shows the estimated male and female mortality rates for South Africa in 2000. By 2000, Aids had increased the levels of child mortality and young adult mortality, reducing the gender difference in the adult ages of 15 to 34 years.

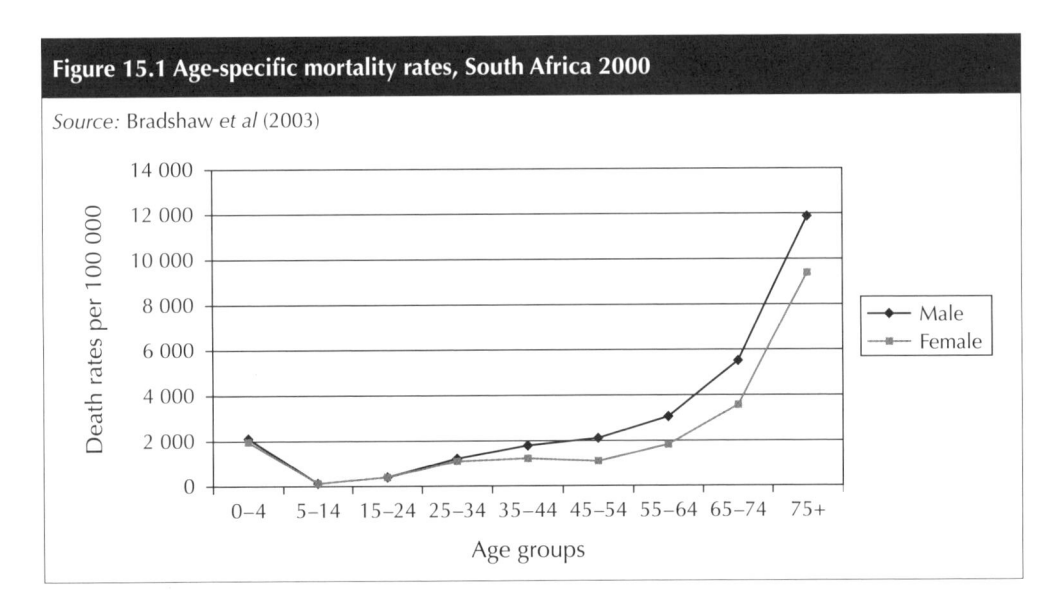

Figure 15.1 Age-specific mortality rates, South Africa 2000

Source: Bradshaw et al (2003)

Standardised rates
(to be read with Appendix I)

When comparing the mortality rates experienced by different populations, it is essential to take account of any differences in the age and sex structure of the populations. A comparison of the *crude* (unadjusted) mortality rates might reflect differences in the age and sex distribution of the populations rather than differences in the actual levels of mortality. Whenever possible, it is advisable that the mortality rates for each of the different age and sex groups of the populations be compared. These are known as *age- and sex-specific rates*.

Alternatively, standardisation can be used to make the rates comparable. A *directly standardised* rate is the overall rate that would be observed in the study population if the study population were to have the age and sex distribution of a selected reference or *standard* population. It is important to specify what age standard is used when calculating the age-standardised rates.

In contrast, the *standardised mortality ratio* (SMR) is based on *indirect standardisation* and is used when the category-specific rates (for example, age- and sex-specific rates) cannot be calculated for the study population. The SMR is calculated by taking the number of observed deaths divided by the number that would be expected if the category-specific rates of some reference population were to occur in the study population.

Directly standardised rates have the advantage that when the same standard population has been used for the standardisation in two or more populations, the rates may be compared to one another. This is because the age and sex distribution for each standardised rate has been adjusted in the identical way. The *comparative mortality factor* (CMF) is the ratio of directly standardised rates in two populations. In contrast, even when the same standard population is used as the reference for indirect standardisation, the SMRs of different populations are *not* comparable to one another as the age and sex distributions have been adjusted differently for each SMR.

The confidence interval of the SMR is generally narrower than that of the CMF (because only the total number of deaths needs to be estimated for the SMR whereas all the specific rates have to be estimated in the case of the CMF). This makes the SMR a useful index when the numbers of deaths in the categories of interest are relatively small.

Key mortality rates

The *infant mortality rate* (IMR) is a valuable age-specific mortality indicator. It is usually calculated from the number of deaths of children under the age of 1 year divided by the number of live births in that year. (It is therefore strictly a *ratio*, not a rate, but is generally used to approximate the risk of mortality in the first year of life.) It is used not only as an indicator of the health status of children under one year of age but also to reflect the health status of the whole population. Clearly it is easier to monitor this rate than the mortality rates over all ages. However, since in South Africa many births and deaths are not registered, routinely available data cannot be used to calculate nationwide IMRs.

Methods of estimating the IMR

Household surveys such as the *South African Demographic and Health Survey* (Department of Health et al, 2001) collect data from a representative sample of women on all the children they have borne, the date of birth and, if the child has died, the date of death. The dates of birth and age at death are grouped into birth cohorts and the probability of dying in each time-period is calculated by age group. This is known as a *life-table analysis*, and is used to estimate childhood mortality rates such as the IMR.

In addition, the survey collects information for the *neonatal mortality rate* (under 28 days) and the *post-neonatal mortality rate* (1 to 12 months). The mortality for older children is also collected and the *child mortality rate* (the probability of a 1-year old child dying before the age of 5 years) and the *under-5 mortality rate* (the probability of a child dying before the age of 5 years) estimated. Although the IMR is a widely used indicator, many demographers suggest that the under-5 mortality rate is a better index to estimate as it is less subject to error than the IMR.

Surveys can also collect information which can be used to estimate the IMR through *indirect demographic techniques*. Such surveys depend on the relationship between some more easily obtained data and the desired mortality indicator. The most commonly used example of an indirect method, the Brass method, is applied by doing a survey of a sample of women and asking them how many children they have ever borne, and how many of those children have died. The proportion of those dead can be converted, according to the age of the mother, into an infant mortality rate on the basis of model life tables. The advantage of the Brass method is that it does not require the dates of birth or death of the children, but relies rather on the mother's age. One of the drawbacks of indirect methods is that they provide estimates that relate to a prior period. Both direct and indirect methods are subject to recall bias and should avoid proxy reporting (some household members may not be aware of infant deaths which occurred a long time ago).

In another indirect method, the McCrae and Brass method, women are asked at the time of delivery about the outcome of their previous delivery. The proportion of the previous children who have died can be used with model life tables to estimate the IMR. This clinic-based approach is more practicable than a field survey and has been applied in antenatal care clinics as well as immunisation clinics. The potential biases in this method are unknown in these settings. However, they could provide useful data to monitor trends.

In South Africa, the importance of *adult mortality* has increasingly become apparent. The *45Q15* is a useful summary index of adult mortality. Based on a life table calculation, it estimates the probability of a 15-year-old individual dying before reaching the age of 60 years. In 1985, it was estimated that 40% of 15-year-old South African males and 23% of 15 year-old South African females would die before the age of 60 years. These rates of adult mortality are extremely high, and are comparable to those in the rest of sub-Saharan Africa. As the HIV/Aids epidemic takes its toll, the 45Q15 has increased further. Originally projected to increase to levels of 80% in both males and females, current projections that include the provision of Aids treatment in the public sector suggest that the 45Q15 will reach levels of 60%.

Cause of death statistics

In order to reduce the burden of disease, it is important to know what the causes of death are. Great strides have been made in improving the cause of death statistics in South Africa through legislation to ensure the registration of deaths and the collection of cause of death information. Every death must be registered with the Department of Home Affairs. Doctors are required to provide details about the *immediate cause* of death as well as the chain of conditions and diseases that they consider led to this cause, *the underlying cause(s)*, on the second page of the death notification form. This form must be submitted to the Department of Home Affairs in a sealed envelope to maintain confidentiality. It is also possible for a headman in a rural area to notify a death and provide information about the cause in cases where it is known by the family members. The death notification forms are then submitted to the national statistical office where the causes of death are coded according to the International Classification of Diseases, now in its tenth revision and known as ICD-10 (WHO, 1992). The underlying causes of death are of public health importance, since they are the causes at which prevention should be aimed. An automated programme to select the underlying cause using the rules of ICD-10 classification has been implemented in recent years.

Enormous efforts have been made to improve death registration in South Africa but there is still evidence of under-registration of events and inadequate recording of cause of death details, resulting in relatively high proportions of the deaths being classified as 'ill-defined' causes. Analysis of trends in the cause of death data suggests that HIV as an underlying cause is greatly under-reported, resulting in such cases in the misclassification of the underlying cause of death as some other cause. Therefore we need careful interpretation of the reported cause of death statistics that takes these inadequacies into account.

Provision is made for the recording of the socioeconomic status of the deceased, but such details are often not completed on the death certificate, making it impossible to analyse mortality data according to socioeconomic class. Information on population group (race) could previously be used as a proxy measure for socioeconomic class, providing valuable insights into mortality differences. Between 1991 and 1998, the population group of the deceased was not included on the death notification form. Population group was reintroduced in 1998 so as to be able to monitor progress in reducing racial disparities. However, about 20 percent of the death certificates still have this detail missing.

Analysis of cause of death

Analysis of cause of death statistics is ideally based on age- and cause-specific rates, or age-adjusted rates by cause. However, if the denominator (that is, population figures) is not known or is unreliable, rates cannot be calculated. It is, however, possible to assess the relative importance of different causes of death by considering the *proportional mortality*. As in the case of mortality rates, the cause of death pattern is influenced by age and sex. For comparative purposes, it may therefore be necessary to calculate the proportion of deaths owing to a particular cause within each age and sex group. When there are numerous age/sex categories, a method of summarising the information is needed.

One such index is the *Proportional Mortality Ratio* (PMR) based on a standard population. This is calculated by taking the total number of observed deaths due to a particular cause, and dividing it by the total number of deaths that would be observed due to that cause if the *proportion* for each age/sex group were that of the standard population. Caution is needed in interpreting the PMR for any disease. For example, if the PMR increases for a particular cause of death, it may be either because the death rate due to this cause has increased, or because the rate of some other important cause of death has declined. For example, in recent years the PMR for most causes has declined because the PMR for Aids has risen so fast.

Potential years of life lost (PYLL) is another summary index that can be used without data for the population denominator. The total number of years of life lost by a population can be calculated by totalling the years by which each death is 'premature' (for example, the number of years lost before the age of 65 years, or any other selected age cut-off point). In order to calculate the total PYLL, the number of deaths at a particular age is multiplied by the difference between that age and the selected age cut-off. In South Africa, it is reasonable to consider 65 years as a suitable cut-off age, as this is close to the life expectancy at birth. Mathematically, the PYLL is expressed as:

$$PYLL = \sum_{x=0}^{64} d_x(65 - x)\text{, where } d_x \text{ is the number of deaths occurring at age x}$$
$$\left[\sum_{x=0}^{64} = \text{sum of all ages from 0 to 64 years}\right]$$

The total potential years of life lost can be divided according to the underlying cause of death, and the relative importance of different causes of death can be measured by taking the potential years of life lost for a particular cause relative to the total potential years of life lost. In this index, it is clear that the deaths that occur in younger age groups are given greater weighting than the deaths that occur in older age groups.

This gives the PYLL importance in public health, where there is a particular emphasis on preventing premature mortality.

The *years of life lost* (YLL) is a generalised formulation of the potential years of life lost that uses a standard life expectancy approach rather than a fixed cut-off age. The YLL measure can also be calculated using age weighting and discounting. However, the basic calculation is expressed as follows:

$$YLL = \sum_{x=0}^{95+} d_x e_x,$$ where d_x is the number of deaths occurring at age x and e_x is the standard life expectancy at age x.

The *disability adjusted life year* (DALY) is a relatively new index that combines (a) the years lived with a disability (YLD) weighted according to severity of the outcome and (b) the years of life lost (YLL) owing to premature death. The DALY therefore adds together the extent of premature mortality and the disability from a disease or injury, using time lost as a measure of equivalence. This yields a measure of the disease burden reflecting more than just mortality. Calculation of YLD uses a weighting factor for the severity of the disability to establish equivalence to time lost from premature mortality. For example, a severe disability such as quadriplegia will have a high severity weighting while the consequence of a mildly disabling respiratory condition will have a low severity weighting. One healthy year lost as a result of death is equivalent to two years lived with a condition that has a severity weight of 0.5. Similarly, five years lived with a condition with a severity weight of 0.2 is equivalent to 20 years with a condition with severity weight of 0.05.

A DALY can be considered as a year of healthy life lost. In using the DALY as an outcome of a preventative strategy, we would speak of 'DALYs avoided' as being the measure of that strategy's effectiveness.

The introduction of the DALY means that value judgements are made in the selection of weights to measure the burden of disease. Although contentious, this process has been helpful in clarifying the explicit role of subjective values in measuring burden. Especially when combining non-fatal and fatal outcomes, it is inevitable that we make value judgements.

It is also important to note that in a ranking exercise, the level of grouping of diseases influences the resulting ranking. If, for example, all cancers are considered as a single group, they will rank higher than if they are considered separately by cancer site.

Determining geographic variations

Researchers often investigate the geographic variation in mortality to identify factors related to a disease. For years up until 1996 the magisterial district of residence of each decedent (person who has died) was available from routinely collected mortality data. This allowed researchers to calculate rates over the whole country at the level of magisterial district. An example of such a study indicated that the rates of certain cancers were unusually high in the areas around Prieska in the Northern Cape, where asbestos is found, consequently implicating asbestos as a cause of these cancers (Botha *et al*, 1986).

Indirect standardisation is often incorrectly applied in such analyses. If the population data on age- and sex-specific cause of death are available for each district, it would be better to use direct standardisation, as the SMR for one magisterial district is not comparable to the SMR for another.

Determining trends over time

It is important to assess whether mortality levels change over time. The first step in such an analysis is to examine graphs showing the mortality rates over time. If possible, age-specific rates or standardised rates should be investigated to ensure that apparent changes in mortality rates are not due to changes in the age structure over time.

As an example, directly standardised cervical cancer mortality trends for white and coloured women in South Africa from 1949 to 1990 are shown in Figure 15.2 (Bailie et al, 1996). The world age standard was used as standard population. It can be seen that the age-standardised rate for white women declined after the mid-1960s, while that of coloured women rose. Different factors are related to changes in cervical cancer mortality, but the introduction of cytological screening (Pap smears) during the 1960s and 1970s had an impact on mortality in many developed countries. One of the possible explanations for the trends in the data in Figure 15.2 is that white women had better access to such screening than coloured women.

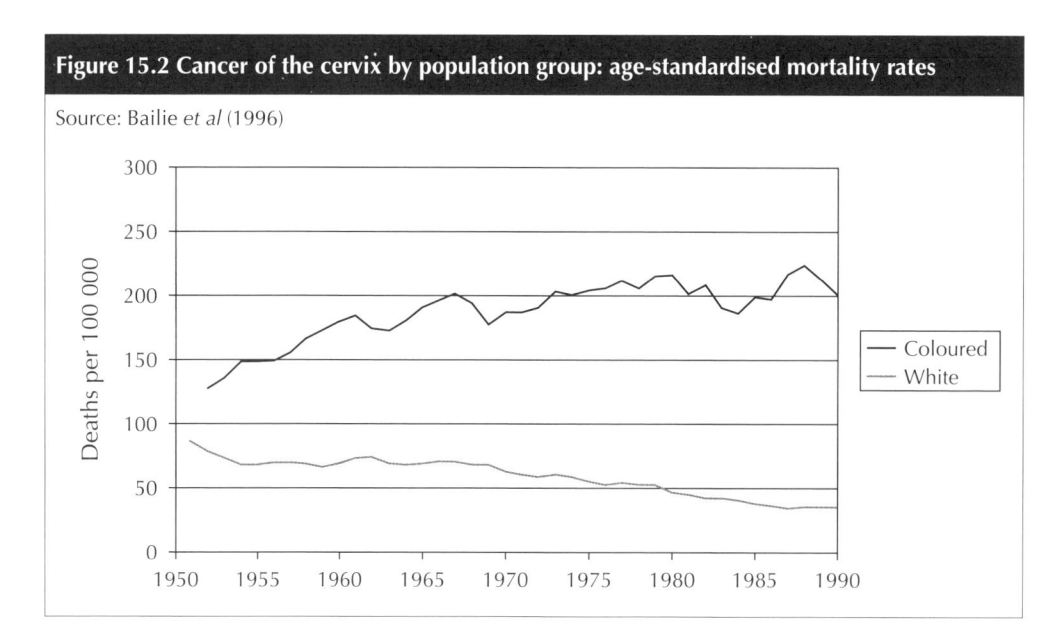

Figure 15.2 Cancer of the cervix by population group: age-standardised mortality rates

Source: Bailie et al (1996)

A *cohort analysis* of the cervical cancer mortality data for white women is shown in Figure 15.3 for successive cohorts of women born in 10-year intervals starting in 1871–1880. Each cohort curve reflects the 'lifetime experience' of women of approximately the same age with regard to cervical cancer mortality. The age effect can be seen in the rise in mortality rate with age within each birth cohort. However, the level of mortality in *successive* birth cohorts has dropped. This can be seen clearly, for example, at age 50 years. This pattern is consistent with a reduction in cervical cancer mortality in this population following the advent of cytological screening in the 1960s.

When considering trends over time it is important to be aware of possible changes in coding practices which might account for changes in the mortality level. One must also allow for seasonal variation. For example, the analysis of the trend in diarrhoea

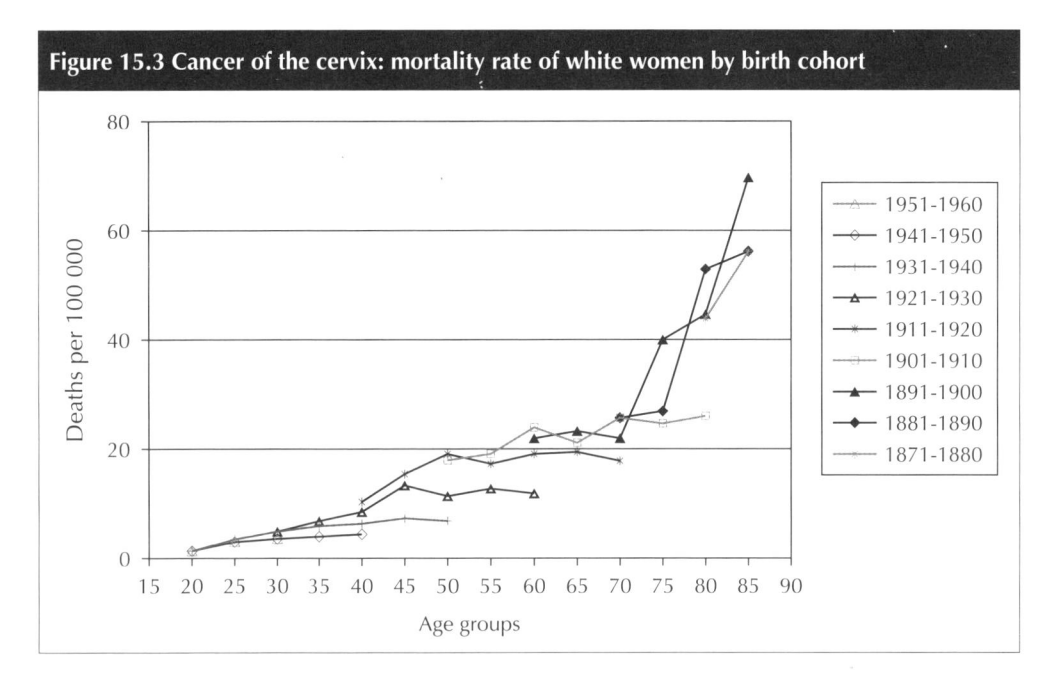

Figure 15.3 Cancer of the cervix: mortality rate of white women by birth cohort

will require the researcher to take the seasonal variation (high summer rates, low winter rates) into account, through a statistical procedure called time series analysis. Comparisons of proportions over time are very difficult to interpret, as apparent changes in one cause may be due to changes in a different cause. For example, the proportion of deaths owing to circulatory diseases in white males dropped between 1970 and 1984, but this could have been due to an increase in the number of injury-related deaths rather than to a decrease in the incidence of circulatory diseases.

EXAMPLE 15.1

Estimating the infant mortality rate

A survey was conducted in the Hewu district of the Eastern Cape during May 1986 to obtain an estimate of the infant mortality rate (IMR), as it was known that the death and birth registers were incomplete. Some 5 102 households were included in the survey, and data were collected from 7 792 women of child-bearing age. From the replies to questions about their children born in the preceding five years, it was estimated that 41 per 1 000 liveborn infants died in the period 1981–1986. Using information on all children ever born, Brass's indirect demographic technique (see above) indicated that for the same period, the IMR ranged from 80–100 per 1 000 live births. The discrepancy in the estimates could be attributed to recall bias, to bias owing to proxy reporting (in the case of the survey), or to the model life table being inappropriate (in the case of the indirect estimate).

Reference:

Yach, D, Katzenellenbogen, J & Conradie, H. 1987. Ciskei infant mortality study: Hewu district. *South African Journal of Science*, 83(7):416–21.

> **EXAMPLE 15.2**

The Initial National Burden of Disease Study for South Africa, 2000

The Initial National Burden of Disease Study for South Africa involved extensive analysis of available mortality data to derive best estimates of the level and causes of mortality in South Africa in the year 2000. In most burden of disease studies, the causes are divided into three broad types. Infectious diseases together with conditions related to maternal problems, perinatal problems and under-nutrition make up Type 1. These conditions are traditionally associated with under-development. Non-communicable diseases such as cardiovascular disease and cancers constitute Type 2 and injuries make up Type 3. As a population becomes more developed, there is usually a shift from a profile dominated by Type 1 conditions to one dominated by Type 2 conditions.

Middle income countries often have a period when there is a double burden, with the population experiencing both types of conditions simultaneously. In the case of South Africa, social factors have led to a large injury burden and an extremely high HIV/Aids burden, resulting in a *quadruple burden* of disease, as demonstrated by the YLL estimates in the 2000 South African National Burden of Disease Study (Figure 15.4).

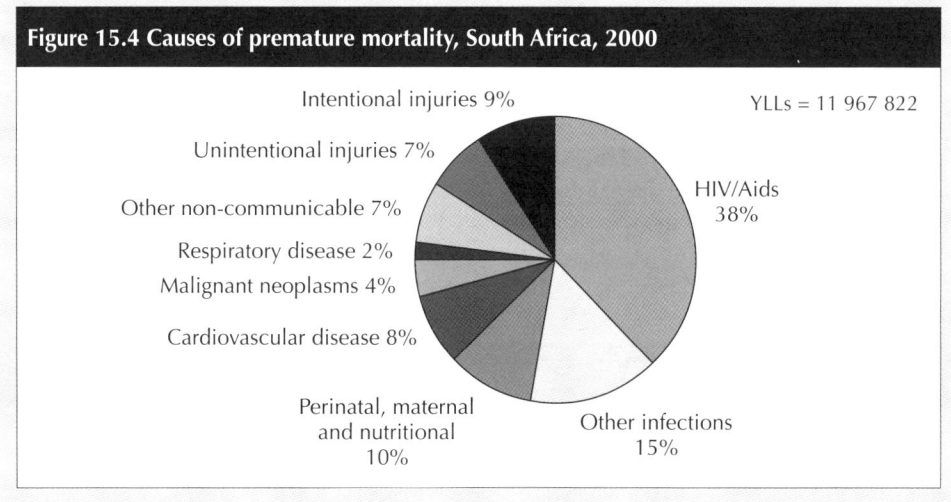

Figure 15.4 Causes of premature mortality, South Africa, 2000

- Intentional injuries 9%
- Unintentional injuries 7%
- Other non-communicable 7%
- Respiratory disease 2%
- Malignant neoplasms 4%
- Cardiovascular disease 8%
- Perinatal, maternal and nutritional 10%
- Other infections 15%
- HIV/Aids 38%

YLLs = 11 967 822

The South African Burden of Disease Study made use of the Actuarial Society of South Africa (ASSA) demographic and Aids model to estimate the total number of deaths and the number resulting from Aids in the year 2000. The cause of death profile from 1996 was used to estimate the profile of the non-Aids natural deaths while the *National Injury Mortality Surveillance System* (NIMMS) was used to obtain the injury profile. This has recently been extended to provide estimates of DALYs for all the causes on the list. Further details about the estimation procedures used are available in a technical report (Norman *et al*, 2006).

A burden of disease study should be accompanied by a risk factor assessment to quantify the burden attributable to selected modifiable risk factors on the one hand, and cost-effectiveness assessments of potential interventions on the other. (See Chapter 27.) Such studies require epidemiological, demographic and economic modelling and provide important information for policy makers to identify the risk factors that should be targeted as well as information on the most cost-effective of the intervention options.

References:

Bradshaw, D, Groenewald, P, Laubscher, R, Nannan, N, Nojilana, B, Norman, R, Pieterse, D & Schneider, M. 2003. *Initial burden of disease estimates for South Africa, 2000*. Cape Town: MRC.

Norman, R, Bradshaw, D, Schneider, M, Pieterse, D & Groenewald, P. 2006. *Revised burden of disease estimates for the comparative risk factor assessment, South Africa 2000*. Cape Town: MRC.

Useful readings

Lopez, AD, Mathers, CD, Ezzati, M, Jamison, DT & Murray, CJ. 2006. Global and regional burden of disease and risk factors, 2001: systematic analysis of population health data. *Lancet*, 367(9524):1747-1757.

Mathers, CD, Vos, T, Lopez, AD & Ezzati, M. 2001. *National burden of disease studies: a practical guide*. 2nd ed. Geneva: World Health Organization Global Programme on Evidence for Health Policy. [Online]. Available: http://www.who.int/evidence/nbd. [25 February 2007].

Useful web sites

Burden of Disease Research Unit, Medical Research Council of South Africa. [Online]. Available: http://www.mrc.co.za/bod/bod.htm. [9 April 2007].

Disease Control Priorities Project. [Online]. Available: http://www.dcp2.org/main/. [25 February 2007].

Statistics South Africa: Mortality Reports. [Online]. Available: http://www.statssa.gov.za/publications/statsabout.asp?PPN=P0309.3&SCH=3659. [25 February 2007].

World Health Organization. Burden of Disease Statistics. [Online]. Available: http://www.who.int/healthinfo/bod/en/. [25 February 2007].

World Health Organization. International Classification of Diseases (ICD). [Online]. Available: http://www.who.int/classifications/icd/en/index.html. [25 February 2007].

World Health Organization. World Health Statistics and Health Information Systems. [Online]. Available: http://www.who.int/healthinfo/en. [25 February 2007].

References used in this chapter

Bailie, RS, Selvey, CE, Bourne, D & Bradshaw, D. 1996. Trends in cervical cancer mortality in South Africa. *International Journal of Epidemiology*, 25(3):488–93.

Botha, JL, Irwig, LM & Strebel, PM. 1986. Excess mortality from stomach cancer, lung cancer, and asbestosis and/or mesothelioma in crocidolite mining districts in South Africa. *American Journal of Epidemiology*, 123(1):30–40.

Department of Health, Medical Research Council & ORC Macro. 2001. *South African demographic and health survey, 1998*. Full report. Pretoria: Department of Health.

World Health Organization. 1992. *International statistical classification of diseases and related health problems*. 10th rev ed. Geneva: World Health Organization.

16

Social epidemiology

Landon Myer Rodney Ehrlich

> **OBJECTIVES OF THIS CHAPTER**
>
> **The objectives of this chapter are:**
> - to define social epidemiology
> - to identify ways in which the associations between poverty and health can be studied
> - to describe an approach to measuring socioeconomic status in epidemiological research in developing country settings
> - to introduce the potential influences that social networks may have on health
> - to describe different ways in which race and ethnicity are defined in the study of health and to provide an approach to using these concepts in epidemiology.

Introduction

Social epidemiology focuses on how social and economic characteristics influence states of health. Different social and economic determinants that are of interest include wealth and poverty, social relationships, racial categories and processes of discrimination. These characteristics are of interest for their impact on individual

Table 16.1 Terminology in social epidemiology	
Discrimination	The processes by which certain individuals or groups are placed at a systematic social and/or economic disadvantage on the basis of race, gender, sexual orientation or other characteristics
Social position	The social identity which an individual has within a society, such as those influenced by gender roles or occupation
Socioeconomic status	The overall economic and social situation of individuals or populations, often measured by their income, education and occupation
Social networks	The number and quality of interpersonal relationships which an individual has that may influence health for better (e.g. through social support) or worse (e.g. by exposure to infectious agents)
Social capital	The set of resources and benefits which individuals may access through membership in communities and other social groupings

health and population health. For example, an individual's social support system may influence his or her health. At the population level, communities with increased levels of social capital may have better health profiles than those with lower levels of social capital. Table 16.1 defines some of the important terminology in social epidemiology.

Using different epidemiological study designs (see Chapter 7), social epidemiologists try to determine whether and how these kinds of social and/or economic factors are associated with disease and death in different settings. As in other areas of epidemiology, social epidemiological research seeks to distinguish true causal effects from those that are due to bias or confounding or have other explanations. An understanding of how social and economic factors influence morbidity and mortality is regarded as increasingly important in epidemiology and public health policy. These perspectives are particularly important to understanding the distribution, determinants and prevention of disease in South Africa and other developing countries.

The history of social epidemiology in South Africa

Social epidemiology has particularly strong historical roots in South Africa. As outlined in Chapter 1, several of the earliest social epidemiological studies in South Africa were conducted by Sidney Kark, who is also known as an influential figure in the Primary Health Care movement. During the 1940s and 1950s, Kark worked at the Pholela health centre in rural KwaZulu-Natal. His research here demonstrated that the socioeconomic conditions of rural communities played a major role in shaping their morbidity profile. In one study, Kark used cross-sectional surveys and disease notification data to show how the transmission of syphilis (then a major cause of morbidity and mortality) between urban and rural areas was promoted by the migrant labour system. Based on this analysis, he referred to the migrant labour system as a 'social pathology', one that could be addressed by allowing black South Africans access to urban family housing to replace the migrant labour system (Kark, 1949). Several of Kark's South African students later played a major role in the development of social epidemiology in the US and Europe.

Social and economic factors remained prominent for many South African epidemiologists through the 1970s and 1980s. Research by Cyril Wyndham, Les Irwig and others based at the Medical Research Council during this period sought to compare the mortality of different race groups. These investigations confirmed a social gradient in mortality rates, with a large disadvantage in all-cause mortality, and particularly infant mortality, among blacks and coloureds relative to whites (with rates among Asians in between) (Wyndham & Irwig, 1979; Wyndham, 1981). During the 1980s, epidemiological methods were also directed to demonstrate the health effects of political unrest. Derek Yach and others used community-based surveys to measure the impacts of political violence on the provision of services such as water and transport, on access to health services, and on injury rates in affected township areas (Yach, 1988). Other commentaries from this period focused on the unequal access to health services as a critical pathway through which apartheid policies shaped the health of different race groups. (See also Chapter 1.)

Following these historical precedents, the objective of social epidemiology in South Africa is to understand how health outcomes are patterned according to social and economic conditions, in an attempt to guide health and social policies to alleviate health inequalities.

The epidemiological study of poverty and health

The relationship between poverty and health has received the most attention in social epidemiological research. The major finding here, which has been documented consistently across countries and through time using a range of study designs, is that poorer individuals experience increased disease and death rates compared to wealthier individuals. This general association is most often described as a *gradient* of wealth and health, i.e. increasing socioeconomic status contributes to improved health across all levels of socioeconomic status, in a 'dose-response' manner (Figure 16.1). Incremental increases in wealth are therefore associated with incremental improvements in health, rather than exhibiting a *threshold effect* in which low socioeconomic position is associated with poorer health only below a certain level of wealth.

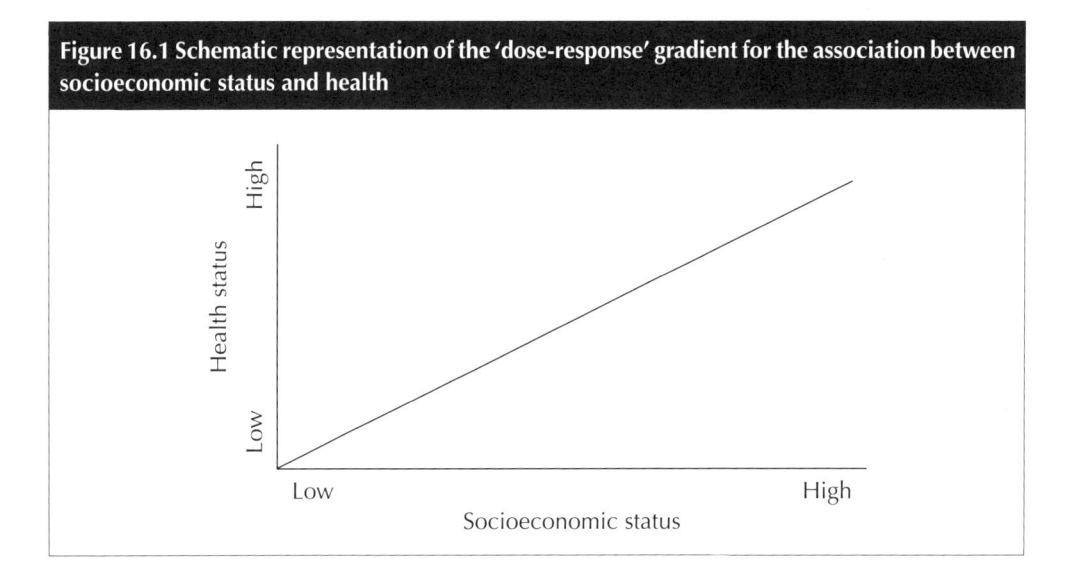

Figure 16.1 Schematic representation of the 'dose-response' gradient for the association between socioeconomic status and health

For example, an analysis of the 1998 *South African Demographic and Health Survey* (a nationally representative survey of more than 10 000 individuals) (Harling, 2006) found a significant association between poverty and tuberculosis infection: individuals who reported having tuberculosis at some time in the past were, on average, poorer than individuals who did not (Figure 16.2). This association showed a clear gradient, with the poorest group of individuals having the highest levels of tuberculosis, followed by the second poorest group, and so on. This example focuses on one particular infectious disease, but it is important to note that the general association between poverty and ill-health has been demonstrated for a wide range of health outcomes, including both infectious and chronic conditions as well as all-cause mortality.

To any observer of health in South Africa, the idea that people who are poorer experience more morbidity and mortality than people who are wealthy may seem obvious. In addition to demonstrating that social and economic conditions are a cause of specific health outcomes, social epidemiology seeks to explain the diverse pathways (whether sociological, behavioural or biological) involved in the associations between poverty and ill-health. For example,

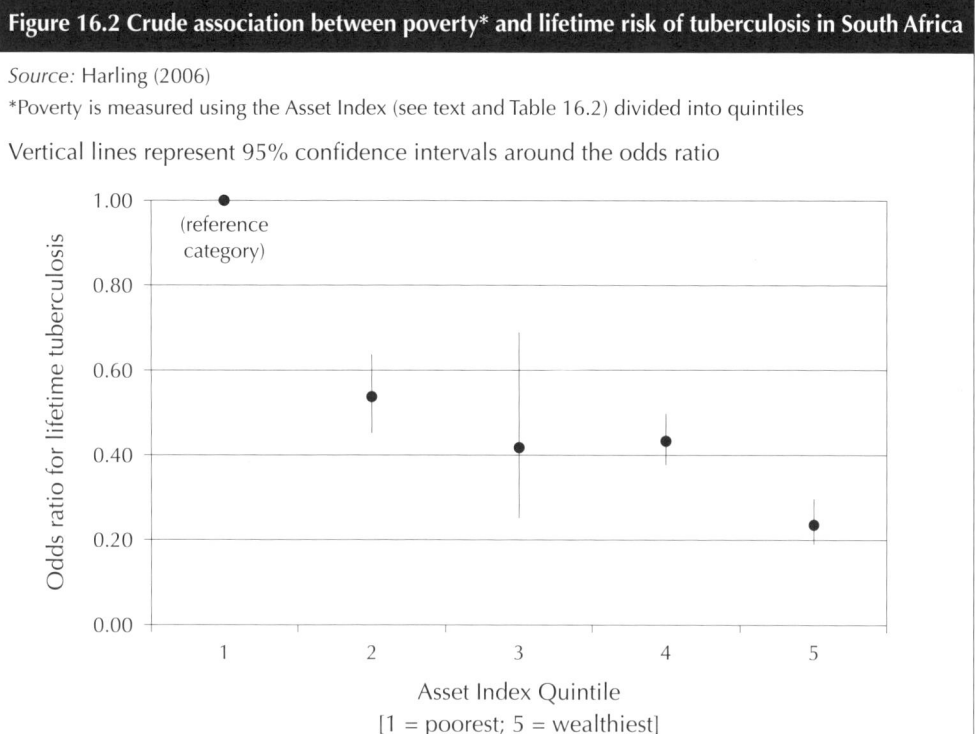

Figure 16.2 Crude association between poverty* and lifetime risk of tuberculosis in South Africa

Source: Harling (2006)
*Poverty is measured using the Asset Index (see text and Table 16.2) divided into quintiles

Vertical lines represent 95% confidence intervals around the odds ratio

sociological mechanisms through which poverty may influence health include patterns of crime in a community which may affect both physical and mental health. Smoking, drinking and sexual activity are prominent behavioural risk factors influenced by poverty, while under- or poor nutrition can be regarded as a biological mechanism.

These pathways are linked and overlap. For example, in the case of tuberculosis, poverty increases the risk of this disease through a number of pathways, including overcrowded housing (increasing the chances of exposure to *Mycobacterium tuberculosis*), poor nutrition (decreasing the ability of the human host to mount an effective immune response once infection has taken place), and reduced access to health services (preventing infected individuals from receiving timely care).

Measuring socioeconomic position

One of the important questions in social epidemiological research is how to measure those aspects of poverty, as well as other social and economic conditions, that are important determinants of health. This question arises whether focusing on poverty as the 'exposure' of interest or carrying out studies in which socioeconomic status may represent a confounding variable for some other risk factor of interest.

Social scientists use the term *socioeconomic status* to refer to the sum of social and economic factors that reflect an individual's position within society. Individuals of low socioeconomic status have fewer social and economic resources that they can draw on to maximise their health, while individuals of higher socioeconomic status have greater access to such resources.

> ### An approach to measuring socioeconomic status
>
> There are several different ways to measure socioeconomic status. The most common approach is by measuring an individual's income, educational level and occupation. In developing a questionnaire, researchers may measure *income* by asking participants how much they or their household earn during a certain time period (for instance, each month or year), or how much money their household spends in a given time period. Measuring *educational level* can be achieved by asking participants about the highest grade they completed at school or their highest tertiary qualification. Questions about *occupation* should begin with asking whether the participant is working, and if so what kind of work they do. Frequently, researchers use this information to create employment categories based on the degree of education and skill required (such as professional versus skilled manual versus unskilled manual labour). Occupation is the specific focus of measures of *social class*, which is a related measure of socioeconomic status.

Socioeconomic status is a widely used concept, and questions regarding income, education and occupation are standard in most research studies. However, in South Africa and other developing countries, using these measures may be problematic, for example in informal settlements and rural areas. Income and expenditure, whether measured for individuals or at a household level, may be inadequate as measures of access to resources where there is trade of resources such as sharing of food and income between families and neighbours. Similarly, education may be an imprecise measure of socioeconomic status in South Africa, where the historical underdevelopment of schools means that relatively few older adults received post-primary schooling.

Given these problems, researchers have developed additional approaches to measuring wealth and poverty in developing countries. Perhaps the most common approach is to ask questions regarding access to services (such as electricity, water and sanitation) and ownership of material goods (such as telephones, cars, or televisions), which may reflect relative wealth within a community

These types of measures can be combined into a composite *asset index* which can then be divided into quintiles (fifths), with the lowest quintile representing the poorest 20% of the population and the highest quintile representing the wealthiest 20%. The asset index has been applied successfully in South Africa to measure poverty and wealth for analysis in health research (for example, in Table 16.2) (Booysen, 2001).

In conclusion, the measurement of socioeconomic status is highly context-specific, and may need to be adapted for research in different populations. For example, the most appropriate measures of socioeconomic status in a rural community may be very different from those used in an urban community, and researchers working in these different settings need to find different ways to measure socioeconomic status.

Social networks and health

A separate area of social epidemiology focuses on how *social networks* influence morbidity and mortality. In different situations, social networks may have positive or negative influences on health. For infectious diseases, social or sexual contacts are an important way of transmitting disease, and in these cases having extensive social networks may be detrimental to health. For non-communicable health conditions, such as mental illness or cardiovascular disease, having strong social support may play an important role in disease prevention

Table 16. 2 Domains used to construct an asset index to measure socioeconomic position in the *South African Demographic and Health Survey, 1998*, with distribution of resources for the poorest 40% and wealthiest 20% of respondents*

Source: Booysen (2001)

Domain	Responses	Distribution for Poorest 40%	Distribution for Wealthiest 20%
Source of drinking water	Piped water in home	3%	96%
	Piped water on site, outside home	16%	2%
	Piped water from public tap	40%	0%
	Surface water from dam or spring or stream	29%	0%
Type of toilet facility	Flush toilet	3%	99%
	Pit latrine	55%	0%
	No toilet facility	29%	0%
Fuels used for cooking and/or heating	Electricity	4%	99%
	Gas	4%	10%
	Paraffin or kerosene	55%	2%
	Wood	58%	1%
Mean number of household members per room in home used for sleeping		2.47	1.65
Main material of floor	Earth floor	40%	0%
	Cement floor	42%	3%
	Vinyl floor	11%	11%
	Carpet floor	5%	55%
Main material of walls	Mud	37%	0%
	Mud & cement	16%	1%
	Corrugated iron	13%	0%
	Plastered walls	15%	94%
Affordability of food	Often goes hungry	19%	1%
	Sometimes goes hungry	50%	3%
	Never goes hungry	25%	95%
Household and individual ownership of specific assets	Electricity in home	18%	100%
	Sheep or cattle	20%	2%
	Car	3%	80%
	Telephone	1%	91%
	Television	18%	98%
	Refrigerator	6%	100%

* Distributions are presented as the percent of households meeting the criterion, with the exception of household members per room in home used for sleeping, which is presented as a mean.

and treatment, for example, in assisting with treatment adherence or maintaining healthy behaviours.

A number of cohort studies conducted in Europe and North America have demonstrated that in older populations where chronic conditions are the dominant cause of disease, individuals with increased social support have lower mortality over long periods of follow-up compared to individuals who are more socially isolated. These associations have been attributed to the ability to get access to material resources and psychological support that comes with stronger social networks. Related to this, there is growing interest in *social capital*, the sum of community social and economic resources which individuals can draw on. There are many ways of measuring social capital, for example through questions about social trust (trusting other people in the community) and participation in community groups, such as churches, *stokvels*, trade unions, sports and youth activities, or civic groups.

Race as a variable in epidemiological studies

Epidemiological studies, both internationally and in South Africa, frequently present or analyse information by 'race'. A consistent feature of such data is the large and enduring inequalities in health outcomes between populations defined by racial categories, although the categories used vary from country to country. In South Africa, where the political and economic system was built on racial stratification and discrimination, it is not surprising that such differences are apparent. However, despite the 'everyday' nature of such observations of difference, the concept of race as a scientific entity is highly contested and the interpretation of such differences a matter of ongoing controversy.

The notion that there are fixed biological entities corresponding to our social definitions of race has been largely discredited on scientific grounds. In evolutionary terms, the single human species shows a wide diversity in appearance, mainly of a superficial nature, reflecting adaptation to different climatic and other conditions through migration and isolation over tens of thousands of years. In modern times, various race classifications have emerged in different settings, and the shifting nature of such classification over time – with political changes, migration and population mixing - demonstrates its dependence of social forces. Population genetic studies are in general agreement that each of the major human 'races' based on continental ancestry (traditionally African, European and Asian) contain within them almost as much genetic diversity as the human population as a whole (Long, 2004). Differences in genetic markers that can be used to predict an individual's group membership or ancestry (which are not necessarily functional genes) make up a relatively small percentage of genetic variability between groups.

On the other hand, race as a way of dividing society politically, socially and economically is deeply entrenched in the modern world. Countries such as South Africa and the United States are dramatic examples of this, but social inequalities according to race can be found in many countries. Almost all the social determinants of health outcomes described in this chapter are correlated with race, particularly socioeconomic status in all of its manifestations. Race is in this sense a proxy for or confounded by these other variables. However, the relationship goes beyond correlation. Race is also 'upstream' to these variables, in that ascribed racial category influences access to resources such as education and jobs and is therefore to a large extent a determinant of social position.

Despite the importance of race as social variable, there is still a strong tendency within the biomedical sciences to view differences in common diseases between races as attributable mainly to fixed genetic inheritance rather than modifiable factors (Williams, 1997). In reaction to this tendency, some researchers have argued that race should as a rule not be used as a category to collect data or describe population health differences in South Africa, as this practice reinforces the 'fixed biology' view and perpetuates a racialised view of the world (Ellison et al, 1997). These authors argued that there are relatively few situations where the use of race categorisation could be justified, and that such justification should be made explicit by the researcher.

However, in South Africa official health data and data in influential national surveys continue to be collected by race, based on South Africa's particular historical four category 'population group' classification into 'blacks', 'whites', 'coloureds' and 'Asians' (or Indians). The generally held justification is that this is an efficient and politically important way to monitor the persistence or reduction of socially generated inequalities in health in South Africa. Along these lines, some researchers have argued not only for the continued collection of data by race but also for the investigation of racist or racialised aspects of society responsible for such differences. For example, in the US context Jones (2001) has postulated three race-linked mechanisms which could lead to ill health and which should be the subject of research: institutionalised racism (e.g. limitation of job opportunity), personally-mediated racism (e.g. belief by others that one is not up to some task, not necessarily explicitly expressed) and internalised racism (acceptance of negative messages about oneself).

Race is therefore still frequently measured in epidemiology, e.g. from records or self-report, and analysed as a descriptive or predictive variable. Kaufman and Cooper (2001) have proposed a classification of the types of study question for which the use of race is likely to lead to interpretations with 'high potential validity' as opposed to those which are likely to have 'low potential validity'. Their schema is summarised in Table 16.3.

Collection of data by race in order to reflect social inequalities as described above consequently has high potential validity in the Kaufman and Cooper schema. Other usages with high potential validity are the use of race as a marker of or proxy for confounding differences between groups (without necessarily understanding what all these differences are), and investigation of race-linked differences in how a given medical condition is managed or treated. By contrast, use of observational studies of race differences to infer a genetic cause for disease or to statistically estimate the proportion owing to 'genetic' versus 'environmental' causes is likely to be of low potential validity. In this regard, studies of disease outcome in people with and without specific genetic markers would have greater potential validity as a means of testing genetic hypotheses.

In summary, race has a potentially useful role to play in understanding the factors underlying disease causation in a society as well as monitoring the effectiveness of social progress in reducing inequalities. However, researchers should define how they measured race in their study and consider the function it serves as a variable in the analysis. Where social variables are postulated to 'mediate' the effect of race, an attempt should be made to measure such variables directly.

Ethnicity

Ethnicity typically describes aspects of group identity beyond appearance such as regional or national affiliation, language and religion. The term 'race or ethnicity' has entered into common use, indicating both the overlap between and the difficulty in defining these concepts. Ethnicity plays a similar role in epidemiology to that of race,

Table 16.3. General guidelines for use of race in observational research

Source: Adapted from Kaufman & Cooper (2001)

Research approach	Example question	Potential validity
Describing inequalities between groups	Are death rates from stroke higher among black women than white women?	High
Effect of race is external to the study participant	Are pregnant black and white women with comparable clinical presentation equally likely to have a caesarian section?	High
Statistical adjustment for race in estimating effect of another variable of interest	What is the association between lead absorption and educational attainment of children after adjusting for race and other potential confounders?	High
Effect of race is internal to the study participant	Is higher eczema incidence among white children relative to black children due to genetic components of race?	Low
'Decomposing effects' i.e. to separate the 'direct' (biological) effects of race from 'indirect' effects via social variables.	What percent of excess risk of hypertension among blacks compared to whites is due to modifiable social factors versus fixed genetic factors?	Low

in that many health inequalities occur between groups that are ethnically defined and such differences are often ascribed to some stable difference between groups, although in this case 'culture' rather than biology. However, as with race, the definition and measurement of ethnicity and the purpose of its measurement in the study need to be explicit. Investigation of cultural factors influencing disease outcomes such as, for example, infant feeding, diet and social norms should be directly studied by developing appropriate measurement tools.

Conclusion

While the social and economic determinants of health are not the specific focus of many research projects, issues of socioeconomic status and race play a role in much health research in South Africa. In all situations, researchers are challenged to think critically about how social and economic factors affect different health outcomes, and the mechanisms that may be involved. In addition, more research using the methods of social epidemiology is needed in South Africa.

EXAMPLE 16.1

Social networks and management of chronic disease

The role of social networks and support in shaping morbidity and mortality risks is gaining increasing attention in South African health research. A cross-sectional study of individuals attending a diabetes outpatient clinic in Pretoria measured social support using questions investigating whether participants felt that the people in their lives provided emotional support and practical support (e.g. assistance in day-to-day activities).

Health outcomes included self-rated health as well as effective control of blood glucose and blood pressure. A total of 263 individuals participated, most of whom had Type-2 diabetes mellitus. The results show that patients with higher levels of social support had better control of blood pressure and rated their health better than individuals with lower levels of social support. In this case, increased levels of social support are probably related to increased support in maintaining healthy behaviours and adhering to long-term treatment, leading in turn to improved health outcomes.

Reference:

Westaway, MS, Seager, JR, Rheeder, P & Van Zyl, DG. 2005. The effects of social support on health, well-being and management of diabetes mellitus: a black South African perspective. *Ethnicity and Health*, 10(1):73–89.

EXAMPLE 16.2

Racial, social and environmental predictors of childhood diarrhoea

Choi (2003) analysed the reported prevalence of childhood diarrhoea from the 1998 *South African Demographic and Health Survey*. The aim of the study was to identify the social and environmental 'mechanisms' of racial differences in disease prevalence. Diarrhoea was defined as the 'passing of liquid, watery or loose stools' in children under 5 years in the two weeks preceding the survey.

The prevalence of diarrhoea overall was 13%. Prevalence by race was blacks 13.5%, coloureds 9.6%, Asians (Indians) 6.7% and whites 1.8%. A number of social and environmental factors were associated with diarrhoea: residence in Mpumalanga or KwaZulu-Natal provinces; residence in a non-urban area; having drinking water sources other than piped or bottled water; toilet facilities other than flush; earth, sand or dung floor in the dwelling; maternal education < 8 years; and lower household wealth.

The author undertook a multiple logistic regression analysis which included race and the above variables, as well as others such as age and sex of the child. The difference between coloureds and blacks disappeared in the model, but the large difference between these groups and whites and Asians persisted even after taking these other factors into account. The author concluded that there may have been a number of other variables relevant to diarrhoea not accounted for in the study, such as storage of food and water, domestic practices in relation to child feeding and defecation, or recall differences in reporting diarrhoea. This 'residual effect' of race after adjusting for potential environmental and social confounders is a common finding in such analyses. This reflects the difficulty of accurately measuring or even identifying these confounders and the complex pathways through which race influences health in a racially stratified society.

Reference:

Choi, SYP. 2003. Mechanisms of racial inequalities in prevalence of diarrhoea in South Africa. *Journal of Health, Population and Nutrition*, 21:264–72.

Useful readings

Berkman, LF & Kawachi, I (eds). 2000. *Social epidemiology*. New York: Oxford University Press.

Marmot, M. 1999. *The social determinants of health*. New York: Oxford University Press.

Myer, L, Ehrlich, R & Susser, ES. 2004. Social epidemiology in South Africa. *Epidemiology Reviews*, 26:112-23.

Useful web sites

Is race real? 2005. A web forum organised by the Social Science Research Council. [Online]. Available: http://raceandgenomics.ssrc.org. [25 February 2007].

MacArthur Foundation Network on Socioeconomic Status and Health. [Online]. Available: http://www.macses.ucsf.edu/. [25 February 2007].

Socioeconomic Determinants of Health: BMJ.com Collection. [Online]. Available: http://bmj.bmjjournals.com/cgi/collection/socioeconomic_determinants_of_health. [25 February 2007].

WHO Commission on the Social Determinants of Health. [Online]. Available: http://www.who.int/social_determinants/en/. [25 February 2007].

References used in this chapter

Booysen, F. 2001. In Bradshaw, D & Steyn, K (eds). *Poverty and chronic diseases in South Africa*. Cape Town: South African Medical Research Council. 15–38.

Ellison, GTH, de Wet, T, IJsselmuiden, CB & Richter, LM. 1997. Desegregating health statistics and health research in South Africa. *South African Medical Journal*, 86(10):1257–62.

Harling, G. 2006. *The social epidemiology of tuberculosis in South Africa: a multilevel analysis*. Unpublished thesis, Master of Public Health. University of Cape Town: Faculty of Health Sciences.

Jones, CM. 2001. Invited commentary: race, racism and the practice of epidemiology. *American Journal of Epidemiology*, 154: 299–304.

Kark, SL. 1949. The social pathology of syphilis in Africans. *South African Medical Journal*, 23:77–84.

Kaufman, JS & Cooper, RS. 2001. Commentary: considerations for the use of racial/ethnic classification in etiologic research. *American Journal of Epidemiology*, 154:291-8.

Long, JC. 2004. Race and genetics in medicine. In Singer, E & Antonnuci, TC (eds). *Proceedings of the conference on genetics and health disparities*. Survey Research Center, Insititute for Social Research, University of Michigan. 11–22.

Williams, D. 1997. Race and health: basic questions, emerging directions. *Annual of Epidemiology*, 7:322–33.

Wyndham, C. 1981. The loss from premature deaths of economically active manpower in the various populations of the RSA. Part I. Leading causes of death: health strategies for reducing mortality. *South African Medical Journal*, 60:411–19.

Wyndham, C & Irwig, L. 1979. A comparison of the mortality rates of various population groups of the Republic of South Africa. *South African Medical Journal*, 55:796–802.

Yach, D. 1988. The impact of political violence on health and health services in Cape Town, South Africa, 1986: methodological problems and preliminary results. *American Journal of Public Health*, 78:772–6.

17

Infectious disease epidemiology

David Coetzee

> **OBJECTIVES OF THIS CHAPTER**
>
> The objectives of this chapter are:
> - to describe the terminology and concepts specific to infectious disease epidemiology
> - to explain how infectious disease occurrence and transmission dynamics are measured
> - to illustrate how various epidemiological study designs can be used to answer questions about infectious disease.

Introduction

Epidemics of infectious diseases have occurred for centuries. Many of the principles of epidemiology have been developed from the investigation of outbreaks of infectious diseases (see Chapter 18). In large areas of the world and particularly the developing world infectious diseases remain endemic and are a major cause of morbidity and mortality. In order to control these diseases we need knowledge of infectious disease epidemiology.

Key concepts in infectious disease epidemiology

Last (2001) describes an infectious disease as 'an illness due to a specific infectious agent or its toxic products that arises through transmission of that agent or its products from an infected person, animal, or reservoir to a susceptible host, either directly or indirectly through an intermediate plant or host, vector, or the inanimate environment'.

Each infectious agent has a reservoir, a vector, vehicle or source of infection and specific dynamics of exposure and transmission. For example, in pulmonary tuberculosis the agent is *Mycobacterium tuberculosis*, it is spread from person to person, and humans are both the reservoir and the source. Exposure to contacts, mixing patterns between the infectious pool and susceptible hosts, and the degree and duration of infectivity and susceptibility are all factors determining the epidemiology of tuberculosis.

> **Factors unique to infectious disease epidemiology**
>
> There are three factors unique to infectious disease epidemiology.
> - The organisms that cause infectious diseases are *necessary causes* (see Chapter 2). Unlike non-communicable disease, exposure to infection is essential for disease to occur.

- Certain organisms may cause infection in an individual without evidence of disease for months or years (*subclinical infection*). The individual may, however, spread the infection as a *carrier*. HIV is a good example of an agent that causes subclinical infection with carrier status for years before disease occurs.
- *Immunity* may be acquired by exposure to certain organisms or through immunisation with vaccines. Examples of agents that cause solid, lifelong immunity following exposure are measles and poliomyelitis.

An understanding of subclinical infection and of immunity is critical to understanding the epidemiology of infectious diseases.

Causation

The classical epidemiological triangle (or triad) is a useful model of causation in infectious disease epidemiology (Figure 17.1). The organisms that cause infectious diseases are referred to as the *agent* – relevant characteristics include virulence, sensitivity to antibiotics and dose. The *host* is the person with infection or disease. Factors that influence the susceptibility of the host to infection include age, sex, customs, occupation, nutritional or immune status, and leisure and travel activities. The *vector*, *vehicle* or *source* is the means by which the person acquired infection. Factors related to the vector, vehicle or source include abundance of the vector or prevalence of the infectious source.

In direct or person-to-person transmission an infectious person is the source and no vector is involved. The environment is the setting in which the transmission of infection occurs and includes factors such as sanitary conditions, overcrowding and poverty. By contrast, in cerebral malaria the agent is *Plasmodium falciparum*, humans are the host, and the vector is the Anopheles mosquito. The environment would be the external conditions necessary for transmission to occur, such as the temperature and humidity required for the mosquito to survive and proximity of the host to water.

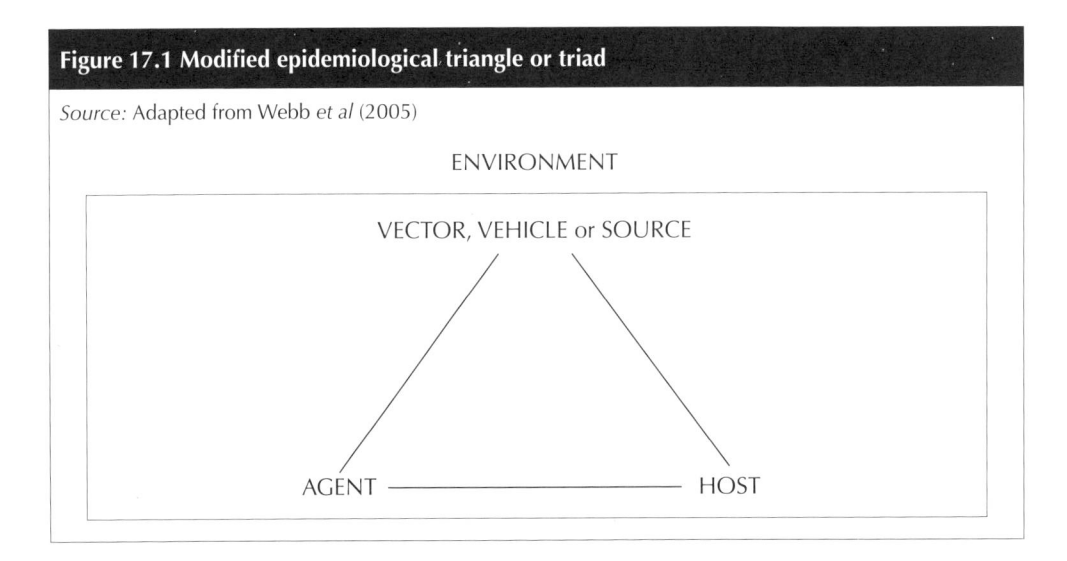

Figure 17.1 Modified epidemiological triangle or triad

Source: Adapted from Webb *et al* (2005)

ENVIRONMENT

VECTOR, VEHICLE or SOURCE

AGENT — HOST

Measuring infectious disease occurrence and transmission

Surveillance of infectious diseases

Much of the surveillance of infectious diseases requires notification by health workers (see Chapter 13). This allows for the collation of information so that epidemics can be identified at the district, provincial and national level. Such surveillance may, however, result in underreporting of cases as less severe cases of disease are not reported to health services. For example, in a measles epidemic many less serious cases of measles may be missed.

In addition the infection may be subclinical, as in the case of HIV. Notification of HIV infection detected by health services would consequently be of little value as the majority of cases remain subclinical for many years. In such a case, active serological surveillance provides a more accurate picture of infection rates of subclinical disease in the community.

Incidence and prevalence

The prevalence of an infectious disease is the product of the incidence and the duration of disease. Many infectious diseases have a short duration and may occur repeatedly, for example diarrhoeal disease. Prevalence is not an important measure in these instances. In the case of infectious agents of a chronic nature, for example hepatitis B, both incidence and prevalence are important measures, with prevalence providing a more accurate measure of risk of infection and the size of the infectious pool. In tuberculosis, each infectious case will infect 10 persons per year and so the prevalence of infectious tuberculosis is central to our understanding of the spread of tuberculosis in the community. Similarly, the seroprevalence of HIV infection in a representative sample of the community provides an accurate measure of the risk of exposure as it is many years before seropositive people show symptoms.

In some epidemics prevalence may be rising, for example when a new treatment is found for an otherwise fatal chronic disease, even as incidence is falling. This is the case with HIV/Aids, where antiretroviral therapy has prolonged life and therefore increased the prevalence of the disease, although the incidence may be decreasing in some populations. Some infectious agents are highly virulent (e.g. the Ebola virus) and result in rapid death in the majority of persons infected. In such instances, the case fatality ratio or probability of dying is high, limiting both the prevalence of potentially infectious cases and the incidence of new cases.

Disease transmission

The *index* or *primary* case is the first case to be identified during an epidemic or outbreak. The persons who are infected by the primary case are called *secondary* cases. The *basic reproductive number*, R_0, is the average number of cases infected by an infectious case during his or her entire infectious period when he or she enters a totally susceptible population. R_0 therefore describes the potential for spread. For example, if R_0 for measles is 15, each primary case of measles will infect 15 secondary cases, who will in turn be infectious.

If R_0 is less than 1, there will be progressively fewer cases of the disease and the disease will eventually disappear. If it is greater than 1, there will be an increasing number of cases, creating an epidemic situation. If R_0 is equal to 1, the number of new cases stabilises and the disease is said to be *endemic*.

D | Epidemiology applied to specific areas

> **More about the basic reproductive number, R_0**
>
> R_0 depends on:
> - The probability of transmission upon contact between an infectious reservoir or source and a susceptible host. For example, the probability of transmission of HIV through a blood transfusion is very high relative to the probability via a single unprotected act of vaginal intercourse.
> - The frequency of contacts and mixing patterns of susceptible persons with the infectious reservoir or vectors of the agent. The frequency of contacts and mixing patterns are the most interesting yet overlooked parts of the determination of the epidemiology of infectious diseases.
> - The length of time transmitters in the infectious pool remain infectious. This is unique to infectious disease epidemiology as the duration of infectivity can be limited by treatment, and is therefore influenced by the recognition of symptoms, health seeking behaviour, quality of care and adherence to treatment.

R_0 can be used to determine the impact of interventions, for example, the impact of a change in risk behaviour such as condom use on the incidence of sexually transmitted diseases, and is the basis of mathematical modelling of infectious disease patterns. Models are important for understanding the population dynamics of transmission of infectious agents and the potential impact of infectious disease control programmes. For example, Hales (2002) used an empirical model to show the potential effect of climatic change on the occurrence of dengue fever. Specifically, he found that climatic change increases the range of the mosquito vector, leading to an increased incidence of the disease. These models are only as good as the assumptions upon which R_0 is based.

Once a particular level of immunity is reached in a population, the probability that an infected person will come into contact with a susceptible person becomes small. If there is random mixing of people within the population, the infected person is more likely to come into contact with immune people. The level of immunity in a population required to prevent epidemics is called *herd immunity* and can be determined from the reproductive number. An example is provided in Table 17.1.

> **Table 17.1 Proportion of persons who should have immunity in order to prevent an epidemic of measles**
>
> There are on average 15 secondary cases for every primary case of measles, so $R_0 = 15$. The level of immunity (p) required in the population to prevent epidemics (herd immunity) presuming random mixing would be:
>
> $$p > 1 - 1/R_0$$
> $$> 1 - 1/15$$
> $$> 0.94$$
>
> i.e. more than 94% of population must be immune in order to prevent epidemics of measles in the population.

Study designs in infectious disease epidemiology

Case reports and case series

As with non-communicable diseases, individual case reports and case series may be used to identify the features of newly identified diseases or to identify factors associated with the acquisition of old diseases that have been rarely seen. These reports may lead to hypotheses about possible causes. For example, Gregg (1941) described a series of cases of congenital cataract and linked them to a large outbreak of rubella six months previously. Through subsequent studies, rubella was established as a cause of congenital cataract.

Descriptive studies (including descriptive cohort or natural history studies)

Descriptive studies of transmission are typically used to identify the natural history of new diseases. The time period from successful infection until the development of infectiousness is referred to as the *latent period*. This is followed by the infectious period when infection can be transmitted to another susceptible host. The *incubation period* is the period between exposure to an infectious agent and the onset of symptoms or signs of infection. For example, studies showed that the latent period for hepatitis B virus (HBV) is relatively short (weeks) compared to the incubation period (months) meaning that HBV transmission can occur long before any signs of disease are apparent. In contrast, the latent period for Severe Acute Respiratory Syndrome (SARS) is longer than the incubation period, implying that if cases of SARS are identified, diagnosed and treated promptly this will reduce the transmission of SARS.

Descriptive cohort studies were also used to determine the natural history of Aids. Medley (1987) followed persons who had acquired HIV through blood transfusions (with known infection dates) and found the incubation period for Aids to be a number of years in most cases.

Hope Simpson (1952), prior to the introduction of a measles vaccine, conducted a descriptive cohort study to measure the infectivity of measles. He identified all children who were exposed to a case of measles and then established how many of these children acquired measles. He found that 80% of children who had not previously had measles and who were exposed to these infectious cases contracted the disease.

Cross-sectional studies

Cross-sectional studies describe the prevalence of infectious disease and identify associated factors, including health service factors. For example Coetzee *et al* (1990) conducted a study in Khayelitsha, Cape Town, to measure childhood disease vaccination coverage and to identify factors associated with coverage. They found that children living in temporary housing had the lowest vaccination coverage.

Although in cross-sectional studies exposure and disease status are measured simultaneously, they can be useful in investigating whether fixed exposures such as genetic make-up or blood group are associated with a particular infection. For example, Glass *et al* (1985) identified in a cross-sectional study that blood group O is associated with more severe disease following infection with cholera. Cross-sectional studies are also typically used in food poisoning outbreaks in order to determine attack rates of diarrhoea or gastroenteritis associated with the consumption of particular foodstuffs (see Chapter 18). Repeated cross-sectional studies on the same population can be used to evaluate the impact of interventions. In this way the annual antenatal seroprevalence studies in South Africa enable us to judge whether preventive measures have had any impact on the Aids epidemic.

Ecological studies

Comparing exposures and infection across entire populations can be used to generate hypotheses on causation. An ecological study design by Bongaarts *et al* (1989) used a database containing information at the population level on rates of circumcision and on HIV seroprevalence in 37 countries in Africa. The correlation between the proportion of uncircumcised males and HIV seroprevalence was high ($r = 0.9$; $p < 0.001$). It was the first study to suggest that circumcision may be associated with HIV transmission. However, the lack of data at the individual level meant that this study could not control for confounders such as the association of religion with both sexual behaviour and circumcision.

Case-control studies

Case-control studies are commonly used in the investigation of disease outbreaks (see Chapter 18). A case-control design is often used for large scale outbreaks when it is not possible to define or to study all people at risk of becoming a case. In this instance, a sample of cases is compared with a sample of controls.

Case-control studies can also be used to identify factors associated with infectious disease. Moodley *et al* (1999) conducted a case-control study to identify risk factors for meningococcal disease in Cape Town. They found that children with meningococcal disease were more likely to have been breast-fed for less than three months (odds ratio = 2.7; 95% confidence interval (CI) 1.5–5.0) and to have lived in overcrowded conditions (odds ratio = 2.8; 95% CI 1.5–5.5) than the children who did not have the disease.

Cohort studies

Cohort studies which start with uninfected people can identify factors associated with subsequent infection. Alternatively, infected people can be followed up over time to identify factors associated with complications of the disease or with survival.

For example, cohorts of families with and without an HIV infected member were followed to identify factors associated with HIV transmission, and were able to demonstrate that HIV was not transmitted via even close contact in the absence of blood, tissue or mucosal exposure. Saracco *et al* (1993) followed a cohort of serodiscordant couples (i.e. in which only one member is HIV positive) and recorded condom use. They showed that the consistent and correct use of condoms prevented HIV transmission from men to women (relative risk = 0.2; 95% CI 0.1–0.5).

Table 17.2 Efficacy of measles vaccine at 9 months of age

If there are 94 cases of measles per 100 children in the unvaccinated group of a vaccination trial of children vaccinated at 9 months of age, and 14 cases per 100 in the vaccinated group, the vaccine efficacy would be:

$$\text{Vaccine efficacy (VE)} = \frac{(\text{incidence in unvaccinated} - \text{incidence in vaccinated}) \times 100}{\text{incidence in unvaccinated}}$$

$$= \frac{(94 - 14) \times 100}{94}$$

$$= 85\%$$

This means the vaccine will prevent disease in 85% of those who are vaccinated at 9 months of age. It is important to note that if vaccination coverage is 80% then only 85% of this 80% (or 68% overall) of children vaccinated will be protected.

Randomised controlled trials

Randomised controlled trials (RCTs) are used to assess new interventions, including new vaccines, treatments or prevention strategies for infectious diseases. An example of an RCT is provided in Example 17.2 below. The efficacy of many vaccines has been evaluated by means of RCTs. *Vaccine efficacy* is the percentage reduction in the incidence of disease as a result of vaccination (Table 17.2).

Vaccine effectiveness, on the other hand, is a measure of the overall effect of vaccination programmes and incorporates both the direct and indirect effects of vaccination. Vaccine effectiveness is usually determined through observational studies but can also be assessed through surveillance of disease.

> ### EXAMPLE 17.1
>
> **A cross-sectional study to determine age-specific occurrence rates of measles in urban, peri-urban and rural areas of KwaZulu-Natal**
>
> A community survey was conducted in KwaZulu-Natal in urban, peri-urban and rural areas to determine the relationship between population density and the occurrence of measles in children under 8 months of age, as mortality from measles is high in infancy. The results showed that in urban areas 45% of children acquired measles before 8 months of age, compared to 15% in peri-urban areas and 10% in rural areas. The percentage diminished as population density decreased. It was concluded that the serious overcrowding which is a feature of populations migrating from rural to urban areas in developing countries may be responsible for the early spread of the disease. Furthermore, if measles vaccination programmes are to be successful, effective immunisation under 8 months of age is required.
>
> *Reference:*
>
> Loening, WEK & Coovadia, HM. 1983. Age-specific occurrence rates of measles in urban, peri-urban, and rural environments: implications for time of vaccination. *Lancet*, 345:324–6.

> ### EXAMPLE 17.2
>
> **A randomised controlled trial of Vitamin A supplementation in children with severe measles**
>
> A randomised double-blind controlled trial was conducted in 1987 at the City Hospital for Infectious Diseases in Cape Town to determine the effect of vitamin A supplementation on measles morbidity and mortality in 187 children hospitalised with severe measles. The children were randomised to receive either vitamin A or placebo. As compared with the placebo group, the children who received vitamin A recovered more rapidly from pneumonia and diarrhoea and had less croup. In the group treated with vitamin A, the risk of death was half that of the control group (relative risk = 0.51; 95% CI 0.35–0.74). The researchers concluded that vitamin A supplementation reduced morbidity and mortality in children with severe measles.
>
> *Reference:*
>
> Hussey, GD & Klein, M. 1990. A randomized, controlled trial of vitamin A in children with severe measles. *New England Journal of Medicine*, 323:160–4.

Useful readings

Giesecke, J. 2002. *Modern infectious disease epidemiology*. London: Arnold.

Kenrad, E & Nelson, MD. 2004. *Infectious disease epidemiology*. New York: Jones and Bartlett Publishers.

Useful web sites

Centers for Disease Control and Prevention, USA: regular updates on endemic infectious diseases as well as epidemics and outbreaks worldwide. Includes training and technical reports on infectious disease epidemiology. [Online]. Available: http://www.cdc.gov/. [25 February 2007].

National Institute for Communicable Diseases: regular updates on epidemiology of infectious diseases in Southern Africa. [Online]. Available: http://www.nicd.ac.za/. [25 February 2007].

World Health Organization: regular updates on endemic infectious diseases as well as epidemics and outbreaks worldwide. [Online]. Available: http://www.who.int/. [25 February 2007].

References used in this chapter

Bongaarts, J, Reining, P, Way, P & Conant, F. 1989. The relationship between male circumcision and HIV infection in African populations. *AIDS*, 3:373–6.

Coetzee, N, Yach, D, Blignaut, R & Fisher, SA. 1990. Measles vaccination coverage and its determinants in a rapidly growing peri-urban area. *South African Medical Journal*, 78:733–7.

Glass, R, Hulmgren, N, Haley, CE, Khan, MR, Svennerholm, A, Stoll, BJ, Belayet Hossain, KM, Black, RE, Yunus, E & Barua, D. 1985. Predisposition for cholera of individuals with O blood group possible evolutionary significance. *American Journal of Epidemiology*, 121:791–6.

Gregg, NM. 1941. Congenital cataract following German measles in the mother. *Transactions of the Ophthalmological Society of Australia*, 19:267–76.

Hales, S, de Wet, N, Maindonald, J & Woodward A. 2002. Potential effect of population and climatic changes on global distribution of dengue fever: an empiric model. *Lancet*, 360:830–4.

Hope Simpson, RE. 1952. Infectiousness of communicable diseases in the household (measles, chickenpox and mumps). *Lancet*, 2:549–54.

Last, JM. 2001. *A dictionary of epidemiology*. New York: Oxford University Press.

Medley, GF, Anderson, RM, Cox, DR & Billard, L. 1987. Incubation period of Aids in patients infected via blood transfusions. *Nature*, 328:719–21.

Moodley, JR, Coetzee, N & Hussey, G. 1999. Risk factors for meningococcal disease in Cape Town. *South African Medical Journal*, 89:56–9.

Saracco, A, Musicco, M, Nicolosi, A, Angarano, G, Arici, C, Gavazzeni, G, Costigliola, P, Gafa, S, Gervasoni, C & Luzzati, R. 1993 Man-to-woman sexual transmission of HIV: longitudinal study of 343 steady partners of infected men. *Journal of Acquired Immune Deficiency Syndrome*, 6:497–502.

Webb, P, Bain, C & Pirozzo, S. 2005. *Essential epidemiology. An introduction for students and health professionals*. Cambridge: Cambridge University Press.

18

Outbreak investigation

David Coetzee Carol Metcalf Nicol Coetzee

> **OBJECTIVES OF THIS CHAPTER**
>
> The objectives of this chapter are:
> - to describe the purpose of outbreak investigation
> - to explain the terminology used in outbreak investigation
> - to set out in detail the steps involved in outbreak investigation.

Introduction

The development of epidemiology is intimately linked with the investigation of disease outbreaks. Outbreaks and epidemics are part of the human record and literature is full of narratives set against the background of infectious disease epidemics such as influenza, small pox and the plague. John Snow, an English physician, conducted one of the first outbreak investigations, of a cholera outbreak in London in 1854, before the microbiological cause of cholera was known. Agents other than infectious organisms may cause disease outbreaks, for example, episodes of organophosphate poisoning in farm workers exposed to pesticides. These should be investigated in the same way as outbreaks of infectious diseases.

Essential terminology in outbreak epidemiology

Disease outbreaks are investigated because someone has noticed either the appearance of a new disease or an increase in the incidence of an old disease in excess of what would normally be expected. An *epidemic* is the occurrence of cases of disease in a community or region at a level that is clearly in excess of the background incidence of disease for this defined group during a particular season and time period. (Season is included, as many infectious diseases show seasonal variation in incidence rates, e.g. seasonal malaria in summer or influenza in winter.) An *outbreak* generally refers to a localised increase in the incidence of disease in which two or more cases are epidemiologically linked in some way. An outbreak is usually of shorter duration than an epidemic, and is localised within a geographical area.

The term *endemic* is used to describe the presence of a level of disease that is constant in the population. For example malaria may be described as endemic in an area where the incidence rate is constant over a number of years, but after heavy rains there may be more cases than usual and this can be described as an epidemic in an endemic area.

> A *cluster* in outbreak epidemiology refers to a group of cases of disease, believed or perceived to be greater than expected, that are associated in time and space. A cluster should be investigated in the same way as an outbreak. (Note that 'cluster sampling' has a different meaning – see Chapter 8.)

Deviation from the normal is the basis of disease outbreak investigations. In order to implement interventions that will control and prevent further disease, we need to identify factors that are associated with the source or cause of the outbreak. The investigation may uncover new risk factors for known diseases or even discover new diseases. Outbreak investigations should lead to better understanding of the reasons that control programmes such as vaccination have failed, and should inform public health policy.

The mode of transmission of the agent and the source or reservoir of the agent are the two key factors we should consider in an outbreak investigation. Exposure to the source may be continuous and require urgent identification and elimination. Alternatively, the exposure may be recurrent (for example, contamination of the water supply during heavy rains).

Any increase over the expected number of cases of a disease should be investigated. In outbreaks of diseases with high morbidity and/or mortality (for example, viral haemorrhagic fever or certain types of pesticide poisoning), one or two cases are enough to require a rigorous outbreak investigation.

In order to achieve the above aims a systematic problem orientated approach to outbreak investigations is advocated and presented in Table 18.1. It should be noted that in practice the investigation carries a sense of urgency, and steps are often undertaken concurrently and repeated as more information becomes available.

Table 18.1 Steps involved in outbreak investigation

- Confirm that an outbreak has occurred and prepare for field work
- Establish a case definition
- Describe the outbreak
- Generate an hypothesis
- Test the hypothesis
- Implement control measures

Steps in outbreak investigation

1. Confirm that an outbreak has occurred and prepare for field work

Outbreaks of diseases can be recognised in a number of ways. There is a statutory obligation for health workers to notify certain conditions to health authorities (so-called notifiable diseases, e.g. measles – see Chapter 13). Notification depends on the uniform and timely filling in of forms and communication of urgent information to the relevant authority. The review of routinely collected clinical and laboratory surveillance data may also identify outbreaks. For example, in 1981 an epidemiologist in the United States noted from the surveillance systems in place an increase in the number of cases of atypical pneumonia (*Pneumocystis carinii*). He noted further that these cases were in young homosexual men from a number of large cities, and much less common in the general population. Investigations led to the identification by health authorities of a new disease, later called Aids.

Confirmation of an outbreak, and steps to be taken immediately

It is important to confirm the existence of an outbreak. Are there more cases than would normally be expected in the particular area and season? Initial reports may be unreliable. Apparent increases may be due to increased clinical awareness with improved case detection, changes in the diagnostic criteria, improved reporting or changes in population size or composition. For example, if a less specific diagnostic test is introduced in an area, one may see an outbreak of that particular disease, as there will be more false positive cases. All available evidence should be used to confirm that an epidemic has in fact occurred. Validating the diagnostic criteria used for case identification is a key step in this process.

Once the outbreak is confirmed, a multi-disciplinary team should be constituted and responsibilities assigned. The team should try to include field epidemiologists, medical microbiologists, infectious disease clinicians, public health specialists and environmental health officers, and other local health service personnel. Regular progress meetings should be held. It is important to have good communications with the affected community as well as the media, as outbreaks may be reported sensationally in the press, creating unnecessary alarm.

2. Establish a case definition

In all outbreaks a case definition should be formulated. A case definition ensures that there is uniformity in the identification and counting of all cases. The case definition should be as sensitive and specific as possible while being easy to apply. In order to establish a case definition, it is important to look for all cases, as the first cases identified may not be representative of all cases. This is because known cases may be only a fraction of the total, and may differ from other cases in important attributes, which could misdirect the course of the investigation. For example, initial reports may be from hospitals, but there may be many less severe cases in the community. All sources of information should be examined, including clinic attendance records, general practice records, school absenteeism records, disease notification and death records. This will also involve taking good clinical histories, including travel and leisure histories from affected people, examining patients, and obtaining relevant laboratory test results.

Depending on the cause of the outbreak the case definition may be broad or strict. Broad or lenient definitions will have greater *sensitivity* but lower *specificity* (see Chapter 9 for definitions of these terms). A broad clinical case definition usually includes clearly defined symptoms and signs, e.g. more than three watery stools in 24 hours following a particular function where food was served, or diarrhoea and abdominal pain with fever greater than 38.5 °C in a resident of town X. This type of broad case definition will identify all potential cases but include many that are not truly cases. As more information is obtained, a more specific case definition may be used. A strict definition could be based on specific laboratory confirmation, e.g. evidence of typhoid in the blood confirmed on microbiological culture. Although this will reduce false positives, such specificity is often not warranted, as the additional burden and costs of collecting specimens and testing may be high. For serious life-threatening diseases there is greater emphasis on a sensitive rather than a specific case definition. In many outbreaks the initial cases may have the diagnosis confirmed by laboratory testing, with subsequent cases defined using a clinical definition. A system of classification into 'probable' and 'confirmed' cases is often used.

Investigators should consult published material and clinical and epidemiological texts once a presumptive diagnosis of early cases has been made, including reviews of the clinical condition, basic epidemiology of the condition being considered, and accounts of similar outbreak investigations. A thorough understanding of the epidemiology of the disease helps investigators to ask relevant questions and conduct appropriate and relevant environmental and laboratory investigations, based on the most likely sources and modes of spread.

3. Describe the outbreak

As active case-finding proceeds the investigators should produce a detailed description of all cases or a representative sample of cases. This involves describing the cases according to person, time, and place. This summary of cases is useful for defining who is at risk of contracting disease, as well as formulating hypotheses as to the likely sources of exposure and modes of transmission of the disease.

Person

Cases should be summarised on key factors such as age, sex, occupation, ethnicity, socioeconomic status, and immunisation status (as well as other relevant disease-specific exposures). For example, a population pyramid of cases may yield valuable information.

Figure 18.1 shows that women aged 16 to 40 years and boys and girls younger than 5 years of age were at risk of diarrhoea in this outbreak. This epidemic may be related to commercially available processed infant feeds. If, for example, mothers taste the feed before giving it to their babies, this would explain why only women of childbearing age and young children of both sexes are affected.

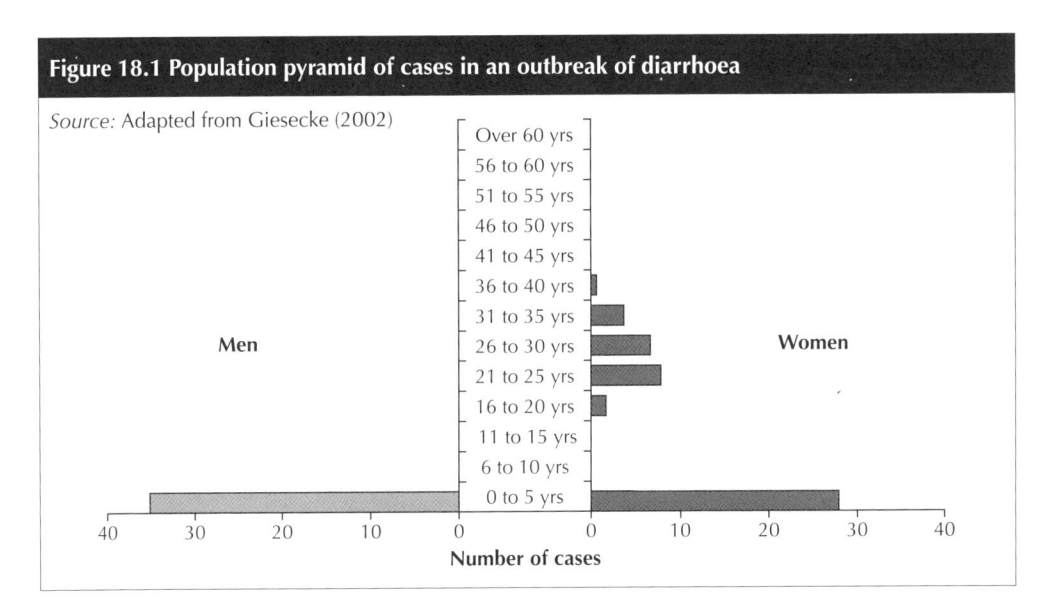

Figure 18.1 Population pyramid of cases in an outbreak of diarrhoea

Source: Adapted from Giesecke (2002)

Time

The time course of the epidemic should be studied by drawing an *epidemic curve*, that is, a histogram with the date on which each case occurred plotted on the X axis and the number of cases plotted on the Y axis. The shape of the epidemic curve is useful in determining the nature of the source of infection, patterns of spread, the magnitude of the epidemic, outliers, time trends and exposure or the incubation period. The *incubation period* is the period between exposure to an infectious agent and the onset of symptoms or signs of infection. The shape of the epidemic curve may therefore provide evidence of the type of epidemic. The *primary case* is the first case to be identified during an epidemic or outbreak. The persons who are infected by the primary case are called *secondary cases*.

A *common source* epidemic may be limited to one point in time or be continuous. A common exposure at a single point in time ('point source' epidemic) results in an epidemic curve with a steep upward curve with a well-defined peak and a relatively short time course (Figure 18.2). The first case occurred on the 4th day of the month, the highest incidence was on the 10th day and the last case was on the 14th of the month, with no further cases. This pattern is typically seen when drinking water is contaminated for a short period of time, e.g. in a cholera or typhoid outbreak.

Figure 18.2 Example of an epidemic curve of a point source outbreak

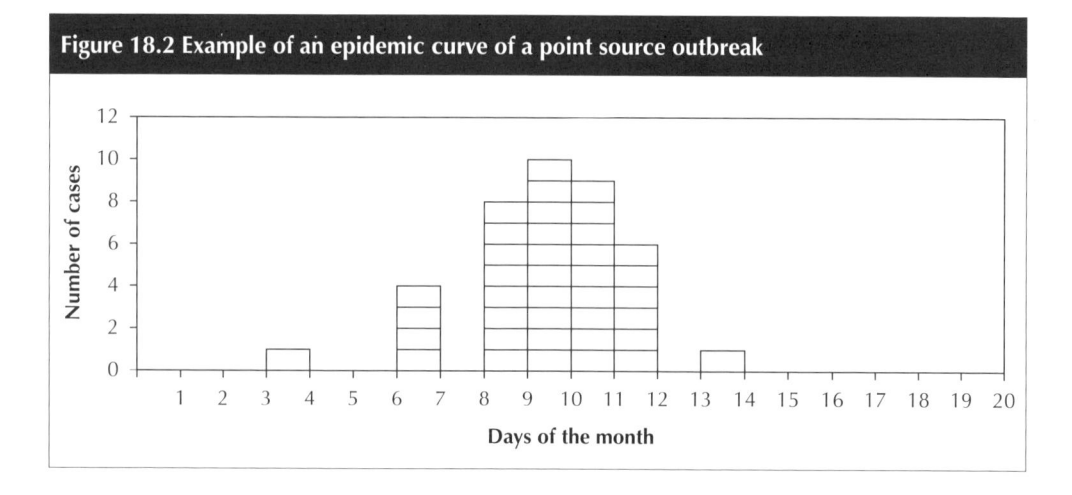

A common exposure may lead to a 'continuous common source' epidemic if individuals continue to be exposed. There is a steep rise with the first exposure but there is little or no sustained decline as individuals are continually exposed (Figure 18.3). This pattern is typically seen if there is ongoing exposure to contaminated water.

Figure 18.3 Example of a common source outbreak

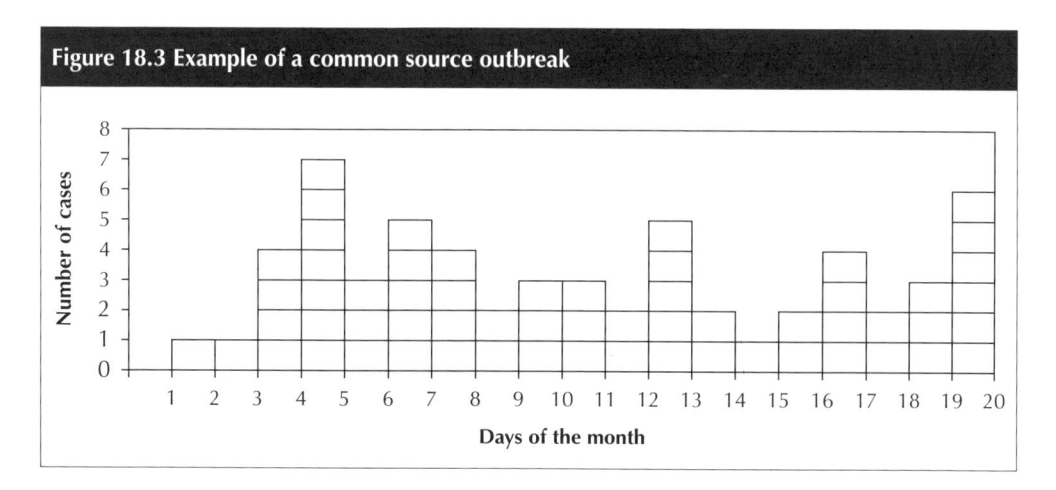

D | Epidemiology applied to specific areas

In contrast to the above, exposures occurring over a period of time causing conditions which are readily spread from person to person are characterised by successive waves of cases, roughly one serial period (often the incubation period) apart, occurring over a protracted period of time (Figure 18.4). These are called *propagated outbreaks*. The first case on the first day probably infected the group of people who fell ill from the 6th day, and they in turn infected the group who fell ill around the 14th day of the month. Propagated epidemics may last longer than common source epidemics. This pattern is typically seen with measles epidemics.

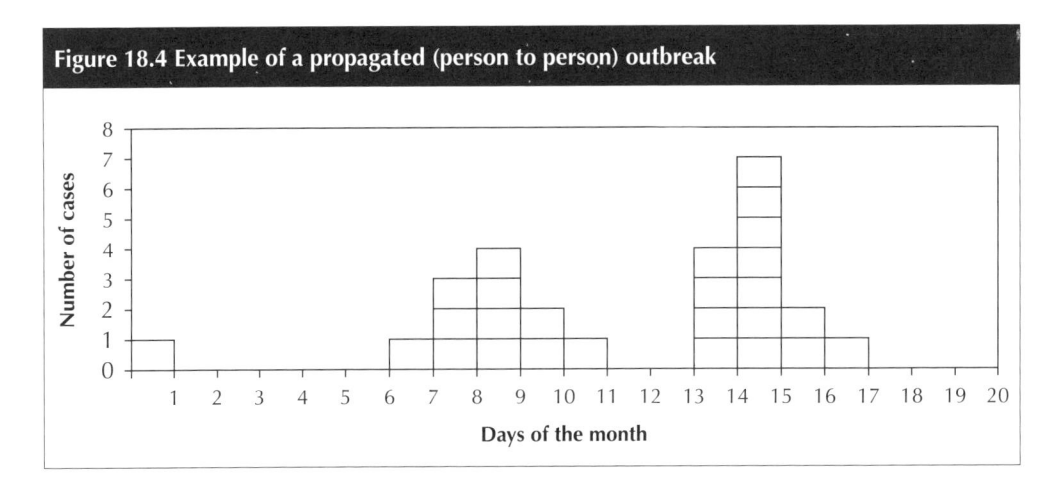

Figure 18.4 Example of a propagated (person to person) outbreak

Some diseases may result in both common source and propagated epidemics. For example, typhoid may initially be spread through a common water source but later it may be spread from person to person by unhygienic practices of food handlers infected with typhoid.

Cases that do not appear to relate to the epidemic are called *outliers* and may also provide valuable information. They may be part of the normal background incidence of the disease, the source case for the epidemic, or someone who was exposed earlier than most of the cases, for example a cook who tasted the contaminated food a number of hours before the guests were served. Late cases, by contrast, may be secondary rather than primary cases.

It is important to separate primary and secondary cases when plotting epidemic curves in order to estimate the incubation or serial period. If the serial interval is short, secondary cases may appear while there are still primary cases becoming ill. It should also be noted that with some diseases different modes of spread of the organism may produce different incubation periods.

The date of any community events that could be related to the exposure should also be shown on the X axis of the epidemic curve, as this may yield important clues to the point at which infection was introduced into the population. This may in turn provide clues to the source of exposure. For example, if the epidemic curve of an outbreak of typhoid showed a peak one to two weeks after a public funeral was held for a leader in the community, one would suspect that food prepared at the funeral was contaminated.

The epidemic curve can also be used to evaluate the course of the epidemic. It will show whether the number of new cases is still on the rise or whether it is declining, and this will help to indicate the urgency of instituting control measures. It is not uncommon to find that the outbreak is already on the decline, in which case the investigation may be less urgent, and additional control measures may not be needed.

Place

Data collected should include home address of cases, address at work or school, location of any function attended, and recent travel or leisure history. If the outbreak is in an institution such as a school or hospital, or limited to a small geographic area, it is useful to plot the spatial location of cases on a spot map. This may indicate if there is evidence for clustering of cases by place and may provide clues to the source of exposure.

Geographical Information Systems (GIS) are increasingly used to track location. They can be used to locate cases of diseases as well as track water and sanitation systems or transport systems. With extensive movement of people today it may be difficult to decide which place should be plotted, for example home or workplace. In an outbreak of typhoid disease in 1993 in the Delmas/Botleng area of Mpumalanga, the spot map of cases showed that only one family who lived in the Delmas area contracted typhoid and all other cases lived around Botleng. The family lived on a smallholding and on investigation it was found that their borehole pump was not working and they were collecting their water in containers from the contaminated source, which was close to their workplace in Botleng (Waner et al, 1998).

The scale of the spot map depends on the investigation and the geographical extent of the epidemic. If the cases are associated with an institution such as a school or hospital, they should be plotted by location within the building (that is, classroom or ward). If they are confined to a geographic area, they should be plotted on a large scale map showing features such as roads and travel connections and the location of potential sources of exposure to infection, such as sources of drinking water and ablution facilities.

In the clinical management of cases, laboratory investigations should be conducted (e.g. of stool or sputum specimens). As part of the epidemiological investigation these may also be collected from controls. In addition, environmental and microbiological investigations may be conducted depending on the nature of the outbreak and whether or not the microbial agent responsible is normally endemic in the population affected by the outbreak. Evidence from environmental investigations complements epidemiological findings, and may confirm the source of infection. Environmental specimens of possible sources of infection (e.g. food, drinking water, swimming water) should be taken as soon as possible after the outbreak is identified, and sent for microbiological investigation (see Example 18.2 at the end of this chapter).

In South Africa the National Institute for Communicable Diseases and a number of Health Sciences Faculties have specialised research laboratories where tests using molecular biology techniques (for example, 'DNA fingerprinting') may be requested to characterise the organism in specimens from patients and environmental specimens. The use of this 'molecular epidemiology' may be useful in confirming or refuting epidemiological links between cases, and in confirming environmental sources of the strain of the organism causing the outbreak.

4. Generate a hypothesis

The investigators should review all existing data, and scrutinise the list of cases for common characteristics and exposures, as well as unusual characteristics or occurrences, as both can provide important clues about the source of exposure. They may generate a number of different hypotheses. In

Example 18.1 below six of seven hospital-acquired cases of Legionnaire's disease had been ventilated in intensive care units, prompting the hypothesis that patient ventilators were the source of infection. In this case, the common exposure led to this hypothesis.

Investigators should use the descriptive information, combined with knowledge of the epidemiology and clinical course of the disease or condition, to formulate hypotheses as to the cause and the most likely reservoir or source of exposure and mode of transmission. Knowledge of the incubation period is invaluable in determining the source of the disease and generating hypotheses as to the mode of spread.

5. Test the hypothesis

Discovering that an exposure is common among cases does not implicate it with certainty. This exposure may be common among non-cases as well. It is therefore necessary to consider an analytical study comparing risk factors and exposures of interest in both cases and non-cases. There are often a number of exposures to consider. While the case-control study design is often used to test the hypothesis, it is worth considering retrospective cohort and cross-sectional studies as they may be as appropriate.

Cohort design versus case-control design

A cohort design is often used when the outbreak is confined to a clearly-defined group of exposed people and it is feasible to obtain a list of all people at risk of becoming cases (see Example 18.2). A point-source food poisoning outbreak that follows a meal or a gathering of people is a good example of the type of situation where it is useful to do a cohort study of the entire population at risk. All people (or as many people as possible) who ate at the suspected place or function during the suspected exposure period should be interviewed so that the specific attack rate and the relative risk (rate ratio – see page 79) associated with eating each food item can be calculated.

A case-control design is often used for large scale outbreaks when it is not possible to define or to study all people at risk of becoming a case. Cases are then compared with a sample of controls. A number of sources may be used to select appropriate controls including, for example, people attending the same health facility or family practice, pupils from the same school, or people from the same workplace or neighbourhood as the cases. Controls should be free of the condition in question, and should have the same *potential for exposure* to the risk factors under investigation as the cases. (Their actual exposure should be determined only once they are chosen.) If the disease is strongly associated with certain characteristics such as age and sex, it may be useful to match cases and controls to ensure that confounding by these factors can be efficiently controlled in the analysis. The obvious advantage of the case-control study over the cohort design is the speed with which a sample of cases and controls can usually be found. This design is also more efficient and less expensive in the collection of data and conduct of the study than cohort studies.

Many outbreaks produce only a small number of cases, and it may be difficult to show a statistically significant result. In these situations it may be useful to have more controls than cases to improve the precision of the odds ratio estimates (i.e. to get a narrower 95% confidence interval). Up to four controls (matched or unmatched) may be selected for each case.

As with interpreting all hypotheses, even if the result is statistically significant, there is still the possibility that the difference found between cases and controls is due to chance. For example, even if the 95% confidence interval for the odds ratio does not include one (i.e. excludes the null hypothesis or 'no effect' level), five percent of the time the result will be due to chance, i.e. there is really no difference between the groups. On the other hand, in small outbreaks a lack of statistical significance should not deter one from inferring that an exposure is causally linked to cases if the magnitude of the exposure-disease association (either the rate ratio or the odds ratio) is large in relation to these other exposures considered. Evidence of a dose-response effect (the greater the exposure, the greater the risk of being a case) may also assist in confirming the source.

If the outbreak is due to one of the Expanded Programme on Immunization (EPI) target diseases against which infants are routinely immunised (for example, poliomyelitis, measles, whooping cough), one should investigate the possibility that the outbreak is due to inadequate vaccine coverage and/or vaccine failure. (See Chapter 17.)

Data collection and analysis to test hypotheses

If feasible, the investigating team should interview each case and control (or family member of each case, if the case is a child or has died) or all relevant persons exposed or not exposed, using a standardised questionnaire. In order to limit recall bias, questionnaires should be completed as soon as possible, as recall bias may lead to the misclassification of exposures. It is imperative that the method of data collection is uniform among cases and between cases and controls. For example, personal interviews of cases and telephonic interviews of controls could differentially influence the replies to questions. For the same reason, a structured questionnaire is essential, as the actual questions asked and the way they are asked may affect the answers given. Items to consider in drawing up the questionnaire are listed in Table 18.2. Items should be selected from this list by considering what is known of the epidemiology of the condition being investigated, omitting items which are not potentially relevant to the investigation.

Table 18.2 Items and questions to consider in developing questionnaires for outbreak investigation

- Symptoms, and particularly those that relate to the case definition (a checklist is often used with a yes or no response for each item on the checklist)
- Precise date of onset (rather than date of first visit to health facility or health worker)
- Important demographic characteristics (date of birth, sex, home or work address)
- Events attended or places visited that could be related to source of exposure
- Time and place of contact with other possible cases
- Source of water for drinking and washing
- Leisure activities (fishing, hiking, camping, water sports)
- Sexual history
- Recent travel history (work and leisure)
- Occupational history (and particularly exposure to chemicals or animals)
- Contact with animals
- Signs or symptoms of bites or rashes
- Immunisation history and history of previous infectious diseases
- Medical history of diseases or conditions that may affect the immune system

Medical records are generally not a suitable substitute for case interviews as they are clinically orientated and epidemiologically relevant information on exposures of interest is often absent from the record. Some clinical information may be required from the records in order to decide if a subject fits the case definition or not. These records also provide the results of diagnostic tests and procedures that may be used in confirming cases.

Descriptive information should be entered onto a computer programme such as Epi Info, Excel or Access as soon as possible in order to create a basic list summarising key attributes of cases (e.g. age, sex, date of onset, area of residence). A laptop computer is useful if available, especially if the investigation is being done in a rural area. This means that information can be entered and analysed on the spot while the investigation is in progress.

The computer programme Epi Info is specially designed for use in outbreak investigations and is relatively easily mastered by people with limited computer experience. It is available at http://www.cdc.gov/epiinfo/Epi6/ei6.htm.

As part of the analysis the investigators should calculate *attack rates*. These are usually stratified by particular risks (risk-specific attack rate). This represents the number of persons who were exposed to a specific risk factor and who became ill as a proportion of the total number of persons who were exposed to the specific risk factor. The investigators can then compare attack rates obtained for different strata or groups.

For example (Table 18.3), in an outbreak of diarrhoea following a wedding attended by 1 100 persons, 810 people got diarrhoea. If 1 000 persons ate the fish course and 800 of these people developed diarrhoea, the risk-specific attack rate for those who ate the fish course would be 80%. The risk-specific attack rate for those who did not eat the fish course would be 10% (10 out of 100). Further analysis should include the calculation of rate ratios (or odds ratios) for those exposed to different factors. Appropriate statistical procedures should be performed to obtain confidence intervals (or *p*-values) to evaluate the probability that the result could be due to chance alone. If there are many exposures as well as possible confounders, the analysis may be complex and it may be necessary to perform multiple logistic regression. The assistance of a statistician should be sought for this purpose.

Table 18.3 Outbreak of diarrhoea following a wedding

		Diarrhoea		
		Yes	No	
Ate fish course	Yes	800	200	1000
	No	10	90	100
Total		810	290	1100

Attack rate among those eating fish course: 800/1000 = 80%
Attack rate among those not eating fish course: 10/100 = 10%
Rate ratio: 80/10 = 8 (95% CI 4.44 – 14.41)
Those who ate the fish were 8 times as likely to develop diarrhoea than those not eating the fish (with a margin of uncertainty of 4.4 to 14.4 times)

6. Implement control measures

The investigators should test all hypotheses, and make a decision as to the most likely causative agent, vector(s), source(s), and mode(s) of transmission. These would include exposure factors relating to the host (for example, lack of immunisation) or environmental factors (for example, floods resulting in contaminated water) which may have been conducive to the outbreak of the disease under investigation. Based on this information, recommendations can be made on specific measures that can be implemented to control the outbreak.

The investigating team should communicate all findings and recommendations to health services involved in controlling the outbreak as well as to the community affected. They should write a summary report including recommendations that are clear and practical, given local circumstances and resources available. Both short- and long-term control measures should be recommended.

Short-term measures

Short-term measures can often be implemented immediately. For example, in the case of a cholera or typhoid outbreak as a result of contaminated water supplies, clean water can be provided by tanker or chemicals can be distributed in order to ensure a clean source of drinking water. This should prevent further new cases from developing and prevent exposure to the source and/or break the chain of transmission. It is often necessary to take interim control measures based on preliminary information, before all likely hypotheses have been tested.

Long-term measures

Once investigations are complete a full report should be written as soon as possible, documenting the outbreak, the investigation, and hypotheses considered and tested, including laboratory evidence, the actions taken and the final outcomes. These findings should detail why the outbreak occurred, why surveillance procedures were insufficient to prevent the outbreak, and what long-term measures should be taken to prevent future outbreaks.

The report should be submitted to the authority requesting the investigation, for example, district, provincial or national health authorities, and other interested parties.

Throughout the investigation the community in which the outbreak occurred should be kept informed of the results of the investigation to allay rumours and unnecessary fears, as well as to gain their co-operation with control measures. This can be done by presentation at community meetings or through press releases or radio.

The investigation should be published as the findings may be used to identify the potential for similar outbreaks in other localities, and innovative epidemiological detective work and analytical study designs may be used to 'solve' similar outbreaks.

Conclusion

Outbreaks provide opportunities to use epidemiological methods to gain practical and useful information about agents of disease, the source or vector of disease, factors relating to the susceptibility of hosts and conditions in the environment conducive to outbreaks. A thorough outbreak investigation should be well planned and include a systematic series of steps relating to data collection, analysis and dissemination of information.

EXAMPLE 18.1

An investigation of Legionnaire's disease in a Johannesburg hospital

Between November 1985 and February 1986, 12 cases of Legionnaire's disease, an infectious lung disease, were identified at a Johannesburg hospital. Based on the knowledge that the incubation period is two to 10 days, it was determined that two cases definitely acquired the disease in hospital, while five other cases might have acquired the disease in hospital. Investigations were carried out to locate a hospital source. A spot map was drawn of all hospital cases by ward, and as water is known to be a reservoir for *Legionella (L.) pneumophila*, the causative agent, water, was cultured from all hot water outlets in the hospital.

Although *L. pneumophila* was cultured in water from three outlets, the distribution of these outlets did not correspond to the distribution of cases, so they were disregarded as the source. It was noted that six of the seven potentially hospital-acquired cases had been ventilated.

Attack rates in intensive care unit (ICU) patients were calculated according to whether or not they had been on a ventilator. The attack rate was 35% in ventilated patients, compared to 2% in ICU patients who were not ventilated. This implicated ventilators as the most likely source of cases who acquired the disease in hospital, a finding in keeping with known modes of transmission of this condition.

Reference:

Strebel, PM, Ramos, JM, Eidelman, IJ, Tobiansky, L, Koornhof, HJ & Koestner, HG. 1988. Legionnaires' disease in a Johannesburg teaching hospital: investigation and control of an outbreak. *South African Medical Journal*, 73:329–33.

EXAMPLE 18.2

An outbreak of food poisoning among children attending an international sports event in Johannesburg

An acute outbreak of illness occurred amongst 578 children participating in the opening ceremony of a major international sports event. Only one meal was eaten by the entire group of children. Shortly after eating the meal a large number of children developed an ill-defined vomiting illness. Two to three days later reports of diarrhoeal illness from a number of children were also received.

Questionnaires were distributed to 578 children and 361 were returned completed (response rate 62.5%). Two case definitions were used. Case definition A was defined as the onset of nausea or vomiting within 6 hours of eating the meal, and case definition B as development of diarrhoea at any stage.

A case-control study was conducted. A list was made of all the food consumed. Children with case definition A were significantly more likely to have consumed fruit juice (odds ratio (OR) = 11.8) and maize-meal porridge (OR = 3.0). Development of diarrhoea was significantly associated with consumption of maize-meal porridge (OR = 8.8) and chicken stew (OR = 7.3).

Shigella bacterium was isolated from a specimen of maize-meal porridge, while the fruit juice samples were found to have high levels of other bacterial contamination. No bacterial contamination could be found in the chicken stew.

Reference:

Karas, JA, Nicol, MP, Martinson, N & Heubner, R. 2001. An outbreak of food poisoning among children attending an international sports event in Johannesburg. *South African Medical Journal*, 91:417–21.

Useful reading

Kenrad, E & Nelson, MD. 2004. *Infectious disease epidemiology*. New York: Jones and Bartlett Publishers.

Useful web sites

Centers for Disease Control, USA: regular updates on epidemics and outbreaks and relevant investigations in the world and includes training and technical reports on the investigation of outbreaks. [Online]. Available: http://www.cdc.gov/. [25 February 2007].

National Institute for Infectious Diseases: regular updates on epidemics and outbreaks and relevant investigations in Southern Africa. [Online]. Available: http://www.nicd.ac.za/. [25 February 2007].

School of Public Health, University of North Carolina: provides useful training in outbreak investigation. [Online]. Available: http://www.sph.unc.edu/. [25 February 2007].

World Health Organization: regular updates on epidemics and outbreaks and relevant investigations worldwide. [Online]. Available: http://www.who.int/. [25 February 2007].

References used in this chapter

Giesecke, J. 2002. *Modern infectious disease epidemiology*. London: Arnold.

Torok, M. 2004. *Focus on field epidemiology*. North Carolina Institute for Public Health Preparedness. 1:1–7. [Online]. Available: http://www2.sph.unc.edu/nccphp/focus/. [9 April 2007].

Waner, S, Kfir, R, Idema, GK & Coetzee, DJ. 1998. Waterborne outbreak of typhoid fever in Delmas. *Southern African Journal of Epidemiology and Infection*, 13:53–7.

19

Epidemiology of HIV/Aids

Quarraisha Abdool Karim

> **OBJECTIVES OF THIS CHAPTER**
>
> The objectives of this chapter are:
> - to demonstrate the central role of epidemiology, in collaboration with laboratory science, in identifying the emergence, distribution and determinants of HIV/Aids
> - to demonstrate the role of epidemiology in the design of interventions to prevent the further spread of HIV and to treat those with Aids
> - to introduce new researchers to the many important research questions this pandemic poses.

Introduction

Epidemiology, as the study of disease pattern and spread, facilitated the discovery of Acquired Immunodeficiency Syndrome (Aids) in the early 1980s with the observation at the United States Centers for Disease Control of a clustering of *Pneumocystis carinii* cases in gay men in San Francisco and shortly thereafter in Los Angeles and New York City. These early cases led to this new phenomenon being described as GRID (Gay Related Immunodeficiency Disease). In 1983 with the isolation of HIV (Human Immunodeficiency Virus) a causal relationship was established between HIV and Aids.

> **Detection of HIV antibodies: a milestone for epidemiological research**
>
> The development of laboratory assays to detect antibodies to HIV infection was a milestone both at a population level as well as at an individual level. It enabled epidemiological surveys to be undertaken to:
> - measure and quantify the magnitude of the epidemic globally and at a country level
> - monitor temporal trends in the evolving epidemic
> - identify risk factors for HIV transmission; and
> - evaluate the impact of interventions to prevent HIV infection.
>
> In addition, the test allowed individuals to establish their HIV status thereby facilitating studies of the pathogenesis and natural history of infection in those infected with HIV. These pathogenetic studies utilised several epidemiological study designs, the most common of which was the prospective cohort study. These studies also informed the development of anti-retroviral drugs and drug combinations, including HAART (highly active anti-retroviral therapy, also known as triple therapy) for treating Aids. These drugs have transformed Aids from an inevitably fatal disease to a chronic, manageable condition, at least in countries where the drugs are widely available.

The continued spread of HIV infection globally 25 years after the isolation of HIV underscores the importance of finding new ways to prevent HIV infection. For this purpose evidence-based decision-making utilising meta-analysis and randomised controlled trials is critical. To demonstrate the efficacy of new HIV prevention interventions requires multi-site studies in high incidence rate settings involving tens of thousands of participants, randomised to the intervention or control and followed up until seroconversion.

Studying transmission of HIV

Most epidemics, including HIV, are influenced by three factors: (a) the proportion of individuals in the population who are infected (prevalence); (b) the proportion in the population at risk of getting infected; and (c) the incidence rate of infection in the population. Epidemiological measurement of prevalence and of incidence rates has been central to understanding the relationship between these three factors in emerging and evolving epidemics. The development of assays to ascertain HIV infection status has enabled these epidemiological measurements to be generated.

In the case of HIV, epidemiological studies using all of the available study designs (see Chapter 7) have helped elucidate the various modes of HIV transmission. In addition, through mathematical modelling and combining prevalence and incidence rate data we have been able to estimate the probability of acquiring infection with HIV by different modes of transmission, and also to project the potential burden and impact of the epidemic in different settings. Analysing these data by sex and age has helped us establish the influence of these demographic characteristics on the risk of acquiring HIV infection. Epidemiological methods have therefore been critical to our understanding of factors associated with HIV acquisition and transmission, projecting the epidemic trajectory for policy, planning and resource allocation purposes, prioritising where to target interventions and at whom to target them.

Viral load and epidemiological studies

By the mid-1990s, further advances in laboratory techniques had resulted in the development of assays to measure the presence of the virus itself. One of the ways this was used was to advance our understanding of HIV transmission dynamics. This led to the conduct of cohort studies in *discordant couples* that compared the viral load (amount of virus) in those infected with HIV and the probability of transmission to their uninfected sexual partners (Quinn *et al*, 2000). Data from these studies demonstrated that regardless of sex, the higher the viral load in the infected partner, the greater the probability of transmitting HIV to the uninfected partner. This very clear close relationship between amount of virus and probability of HIV transmission led to the development of intervention studies (e.g. in the form of a 'proof of concept' randomised controlled trial that is currently under way) to determine the impact of use of antiretroviral drugs in infected persons to reduce HIV transmission to the uninfected sexual partner.

The next natural history cohort study was to establish viral load during different stages of HIV infection, ranging from days post-infection through to the onset of advanced HIV disease or Aids and death. A study conducted in Uganda established that viral load is highest during early infection with HIV prior to the development of antibodies (also known as acute HIV infection) (Wawer *et al*, 2005). Viral burden is also high during infection with other sexually transmitted infections and during advanced HIV disease (Cohen *et al*, 2005). These observations, together with increasing access to anti-retroviral treatment (ART), have resulted in a major shift in HIV prevention efforts from a focus on HIV uninfected persons to a continuum of prevention that includes HIV uninfected, recently infected, infected and asymptomatic persons and those with advanced HIV disease.

In addition to viral burden, detection of viral presence has been greatly useful in understanding mother-to-child transmission of HIV. A major confounder in studying and diagnosing HIV infection in infants is the presence of circulating maternal antibodies in the infant's blood up to 18 months after birth. Tests to detect the presence of virus have helped identify recent HIV infection in newborn infants. These tests have enhanced our ability to undertake randomised controlled trials to test new interventions to reduce HIV transmission to infants. They are also used in cohort studies to better understand the natural history of infection in newborn infants including, for example, those who are breastfed versus those not breastfed.

Monitoring the evolving HIV epidemic

As the HIV pandemic is a complex mix of changing epidemics, monitoring the evolving epidemic through epidemiological surveillance is an important part of informing decision-making for resource allocation, prioritisation of programmatic activities as well as understanding new dimensions of the pandemic. The HIV pandemic is monitored mainly through the conduct of cross-sectional surveys in selected populations. The reliability of the prevalence estimates generated in these surveys is influenced by a number of factors. These include, among others, the specific populations or groups included in the survey, how often these surveys are conducted, sampling methodology employed (e.g. population versus facilities-based) and whether individuals screened are volunteering to be tested or are being tested anonymously.

In light of the human rights violations experienced by HIV infected persons, several international guidelines such as the WHO and CDC guidelines (World Health Organization, 2001) have been developed for the ethical conduct of surveys for surveillance purposes. In addition, when conducting studies and surveys for monitoring and surveillance purposes it is necessary to reflect periodically on their appropriateness and utility as the dynamics of HIV transmission change.

In South Africa, the national, annual, anonymous antenatal clinic (ANC) surveys conducted since 1990 have provided the most reliable estimates of the evolving HIV epidemic in South Africa (http://www.doh.gov.za). To date 15 such surveys have been conducted using similar methods regarding study population, sampling frame and timing of the survey. This has helped minimise important biases that usually influence the utility of cross-sectional studies. Additionally, as the survey protocol remains constant, any inherent biases are assumed to carry through from year to year. Temporal trends can therefore be reliably observed.

A temporal trend analysis is presented in Table 19.1. Reflecting on the evolving HIV epidemic in South Africa over different time periods is important in understanding epidemic dynamics.

During the early stages of heterosexually transmitted HIV epidemics, as has been the case in South Africa, when the majority of the infections are asymptomatic, monitoring of HIV prevalence in the antenatal clinic population is informative as this population represents one half of a sexually active partnership that is not using condoms. However, as the epidemic becomes more generalised and individuals who were

| Table 19.1 The evolving HIV epidemic in South Africa |||
Year	Phase	Characteristics
Pre-1987	I	1982: first reported cases of Aids Epidemic largely limited to men who have sex with men, transfusion recipients and haemophiliacs Localised Clade (virus subtype) B epidemic
1987–1993	II	Introduction of HIV in heterosexual population Major epidemic: general population and mother to child transmission Clade C Steady growth in HIV transmission Exponential increase: doubling time 15.1 months (95% CI: 12.3–18.1)
1994–1998	III	Generalised epidemic well established High incidence rates Explosive growth in HIV transmission Genetically diverse epidemics coalesce Mortality still low
1999–2006	IV	Generalised epidemic nearing saturation High incidence rates remain HIV prevalence almost static Mortality rising rapidly

infected during the early years of the epidemic start to progress to advanced disease and die, this population becomes less reliable, as does monitoring prevalent infections. Prevalence estimates 'stabilise', masking the dynamic relationship between the increasing overall Aids-related mortality and the rates of new HIV infection i.e. incident infection.

Incidence can be measured using sensitive ribonucleic acid-polymerase chain reaction (RNA-PCR) assays in the absence of antibodies. Incidence rates provide a more sensitive marker of the HIV epidemic as it matures, and are usually generated by establishing large cohorts of uninfected individuals and following them up for fixed time periods until they seroconvert. The population included in the surveillance programme also needs to be expanded to reflect the changing pattern of the epidemic.

Identifying risk factors for HIV infection

Several epidemiological factors influence the sexual spread of HIV in South Africa, as they do elsewhere. These include gender, age, migration, and other sexually transmitted infections. Epidemiological studies are needed to elucidate the relationship between these factors and HIV acquisition. Some examples are provided below.

Age and gender

A striking characteristic of heterosexual transmission is the disproportionate burden of HIV infection in young women compared to men. Women acquire HIV infection at a younger age, at least 5 to 10 years earlier than men. Young boys aged 15 to 19 years have little HIV infection while teenage girls are already close to peak prevalence. Explanatory factors include the coupling of younger women (14 to 24 years) with older men, and the anatomical differences between the male and female reproductive tract and consequently differences in probability of HIV transmission by sex.

Migration

HIV prevalence in mobile couples is 2- to 3-fold higher than in stable couples. A number of epidemiological studies have been undertaken to investigate characteristics and patterns of migration associated with HIV acquisition. These data have been important in designing and testing interventions to reduce HIV infection in these mobile populations.

Other sexually transmitted infections

It is now well established that the presence of other sexually transmitted infections (STIs) is a major factor influencing spread of HIV. Data from several Cochrane analyses (see Chapter 6) clearly demonstrate that STIs increase the risk of HIV transmission about 4-fold on average (Rottingen et al, 2001). The burden of untreated STIs is high in many developing countries and it is biologically plausible that this population burden facilitates the spread of HIV infection.

This evidence was the basis of the design and conduct of three complex randomised controlled trials to test the impact of enhanced STI management on HIV transmission: at Mwanza (Grosskurth et al, 1995), Rakai (Wawer et al, 1999) and Masaka (Kamali et al, 2003). However, these trials have generated inconsistent results. This demonstrates that a 'causal finding' from observational studies does not necessarily translate into a protective effect in interventions. Researchers and decision-makers are therefore left with the difficult challenge of interpreting the implications of these trials for future research and policy formulation.

Studying prevention

For those who are unable to, or fail to, reduce their number of 'discordant' sexual acts (i.e. with an HIV positive partner), the critical prevention goal is to reduce the probability of transmission in discordant sexual acts. In this context, male and female condoms provide a proven prevention option. The use of antiretrovirals for prevention, chemoprophylaxis for herpes simplex virus-2 with the drug acyclovir and male circumcision are potential but as yet unproven prevention options. Additionally, both microbicides and vaccines remain a long-term goal for prevention of HIV infection.

Despite substantial scientific progress in these areas to date, many challenges remain. South African scientists are playing a central role in product development of vaccines and are also at the forefront of testing microbicide effectiveness. The high incidence rates, highly trained staff, and strong laboratory and clinical trial infrastructure make South Africa an attractive site for the conduct of clinical trials. On the other hand the relatively research-naïve populations impose responsibilities in ensuring the ethical conduct of these studies and trials. Ethical and human rights issues and considerations in the conduct of epidemiological research are covered in Chapter 3.

Examples 19.1 and 19.2 below describe the use of epidemiological evidence in responding to the epidemic. The first example addresses the use of a proven HIV prevention intervention, namely male condoms, and the second an unproven intervention, male circumcision.

Conclusion

The HIV/Aids pandemic, of which the South African epidemic is a part, is a dynamic one. Epidemiology provides tools for understanding infection transmission, monitoring the evolution of the epidemic and determining risk factors for infection as well as prognosis among those infected. It also provides researchers with many opportunities to develop and test new forms of intervention and to inform evidence-based public health decision-making.

EXAMPLE 19.1

Are male condoms being wasted?

There are convincing data from several studies collated in a Cochrane review (Weller & Davis, 2002) that consistent condom use reduces HIV incidence by at least 80%, although with varying levels of effectiveness described in different studies. Reliable supplies of condoms are therefore a critical part of consistent condom use. The South African government's public sector condom promotion strategy is a good example of success in increasing distribution. Condom distribution increased dramatically from 250 million units in 2000 to 267 million in 2001 to an estimated 350 million in 2002. This excluded distribution through social marketing and the private sector.

Some have argued that increasing condom distribution does not translate into actual use, or that free distribution of condoms leads to wastage. A prospective cohort study from South Africa followed a nationally representative sample of 384 sequential condom recipients and the 5 528 condoms they obtained from public sector primary care clinics. After 5 weeks 43.7% of the condoms had been used in sex, about 20% were given away to others to use in sex, 8.5% were lost or discarded, and 26% were still available for use. Five weeks after obtaining the condoms, wastage was less than 10%. The authors concluded that condoms obtained in the public sector were mostly being used for their designated purpose.

References:

Myer, L, Mathews, C, Little, F & Abdool Karim, SS. 2001. The fate of male condoms distributed to the public in South Africa. *AIDS*, 15: 789–93.

Weller, S & Davis, K. 2002. Condom effectiveness in reducing heterosexual HIV transmission. *Cochrane Database of Systematic Reviews*, CD003255.

EXAMPLE 19.2

Does male circumcision protect against HIV infection?

Male circumcision is an example of a situation where conflicting epidemiological evidence and biological possibilities make the establishment of causation difficult. A Cochrane analysis of several observational studies suggested a protective benefit of male circumcision in a range of *high-risk* groups (Siegfried *et al*, 2003) (Figure 19.1). Most of the studies included in this analysis were cross-sectional and almost all the effect sizes showed that circumcision had a protective effect. However, there were several important biases and potential confounders in these studies including sexual behaviour, religion, penile hygiene, viral load and immune status.

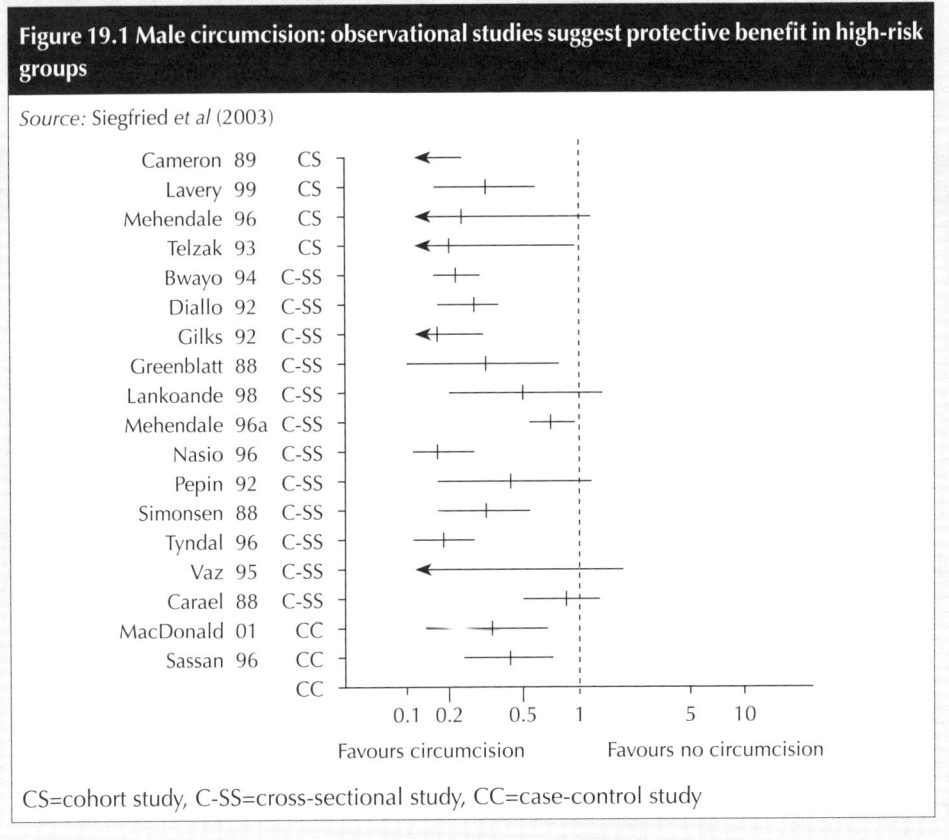

Figure 19.1 Male circumcision: observational studies suggest protective benefit in high-risk groups

Source: Siegfried et al (2003)

Study	Type
Cameron 89	CS
Lavery 99	CS
Mehendale 96	CS
Telzak 93	CS
Bwayo 94	C-SS
Diallo 92	C-SS
Gilks 92	C-SS
Greenblatt 88	C-SS
Lankoande 98	C-SS
Mehendale 96a	C-SS
Nasio 96	C-SS
Pepin 92	C-SS
Simonsen 88	C-SS
Tyndal 96	C-SS
Vaz 95	C-SS
Carael 88	C-SS
MacDonald 01	CC
Sassan 96	CC
	CC

0.1 0.2   0.5   1   5   10

Favours circumcision   Favours no circumcision

CS=cohort study, C-SS=cross-sectional study, CC=case-control study

Recent evidence from a large cohort study of discordant couples in Uganda revealed the HIV incidence was 0% among circumcised men compared to 16.7% in those not circumcised (Gray et al, 2002).

Biological plausibility could work both ways. On the one hand, the foreskin has a high level of immunological Langerhans cells with CD4 and other receptors, providing increased opportunity for HIV acquisition (Szabo et al, 2000; Soto-Ramirez et al, 1996). On the other hand, the inner foreskin has apocrine glands which secrete lysozyme, an enzyme that kills HIV (Patterson et al, 2002).

The Cochrane analysis of 13 observational studies undertaken in the *general* population (Siegfried et al, 2003) showed a lack of association with HIV and male circumcision (Figure 19.2). This lack of agreement in observational studies suggests that randomised trial data are needed to resolve this debate.

Three Phase III (effectiveness) randomised controlled trials were initiated in 1999 by three different study teams in South Africa (Auvert et al, 2005), Kenya (Agot et al, 2004) and Uganda (Gray et al, 2002). All three trials have been stopped prematurely on the basis of an observed 50%–60% protective effect of medical male circumcision. Notwithstanding the consistent results from these 3 trials, a number of additional issues such as acceptability, surgical complication rates and health care delivery infrastructure will need to be carefully considered prior to any public health policy decision on recommending medical male circumcision.

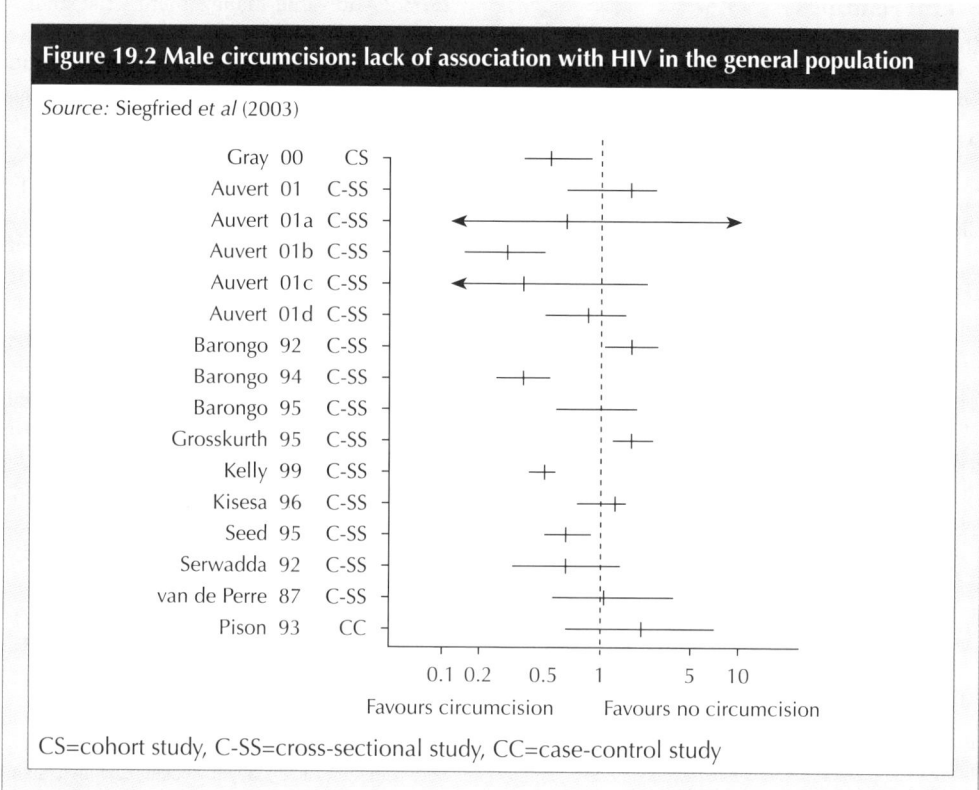

Epidemiology of HIV/Aids

Figure 19.2 Male circumcision: lack of association with HIV in the general population

Source: Siegfried et al (2003)

Study	Type
Gray 00	CS
Auvert 01	C-SS
Auvert 01a	C-SS
Auvert 01b	C-SS
Auvert 01c	C-SS
Auvert 01d	C-SS
Barongo 92	C-SS
Barongo 94	C-SS
Barongo 95	C-SS
Grosskurth 95	C-SS
Kelly 99	C-SS
Kisesa 96	C-SS
Seed 95	C-SS
Serwadda 92	C-SS
van de Perre 87	C-SS
Pison 93	CC

0.1 0.2   0.5   1   5   10
Favours circumcision   Favours no circumcision

CS=cohort study, C-SS=cross-sectional study, CC=case-control study

References:

Agot, K, Bailey, RC, Moses, S, Maclean, IW, Ndinya-Achola, JO & Parker, CB. 2004. A randomized controlled trial of male circumcision to reduce HIV incidence in Kisumu, Kenya; preliminary baseline results. *XVth international conference on AIDS: Bangkok.*

Auvert, B, Taljaard, D, Lagarde, E, Sobngwi-Tambekou, J, Sitta, R & Puren, A. 2005. Randomized, controlled intervention trial of male circumcision for reduction of HIV infection risk: the ANRS 1265 trial. *Public Library of Science Medicine,* 2:e298.

Gray, RH, Wawer, MJ, Kiwanuka, N, Serwadda, D, Sewankambo, NK & Wabwire-Mangen, F. 2002. Male circumcision and HIV acquisition and transmission: Rakai, Uganda. *AIDS,* 16(5):809–10.

Patterson, BK, Landay, A, Siegel JN, Flener, Z, Pessis, D, Chaviano, A & Bailey, RC. 2002. Susceptibility to human immunodeficiency virus-1 infection of human foreskin and cervical tissue grown in explant culture. *American Journal of Pathology,* 161: 867–73.

Siegfried, N, Muller, M, Volmink, J, Deeks, J, Egger, M, Low, N, Weiss, H, Walker, S & Williamson, P. 2003. Male circumcision for prevention of heterosexual acquisition of HIV in men. *Cochrane Database of Systematic Reviews,* Issue 3, CD003362. DOI: 10.1002/14651858. US: Cochrane Collection.

Soto-Ramirez, LE, Renjifo, B, McLane, MF, Marlink, R, O'Hara, C, Sutthent, R, Wasi, C, Vithayasai, P, Vithayasai, V, Apichartpiyakul, C, Auewarakul, P, Pena Cruz, V, Chui, DS, Osathanondh, R, Mayer, K, Lee, TH & Essex, M. 1996. HIV-1 Langerhans' cell tropism associated with heterosexual transmission of HIV. *Science,* 271:1291–3.

Szabo, R & Short, RV. 2000. How does male circumcision protect against HIV infection? *British Medical Journal,* 320:1592–4.

Useful readings

Abdool Karim, SS & Abdool Karim, Q (eds). 2005. *HIV/AIDS in South Africa*. Cape Town: Cambridge University Press.

Department of Health, South Africa. 2005. *National HIV survey of women attending antenatal clinics of the public health services*. Pretoria: Health Systems Research and Epidemiology.

Useful web sites

Alliance for Microbicide Development. [Online]. Available: http://www.microbicide.org. [25 February 2007].

Centers for Disease Control. [Online]. Available: http://www.cdc.gov/. [25 February 2007].

Centre for AIDS Development, Research and Evaluation (CADRE). [Online]. Available: http://www.cadre.org.za/. [25 February 2007].

Department of Health web site with links to Aids and HIV information from South Africa. [Online]. Available: http://www.doh.gov.za/. [25 February 2007].

International AIDS Vaccine Initiative. [Online]. Available: http://www.iavi.org. [25 February 2007].

UNAIDS. [Online]. Available: http://www.unaids.org/en/. [25 February 2007].

References used in this chapter

Cohen, MS & Pilcher, CD. 2005. Amplified HIV transmission and new approaches to HIV prevention. *Journal of Infectious Diseases*, 191:1391–3.

Grosskurth, H, Mosha, F, Todd, J, Mwijarubi, E, Klokke, A, Senkoro, K, Mayaud, P, Changalucha, J, Nicoll, A, ka-Gina, G, Newell, J, Mugeye, K, Mabey, D & Hayes, R. 1995. Impact of improved treatment of sexually transmitted diseases on HIV-1 infection in rural Tanzania: randomised controlled trial. *Lancet*, 346:530–6.

Kamali, A, Quigley, M, Nakiyingi, J, Kinsman, J, Kengeya-Kayondo, J, Gopal, R, Ojwiya, A, Hughes, P, Carpenter, LM & Whitworth, J. 2003. Syndromic management of sexually-transmitted infections and behaviour change interventions on transmission of HIV-1 in rural Uganda: a community randomised trial. *Lancet*, 361:645–52.

Quinn, TC, Wawer, MJ, Sewankambo, N, Serwadda, D, Li, C, Wabwire-Mangen, F, Meehan, MO, Lutalo, T & Gray, RH. 2000. Viral load and heterosexual transmission of human immunodeficiency virus type 1. *New England Journal of Medicine*, 342:921–9.

Rottingen, JA, Cameron, DW & Garnett, GP. 2001. A systematic review of the epidemiologic interactions between classic sexually transmitted diseases and HIV: how much really is known? *Sexually Transmitted Diseases*, 28(10):579–97.

Simon, V, Ho, DD & Abdool Karim, Q. 2006. HIV/AIDS epidemiology, pathogenesis, prevention, and treatment. *Lancet*, 368(9534): 489–504.

UNAIDS/WHO. 2004. *Policy statement on HIV testing*. [Online]. Available: http://data.unaids.org/una-docs/hivtestingpolicy_en.pdf. [25 February 2007].

Wawer, MJ, Gray, RH, Sewankambo, NK, Serwadda, D, Li X, Laeyendecker, O, Kiwanuka, K, Kigozi, G, Kiddugavu, M, Lutalo, T, Nalugoda, F, Wabwire-Mangen, F, Meehan, MP & Quinn, TC. 2005. Rates of HIV-1 transmission per coital act, by stage of HIV-1 infection, in Rakai, Uganda. *Journal of Infectious Diseases*, 191: 1403–9.

Wawer, MJ, Sewankambo, NK, Serwadda, D, Quinn, TC, Paxton, LA, Kiwanuka, N, Wabwire-Mangen, F, Li, C, Lutalo, T, Nalugoda, F, Gaydos, CA, Moulton, LH, Meehan, MO, Ahmed, S & Gray, RH. 1999. Control of sexually transmitted diseases for AIDS prevention in Uganda: a randomised community trial. *Lancet*, 353(9152):525–35.

World Health Organization. 2001. *Guidelines for using HIV testing technologies in surveillance: selection, evaluation, and implementation*. [Online]. Available: http://whqlibdoc.who.int/hq/2001/WHO_CDS_CSR_EDC_2001.16.pdf. [9 April 2007].

20

Environmental epidemiology

Angela Mathee

OBJECTIVES OF THIS CHAPTER

The objectives of this chapter are:
- to describe the public health problems to which environmental epidemiology is applied
- to outline the main methodological concerns in environmental epidemiology, particularly those relating to measurement of exposure
- to provide examples of how different study designs are used in environmental epidemiology
- to describe considerations in the planning of environmental epidemiology studies.

Introduction

During the past three centuries, environmental health and environmental epidemiology have contributed to considerable public health gains from reducing population exposure to contaminants in air, water and soil (Pekkanen & Pearce, 2001). Environmental epidemiology may be defined as *the study of environmental factors that influence the distribution and determinants of disease in human populations*.

Awareness of the environment as a causative factor in disease goes back to ancient civilisations. Modern environmental health has its roots in the public health movement of the nineteenth century (known as the sanitary movement), when basic environmental health interventions such as the provision of better housing, safe water and sanitation were associated with notable public health gains. In recent decades there has been renewed attention devoted globally to environmental health concerns. One of the reasons for this has been a number of disastrous environmental incidents that have taken place, resulting in death, illness and hardship among local residents as well as communities located at considerable distances from the incident. Examples include the nuclear radiation release from the Chernobyl power plant in the Ukraine in 1986 and the gas release following an explosion at the Union Carbide plant in Bhopal, India, in 1984. In South Africa too, several incidents of environmental contamination in recent times have received widespread media attention. For example, the collapse of a mine slimes dam in 1994 at Merriespruit in the Free State province led to the loss of 17 lives, while a sulphur fire at Macassar in Cape Town (see Table 20.1) resulted in three deaths and highlighted how environmental contamination and degradation can adversely affect local communities.

It is currently estimated that around one quarter of the global burden of disease may be attributable to environmental factors (World Health Organization, 1997). This proportion is higher still in developing countries, and especially in Africa, where

> **Table 20.1 Community exposure from a sulphur fire near Cape Town (Macassar)**
>
> Source: Batterman et al (1999)
>
> In December 1995 local bushfires set ablaze a sulphur stockpile of around 15 000 tons at an explosives and chemical plant near Cape Town. An estimated 14 000 tons of sulphur were released over a 20-hour period, seriously affecting nearby urban and agricultural areas. The resulting cloud of toxic sulphur dioxide gas engulfed the town of Macassar, located 2.4 to 4 kilometres downwind, as well as other settlements in the area. Those affected experienced burning or stinging eyes and breathing difficulties. The incident was associated with the deaths of three people, while a further 100 individuals were injured and 2 500 were evacuated.

environmental problems related to underdevelopment occur alongside those associated with rapid industrialisation and chemical pollution. The World Health Organization (WHO) estimates that 90 percent of the burden of diarrhoeal disease, for example, is associated with inadequate water, sanitation and hygiene, while 60 percent of the burden of pneumonia is attributed to exposure to indoor air pollution (World Health Organization, 1997).

Considerations in the planning and design of environmental epidemiology studies

Getting started

While some environmental epidemiology studies may be exploratory in nature, more frequently studies are designed around a particular hypothesis. In this regard, there are important questions that need to be asked in the early planning or design phases of such studies.

> **Useful questions to consider in the design phase of an environmental epidemiology study**
>
> Source: Adapted from World Health Organization (1983)
>
> - **Who** should be studied? Are particular subgroups of the population at risk? How should control groups be selected?
> - **What** should be measured? Can specific environmental agents be identified? Is there a single pathway (for example, via inhalation or ingestion) or have several ways of entry into the body to be considered simultaneously? How are effects on health to be assessed?
> - **Where** should the study take place? Should geographical position, altitude or meteorology be taken into account in selecting a locality? Are there existing environmental monitoring stations or sets of data relating to the environmental factors in question?
> - **When** should the study be carried out? Are seasonal effects likely to be important? Is the available time-span long enough to provide a satisfactory estimate of long-term exposures? Should exposures be averaged over months or years, or are short-term peaks relevant?

A further important consideration is the amount of time and money available to undertake studies. Financial constraints may require a reduction in the sample size by concentrating on those at high risk or changing to a cheaper study design. Prospective cohort studies, for example, are costly relative to case-control studies. An outline of the designs that have been particularly useful in studying the effects of environmental agents on health, and examples from South Africa, are given later in this chapter.

Exposure assessment

When conducting environmental epidemiology investigations, the characterisation of the hazardous environmental agents to which people are exposed is one of the most important steps to plan carefully. The difficulties in accurately identifying and measuring exposures are what set environmental epidemiology apart from traditional epidemiology. People are exposed to a variety of potentially harmful agents in the air they breathe, the liquids they drink, the food they eat, the items they touch and the products they use. On a daily basis people move about in various settings – home, work, school or recreation – with exposure profiles varying greatly from one place to another. Exposure assessment can therefore be a complex exercise requiring analysis of a number of different aspects of contact between people and hazardous substances (Table 20.2). The lack of accurate exposure data has been referred to as the Achilles heel of environmental epidemiology (Perera & Weinstein, 1982).

Table 20.2 Aspects of the contact between people and pollution that are potentially important in environmental exposure analysis

Source: Sexton et al (1995)

Agent(s)	Biological, chemical, physical, single agent, multiple agents, mixtures
Source(s)	Anthropogenic (of human origin) or non-anthropogenic, area or point, stationary or mobile, indoor or outdoor
Transport medium	Air, water, soil, dust, food, product or item
Exposure pathway(s)	Eating contaminated food, breathing contaminated workplace air, touching residential surfaces
Exposure concentration	mg/kg (food), mg/litre (water), µg/m^3 or fibres/m^3 (air), µg/cm^2 (contaminated surface)
Exposure route(s)	Inhalation, dermal contact, ingestion, multiple routes
Exposure duration	Seconds, minutes, hours, days, weeks, months, years, lifetime
Exposure frequency	Continuous, intermittent, cyclic, random, rare
Exposure setting(s)	Occupational or non-occupational, residential or non-residential, indoors or outdoors
Exposed population	General population, population subgroups

We can categorise methods for assessing environmental exposure as one of two general approaches: direct or indirect. Direct approaches include personal exposure monitoring and biological markers of exposure. Indirect approaches include environmental sampling, combined with exposure factor information, modelling and questionnaires.

Defining outcomes

Environmental health outcomes

Health effects from environmental exposures may range from death and coma, defined diseases and disease categories (for example, pneumonia, emphysema and cancer), symptom complexes (coughing and wheezing) through to minor physiological changes. Acute illness may be the result of heavy exposure (for example, a disaster) or may occur as short duration episodes in response to continuing exposure (for example, respiratory infections due to indoor air pollution). Chronic disease may occur as a result of ongoing exposure (for example, chronic obstructive pulmonary disease due to heavy air pollution) or from early life exposure (intellectual impairment from lead poisoning). Some effects, such as cancer of the pleura from exposure to asbestos, may take 20 or more years to develop. Tracing the original populations exposed to hazards with long *induction periods* (the period between exposure to an agent and the onset of disease) may be difficult or impossible.

In environmental epidemiology the diseases of interest usually occur infrequently, the prevalence or levels of environmental exposures are usually low in the general population and the effects are small (odds ratios or rate ratios less than 2.0). There is, in addition, a high probability of measurement error, which in turn results in loss of precision (see Chapter 12) with which to estimate health effects and typically an underestimation (downward bias) of the true effect.

Study designs in environmental epidemiology

The study designs employed in traditional epidemiology are also used in environmental epidemiology, albeit with particular emphasis on exposure characterisation. There are two approaches to framing research questions in environmental epidemiology. The first involves the identification of a *disease* of interest (e.g. breast cancer) followed by the measurement of a variety of environmental exposures that may be implicated in causing that disease. The second approach involves the identification of a potentially hazardous *exposure* (e.g. pesticides) followed by observation of exposed and unexposed groups to detect possible adverse health outcomes.

Case reports

The investigation of a single case may sometimes lead to valuable environmental health action. In 2002, while investigating the extent of lead poisoning amongst South African children in a cross-sectional study, researchers identified a seven-year old girl with a blood lead level of 44.4 µg/dl. Since this level was more than four times higher than the internationally accepted action level (10 µg/dl) for lead in children's blood, and six times higher than the survey mean, the researchers conducted a home assessment. Samples of water, dust, soil and paint were collected for lead content analysis. The paint samples in particular proved to have very high lead concentrations – up to 46 000 µg/g (more than nine times the international safety standard). Interviews with the parents revealed that the girl had a severe pica habit, and had been ingesting paint chips, soil and putty for much of her life (Mathee *et al*, 2003).

Further investigations prompted by these findings alerted the researchers to the ongoing practice among South African paint manufacturers of adding lead to paint, in some instances at alarmingly high concentrations (up to 189 000 µg/g), and the absence of any legislation to control paint lead levels in the country. Following presentation of the findings to the Minister of Health, the Department of Health announced that regulations would be drafted to limit the amount of lead that may be added to paint in South Africa, and also conducted the first-ever nationwide lead awareness campaign.

Ecological studies

Figure 20.1 gives a comparison, by province, of the proportion of households using high risk water sources (dams, rivers, streams, boreholes) with the provincial infant mortality rate. The data on sources of water were obtained from Statistics South Africa, while infant mortality rates were obtained from the Department of Health (2001). From Figure 20.1 it appears that, with some exceptions, those provinces with the highest proportions of households using risky sources of water are also those with the highest infant mortality rates.

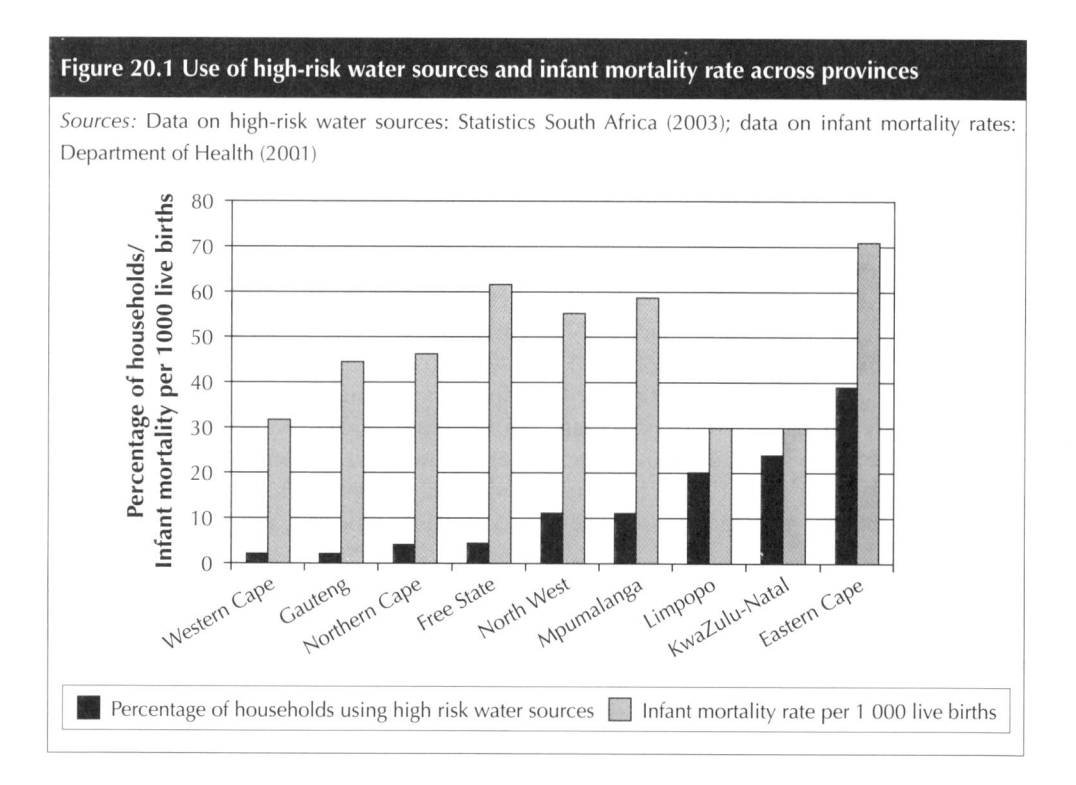

Figure 20.1 Use of high-risk water sources and infant mortality rate across provinces

Sources: Data on high-risk water sources: Statistics South Africa (2003); data on infant mortality rates: Department of Health (2001)

Cross-sectional studies

In 2005 cross-sectional analytical studies of housing conditions and health status were undertaken in the degraded apartheid era Riverlea Extension 1 township to the south-west of central Johannesburg, as well as the relatively new low-cost Braamfischerville housing development in Soweto. Participating dwellings were selected from a database of the Planning Department of the City of Johannesburg. In each area, the first dwelling for inclusion in the study was randomly selected, with every second dwelling being included thereafter. Where no suitable respondent was available after two visits to a particular dwelling, an adjacent residence was selected for inclusion in the study. Information on housing and health was obtained by trained interviewers through the administration of a structured questionnaire.

The results provided informative profiles of the study communities, as well as their living conditions and health concerns. The samples were relatively similar in educational and occupational status, but were very different with respect to population group. Africans were the predominant population in Braamfischerville, while Riverlea residents were mainly Coloured. With higher mean and median numbers of people per dwelling, Riverlea homes appeared to be more crowded than Braamfischerville homes. As expected, a much higher proportion of households had been resident for more than five years in the older Riverlea Township than in Braamfischerville.

Relatively high proportions of households in both communities were affected by diabetes, hypertension, asthma and arthritis. There was a particularly high prevalence of asthma in Riverlea when compared with Braamfischerville (Mathee A, Naicker, N, Barnes, B & Swart, A, unpublished data). The Riverlea community was badly affected by socioenvironmental concerns such as crime, as well as drug and alcohol abuse. In Riverlea, for example, 12%, 21% and 22% of respondents reported that a household member had been respectively raped, shot or stabbed, compared with Braamfischerville, where the respective figures were 2%, 2% and 4%.

The findings from these cross-sectional studies of housing and health status in Riverlea and Braamfischerville should assist city managers in making decisions about the interventions needed to improve quality of life and health status in these and similar communities.

When cross-sectional studies are repeated, they are referred to as *panel studies*. Lead poisoning, which is associated with intellectual impairment, behaviour problems and poor school performance, is possibly the main environmental health problem faced by urban South African children. The Medical Research Council conducts cross-sectional surveys of first grade school children at approximately 5-year intervals to determine blood lead distributions. One such survey was undertaken in 1995 among first grade school children in the suburbs of Alexandra, Soweto, Riverlea, Westbury and downtown Johannesburg (Mathee *et al*, 2002) (Figure 20.2). The 1995 results showed that blood lead levels ranged from

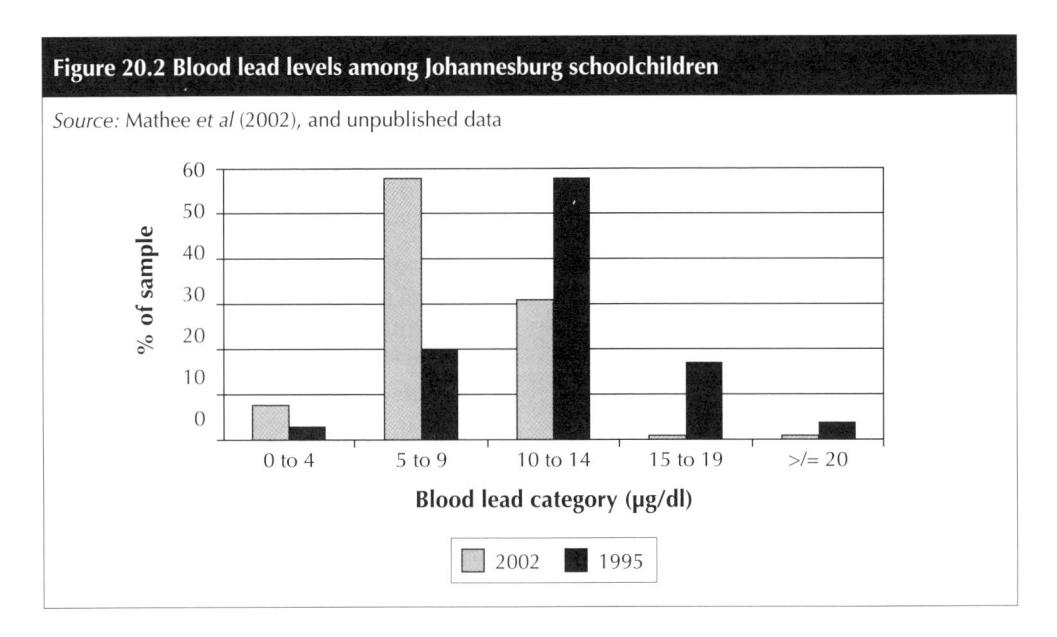

Figure 20.2 Blood lead levels among Johannesburg schoolchildren

Source: Mathee *et al* (2002), and unpublished data

6 to 26 µg/dl (mean = 11.9 µg/dl), and that 78% of the study subjects had blood lead levels equalling or exceeding the action level of 10 µg/dl. By the time the study was repeated in 2002, blood lead levels ranged from 1.0 to 44.4 µg/dl (mean = 9.1 µg/dl) and 35% of the children had blood lead levels equalling or exceeding 10 µg/dl.

The researchers attributed the overall reduction in children's blood lead levels to the reduction in the maximum permissible lead concentration of petrol in South Africa, and the introduction in 1996 of unleaded petrol. We can expect that future cross-sectional surveys of children's blood lead levels in Johannesburg will show further declines in blood lead levels as a consequence of the phasing out of leaded petrol in South Africa as from 1 January 2006.

Case-control studies

A landmark case-control study in the area of indoor air pollution and pneumonia, that continues to be widely cited in international air quality and health publications, was undertaken in the former Natal (now KwaZulu-Natal) in the 1980s. In order to investigate the risk factors for acute lower respiratory infections in children, Kossove (1982) investigated two groups of children – one with and one free of respiratory problems. Of 132 infants with severe lower respiratory tract disease, 70% had a history of daily heavy smoke exposure from cooking and/or heating fires. Only 33% of 18 infants free of respiratory problems had such exposure. Wood smoke was suggested as a potent risk factor in the development of severe lower respiratory tract disease in infants.

Prospective cohort studies

The *Birth to Twenty* study is the largest and longest running cohort study in South Africa. It involves the study of 3 274 children (and their families) who were born between March and June 1990 in the metropolitan area of Johannesburg-Soweto (Richter *et al*, 1995). The study, which has the overarching aim of gaining an understanding of the determinants of child and adolescent health and development within Johannesburg-Soweto, will follow the children over the first twenty years of their lives. Close to 70% of the cohort has been retained after 16 years, and the current focus of the study is on risk factors for sexual, reproductive and non-communicable disease outcomes. Environmental risk factors that have been studied under the umbrella of the *Birth to Twenty* project include lead exposure at birth and in adolescence, housing quality, access to basic environmental health services (water, sanitation and waste), fuel use, and exposure to indoor air pollution (http://www.wits.ac.za/birthto20). In relation to indoor air pollution exposure, for example, the *Birth to Twenty* study has shown higher levels of respiratory and other ill health outcomes amongst children with greater exposure to indoor air pollution.

Intervention studies

In the past the emphasis in environmental epidemiology has been on studies of the causes of disease. In recent years intervention studies have been increasingly used to evaluate the impact of attempts to reduce environmental exposures. Such studies are important since many environmental exposures are associated with industrial or agricultural activities that also bring considerable benefit to communities. Avoidance of such exposures would be costly or achievable only in the long-term. One such intervention study (Example 20.1) has recently been completed in rural villages of the North West province. The purpose was to evaluate the impact of a behaviour change intervention on the exposure of young children to indoor air pollution.

> **EXAMPLE 20.1**

Evaluating the impact of a behaviour change intervention on the exposure of young children to indoor air pollution

Indoor air pollution caused by the indoor burning of biomass fuels (e.g. wood and cattle dung) has been causally linked to acute lower respiratory infections (ALRIs) such as pneumonia amongst young children in developing countries.

The study had a quantitative and a qualitative component. The quantitative evaluation employed a quasi-experimental before-and-after study design with a matched control group. Baseline data were collected in the winter (when exposure to indoor air pollution and levels of pneumonia are highest) of 2003 in the intervention and control groups. Immediately thereafter the behaviour-based intervention (promotion of improved ventilation and keeping children away from domestic fires) was implemented in the intervention group but not in the control group. Post-intervention data were collected from both groups during the winter of 2004.

The villages included in the study were similar in size, population and socio-demographic characteristics. A cohort of 502 eligible children were recruited in the intervention (n = 244) and control groups (n = 258). Data were collected on behavioural risk factors (including location of fires, location of children and ventilation practices), indoor air quality [particulate matter with a diameter $\leq$ 10 microns (PM_{10}) and carbon monoxide (CO)] and health (ALRI morbidity and mortality). The study measured a number of confounding variables (characteristics of the household, caregiver and child) that have been reported to be associated with indoor air pollution, pneumonia or both. Behavioural risk factors were assessed using a questionnaire interview with caregivers. Levels of PM_{10} and CO were measured using standardised air quality measurement protocols and the determination of ALRI was undertaken through caregiver reports and confirmed by health card.

The study results showed a significant decrease in high risk behaviours after the intervention, and an elevated ALRI risk amongst those who remained in the high risk behaviour category. A number of methodological weaknesses were evident. For example, the fact that there was only one community in each arm restricted the strength of the evaluation. In addition, the study suffered a high (albeit random) loss to follow-up, which would have had the effect of widening the confidence interval around the estimates of effect. Behavioural response to the study (for example, to the interview and the indoor air pollution measurement process) was also evident among the control group. The design focused only on children diagnosed within the formal health care system and failed to capture ALRI cases that did not present at the hospital. However, the study did adjust for factors that might bias health-seeking behaviour such as income, distance from hospital and frequency of hospital visits. In conclusion, the study allowed for the first scientific exploration of the associations between behaviours, child indoor air pollution exposure and child ALRIs in developing countries.

References:

Barnes, BR. 2005. Interventions to reduce child exposure to indoor air pollution in developing countries: behavioural opportunities and research needs. *Children, Youth and Environments*, 15(1):67–82.

Barnes, BR, Mathee, A & Moiloa, KR. 2005. Assessing child time-activity patterns in relation to indoor cooking fires in developing countries: a methodological comparison. *International Journal of Hygiene and Environmental Health*, 208(3):219–225.

Conclusion

Environmental epidemiology has proved to be a useful tool in the elucidation of the relationships between environmental agents and health. While many studies have become increasingly sophisticated and costly, especially in exposure assessment, the value of relatively simple descriptive studies in environmental epidemiology has been repeatedly demonstrated, resulting in important observations and policy development. There is a need to increase capacity and resources in environmental epidemiology in South Africa in order to inform future environmental health policy.

Useful readings

Aldrich, T & Griffith, J (with Cooke, C). 1993. *Environmental epidemiology and risk assessment*. New York: Von Nostrand Reinhold.

Beaglehole, R. 1993. *Basic epidemiology*. Geneva: World Health Organization.

Useful web sites

International Society for Environmental Epidemiology: includes debates among environmental epidemiology professionals. [Online]. Available: http://www.iseepi.org. [25 February 2007].

World Health Organization: information on global environmental health concerns and methods in environmental epidemiology, as well as publications. [Online]. Available: http://www.who.int. [25 February 2007].

References used in this chapter

Batterman, SA, Cairncross, E & Huang, YL. 1999. Estimation and evaluation of exposures from a large sulfur fire in South Africa. *Environmental Research*, 81(4):316–33.

Department of Health, Medical Research Council & ORC Macro. 2001. *South African demographic and health survey, 1998*. Full report. Pretoria: Department of Health.

Kossove, D. 1982. Smoke-filled rooms and lower respiratory disease in infants. *South African Medical Journal*, 61:622.

Mathee, A, Rollin, HB, Ditlopo, NN & Theodorou, P. 2003. Childhood lead exposure in South Africa. *South African Medical Journal*, 93(5):313.

Mathee, A, Rollin, HB, von Schirnding, YER, Levin, J & Naik, I. 2006. Reductions in blood lead levels among school children following the introduction of unleaded petrol in South Africa. *Environmental Research*, 100(3):319–22.

Mathee, A, von Schirnding, YER, Levin, J, Ismail, A, Huntley, R & Cantrell, A. 2002. A survey of blood lead levels among young Johannesburg school children. *Environmental Research*, 90:181–4.

Pekkanen, J & Pearce, N. 2001. Environmental epidemiology: challenges and opportunities. *Environmental Health Perspective*, 109(1):1–5.

Perera, F & Weinstein, P. 1982. Molecular epidemiology and carcinogen-DNA adduct detection: new approaches to studies of cancer causation. *Journal of Chronic Disease*, 35:581–600.

Richter, LM, Yach, D, Cameron, N, Griesel, RD & de Wet, T. 1995. Enrolment into birth to ten (BTT): population and sample characteristics. *Paediatric Perinatal Epidemiology*, 9(1):109–20.

Sexton, K, Callahan, MA, Ryan, EF, Saint, CG & Wood, WP. 1995. Informed decisions about protecting and promoting public health: rationale for a national human exposure assessment survey. *Journal of Exposure Analysis and Environmental Epidemiology*, 5(3):233–56.

Statistics South Africa. 2003. *Census 2001: census in brief. Report no 03-02-03 (2001)*. Pretoria: Statistics South Africa. [Online]. Available: http://www.statssa.gov.za. [9 April 2007].

World Health Organization (WHO). 1983. *Environmental health criteria no. 27: guidelines on studies in environmental epidemiology*. Geneva: World Health Organization.

World Health Organization (WHO). 1997. *Our planet, our health – report of the WHO Commission on Health and Environment*. Geneva: World Health Organization.

21

Occupational epidemiology

Rajen Naidoo

> **OBJECTIVES OF THIS CHAPTER**
>
> **The objectives of this chapter are:**
> - to define occupational epidemiology and its uses
> - to outline methodological and ethical considerations in occupational epidemiology
> - to define the healthy worker effect and its consequences
> - to discuss different methods of exposure assessment
> - to outline typical outcomes and study designs in occupational epidemiology.

Introduction

Occupational epidemiology is defined as 'the systematic study of illnesses and injuries that are related to the workplace environment' (Checkoway et al, 2004). The objective of the discipline is to prevent disease among workers and this is achieved by attempting to understand the association between work or workplace exposures and diseases or injuries. The discipline provides the tools for recognition and quantification of health outcomes and allows for the determination of occupational exposure limits.

> **Ramazzini, the 'father of occupational medicine'**
>
> *Source:* Wright (1983)
>
> Bernardino Ramazzini, accredited as the 'father of occupational medicine' (quoted in Wright, 1983) was the first, in the late 17th century, to study systematically the relationship between workplace exposures and disease. He is still widely quoted, for example:
>
> 'When a doctor visits a working-class home he should be content to sit on a three-legged stool, if there isn't a gilded chair, and he should take time for his examination; and to the questions recommended by Hippocrates, he should add one more — what is your occupation?'
>
> 'Medicine, like law, should make a contribution to the well being of workers and see to it that so far as possible they should exercise their callings without harm.'

Occupational epidemiology presents researchers with opportunities not usually found in other branches of epidemiology. Basing studies in a specific factory, workplace or industry provides researchers with an available population, allowing for the conduct of measurements of health outcomes and exposure. In addition, some workplaces may have conducted exposure or health assessments in the past, and this may be available to the researchers, enhancing their pool of data and the ability to answer questions important to prevention.

The occupational epidemiologist is sometimes presented with 'studies of convenience', for example, when called upon to assist with medical assessments of new entrants into an industry or with exit assessments (which may be requested by the labour union) at retrenchment. By carefully constructing measurement instruments prior to the commencement of these assessments, one may be able to conduct a rigorous study without the need for large financial or human resources.

Challenges facing the occupational epidemiologist

We need to be aware that the workplace is traditionally characterised by a conflictual relationship between the employer and workers. For example, denial of access to the workplace by management or lack of support by the labour union concerned about job security may place serious limits on the ability to conduct or complete an epidemiological study.

A related challenge to the occupational epidemiologist is that of research ethics. Use of company premises, data or company commissioned studies may create a sense of obligation on the part of the researcher. However, we must ensure that the study is conducted with due regard for the ethical rights of the study participants, and must retain the right to publish in scientific literature without interference from any stakeholder. We must ensure that there is proper medical management of workers diagnosed with occupational diseases during the course of the research and that the job security or employment benefits of such workers are not compromised. We therefore have a responsibility to consider how (and whether) the research will result in greater protection of the health of workers.

There are a number of methodological issues in occupational epidemiology. These are summarised in Table 21.1 and we discuss them further in this chapter.

Uses of occupational epidemiology

Identification of new hazards or determination of seriousness of known hazards

Workers face myriad hazards on a daily basis. It is estimated that there are over 60 000 chemicals found in working environments throughout the world, with thousands of new ones entering the workplace each year. New technologies are being introduced into the rapidly evolving workplace, from increasing use of non-ionising radiation (such as cellular telephones and video display terminals) to nanotechnology (i.e. the production of materials 1 to 100 nanometres in size, with unique properties and having the potential for a multitude of uses). The health risks have been documented for only a small percentage of these materials. Occupational epidemiology provides the tools to investigate such potential hazards.

Historically, case series by alert observers have discovered adverse health outcomes associated with occupational exposures. A local example is a case series reported in 1961 by a group of South African medical practitioners of 33 cases of a rare form of cancer of the lung pleura, mesothelioma, all of whom had exposure to asbestos in the Northern Cape (Wagner *et al*, 1960). Similarly, at the BF Goodrich Company in the United States in 1967 researchers found that a cluster of cases of the rare

D | Epidemiology applied to specific areas

Table 21.1 Summary of methodological issues in occupational epidemiology

Study design
- Cross-sectional common as case-control and cohort may not be possible or affordable
- Retrospective cohort possible if good exposure data available
- Relatively easy access to control groups an advantage
- Need for more intervention studies recognised

Sampling
- Often not necessary because all employees are studied
- May require studying several workplaces with similar exposures to increase power of the study

Sources of data
- Employment records; factory layout plans; process and production reports; engineers' reports, accidents and incident reports; occupational hygiene and other monitoring data; medical surveillance and biological monitoring data

Exposure assessment
- Better opportunities for precise characterisation of exposure than in community studies
- Need to decide whether current or cumulative exposure better associated with outcomes of interest
- Need to be cautious in use of historical exposure data collected for reasons other than research

Bias and confounding
- As in all epidemiology, unbiased estimation of strength of association depends on accuracy of exposure and outcome data and ability to control biases and confounding
- Biases include healthy worker effect, recall bias for exposure (which can lead to either over- or under-estimation of an effect)
- Potential confounders include smoking and education (e.g. greater prevalence of smokers among working population; lower educational levels in certain groups of workers)

Analysis
- Control for confounding by stratifying can be difficult because of the small sample size
- Multivariate regression models useful in adjusting for multiple covariates

Assessing causality (see Chapter 2)
- Exposure-outcome relationships enable dose response gradients to be assessed
- Consistency assessed by studies in different populations with similar exposures
- Establishing temporality between exposure and outcome not usually a problem, but may be for chronic diseases in cross-sectional studies
- Biological plausibility varies owing to limited toxicological information on many chemical exposures
- Specificity of exposure or disease outcome the exception, e.g. asbestos and mesothelioma; most outcomes, e.g. asthma, have multiple possible causes

cancer, haemangiosarcoma of the liver, was associated with exposure to the chemical vinyl chloride monomer.

For many exposures, however, researchers start with a cross-sectional study design to identify new health hazards or to determine their severity in a particular setting. This design is attractive because of its low resource demands. (See Example 21.2 at the end of this chapter.)

Determining causal relationships or aetiology

Confirming causal relationships between health outcomes and specific exposures is the 'holy grail' of epidemiology. While laboratory studies allow researchers to control exposures and measure outcomes carefully, extrapolating these findings to a human population is complex. Community-based studies often do not permit one to construct exposure measures accurately because of multiple exposure types and sources. Occupational epidemiology, in contrast, allows researchers in many instances to identify specific exposures (chemical, biological or physical) which are confined to the workplace, and to measure levels of exposure or develop models of exposure.

The most useful type of study design for addressing causation is a prospective or retrospective cohort design. Researchers have used the retrospective design to confirm, for example, the causal relationship between lung cancer and asbestos. In the early 1960s, Irving Selikoff conducted a 'prospective study retrospectively carried out' on 632 men with at least 20 years of asbestos exposure. Workers exposed to asbestos had seven times more deaths from lung cancer than the reference US population, providing substantial evidence for a causal relationship (Selikoff *et al*, 1964).

Exposure-response relationships

Many types of work are associated with potentially hazardous exposures. The role of occupational health and safety practitioners is to limit or control these exposures in such a way that they present the smallest possible risk to the health of workers. The role of the occupational epidemiologist is to define the exposure level associated with this 'smallest' risk. We can achieve this by examining exposure (or dose) re-sponse relationships. Exposure-response can be studied in animals in laboratories, but generalising these findings to human beings is fraught with uncertainties. By carefully documenting the exposures of workers associated with a particular outcome, we can establish the presence of a gradient: increasing exposure results in greater disease prevalence or incidence. By extrapolating back 'down the curve' to the point at which no disease is seen, we can identify the corresponding level of exposure at or below which the working environment would be safe for workers in that industry.

Both cross-sectional and cohort studies could provide this information, but unless we have good quality historical exposure data, we cannot adequately assess exposure-response relationships for chronic outcomes in cross-sectional studies. In a study of 520 goldminers from South African gold-mines, Churchyard *et al* (2004) were able to show that despite being exposed to levels of quartz (silica) below that of the occupational exposure limit of 0.1mg/m^3, almost 20% of exposed workers developed silicosis, strongly suggesting that this legal level is not protective of workers' health. However, they based their conclusion on the assumption that quartz exposures had been constant over the previous two decades. Also, the study did not include those miners who had left mining because of silicosis or those who developed silicosis after leaving the industry. (See 'The healthy worker effect' below.)

Intervention studies

A potentially important use of occupational epidemiology is to assess the effectiveness of interventions introduced either to reduce risk or to prevent disease. The intervention could be introduced either by the researcher during the conduct of the study, or by another party (management, state, trade union or any other stakeholder), and be evaluated by the researcher. In a study of approximately 2 000 health care workers at Groote Schuur Hospital in Cape Town, researchers found 182 subjects with sensitisation to latex (natural rubber used in gloves), based on immunological testing

(Potter et al, 2001). The researchers introduced an intervention in which all those sensitive to latex were advised to wear only non-latex gloves and avoid environments where powdered latex gloves were used. They followed up this group 3-6 months later. Almost all of these sensitised workers stopped using latex gloves, and about 80% experienced a reduction in or complete cessation of symptoms, with overall a statistically significant reduction in skin or eye symptoms. This study showed that introducing an intervention such as latex-free gloves in a health care environment may substantially reduce the risk of work-related allergy symptoms among those sensitised to latex.

Prevention of disease and reduction of exposure through optimal medical surveillance

Another form of intervention in occupational medicine is medical surveillance of exposed workers for a specific disease in order to detect early abnormality as a basis for action. Deciding on the most appropriate test or instrument for a medical surveillance programme for a specific health outcome requires evidence of the sensitivity and specificity of the test used to detect the outcome. (See Figure 9.4, Chapter 9.) We can use epidemiological studies to measure these components of validity as well as the cost and usefulness of such surveillance. The use of standardised and validated instruments (such as questionnaires) is important in medical surveillance. Examples of such validated instruments are given under 'Useful readings' at the end of this chapter.

The healthy worker effect

A distinctive problem of occupational epidemiology is the healthy worker effect. Some have described this as a confounder, while others have chosen to characterise it as an effect modifier (Robins, 1989) (see Chapter 12). It can seriously bias the results of an epidemiological study. In studies of mortality, this effect is characterised by the 'lower relative mortality, from all causes combined, in an occupational cohort' (Checkoway et al, 2004), and arises from comparing a working population to a non-working population.

The healthy worker effect consists of three distinct types, each of which is graphically represented below. The first, the *healthy worker survivor* effect, results when workers who become ill are 'selected out' of employment (Figure 21.1(a)). This effect can be particularly strong if the exposures of the working environment contribute to the health outcome under study. For example, if asthmatic workers exposed to dust leave the workforce, through either medical disability or resignation, this will result in reduced risk estimates in a cross-sectional study assessing the relationship between the dust and asthma. (See Example 21.1 at the end of this chapter.)

The second type is the *healthy worker selection* (or hire) effect (Figure 21.1(b)). Here healthier workers are more likely to be given employment than those with a history of health problems, resulting in workers more resistant to adverse outcomes to various pollutants being employed. This could 'mask' the health impact of a potential hazard in a general working population.

The third type occurs particularly in mortality studies and is related to the length of time that the population has been followed up ('*time since hire effect*') (Figure 21.1(c)). The relative risk of death or disease of employed workers compared to the general population is the lowest (protective effect of employment) in the period shortly after employment, slowly reaching estimates of equal risk as the cohort is followed up over time.

The researcher can minimise the healthy worker *survivor* effect by analysing currently employed and formerly employed workers separately. We can offset the healthy worker *selection* effect at least partially by selecting

Figure 21.1(a) Healthy worker survivor effect

Time of hire

Ill workers ending work

Healthier workers continuing work

Sampling for cross-sectional study

Time

Figure 21.1(b) Healthy worker selection effect

Ill workers not selected to work

Time of hire

Healthier workers selected to work

Sampling for cross-sectional study

Time

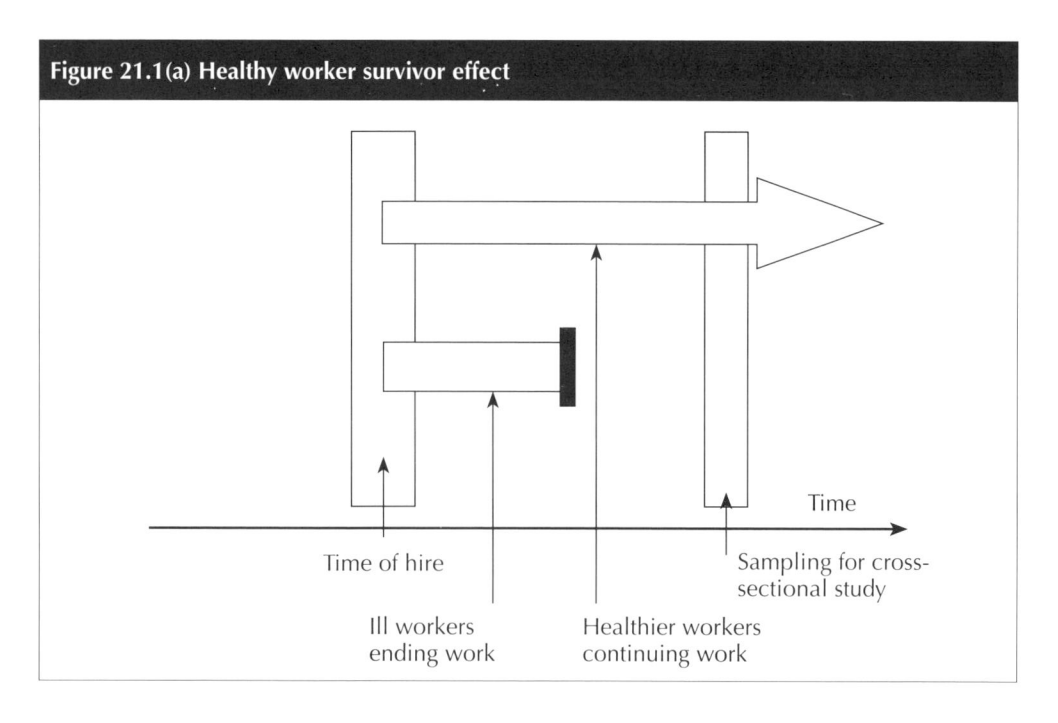

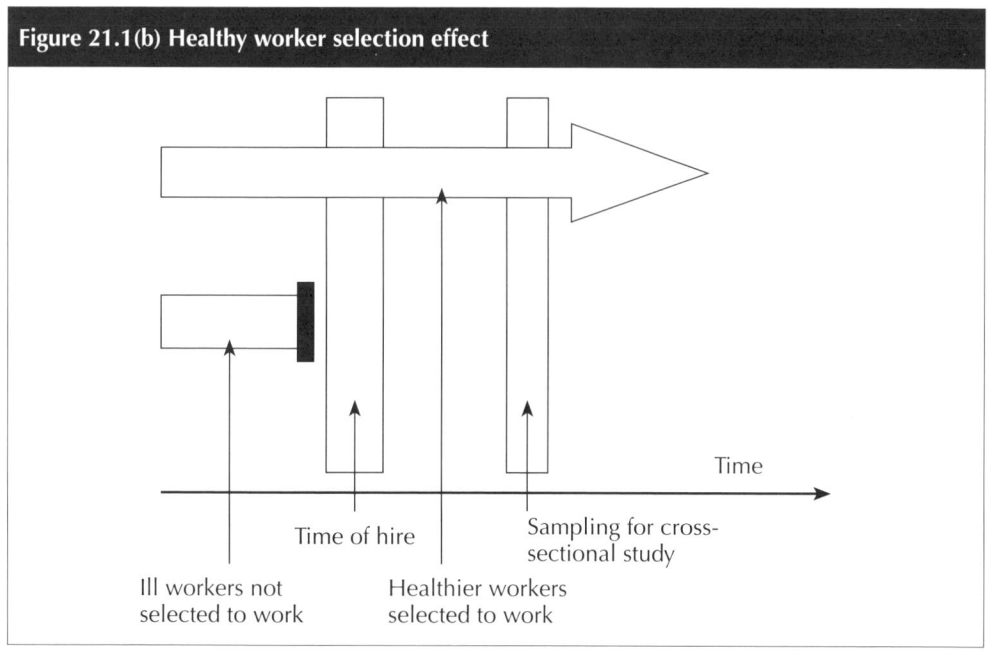

controls having low or no exposure from within the same workforce as the study sample, rather than from an external population. Analytical approaches to controlling 'time since hire effect' are complex and beyond the scope of this text. We direct interested readers to the dedicated occupational epidemiology texts listed in the 'Useful readings' section at the end of this chapter.

Figure 21.1(c) Time since hire effect

Time of hire

Hire of new workers of same age as current workers

Cohort with much larger cumulative exposures

Newly hired cohort with lower cumulative exposures

Sampling for cross-sectional study – similar ages, different cumulative exposures

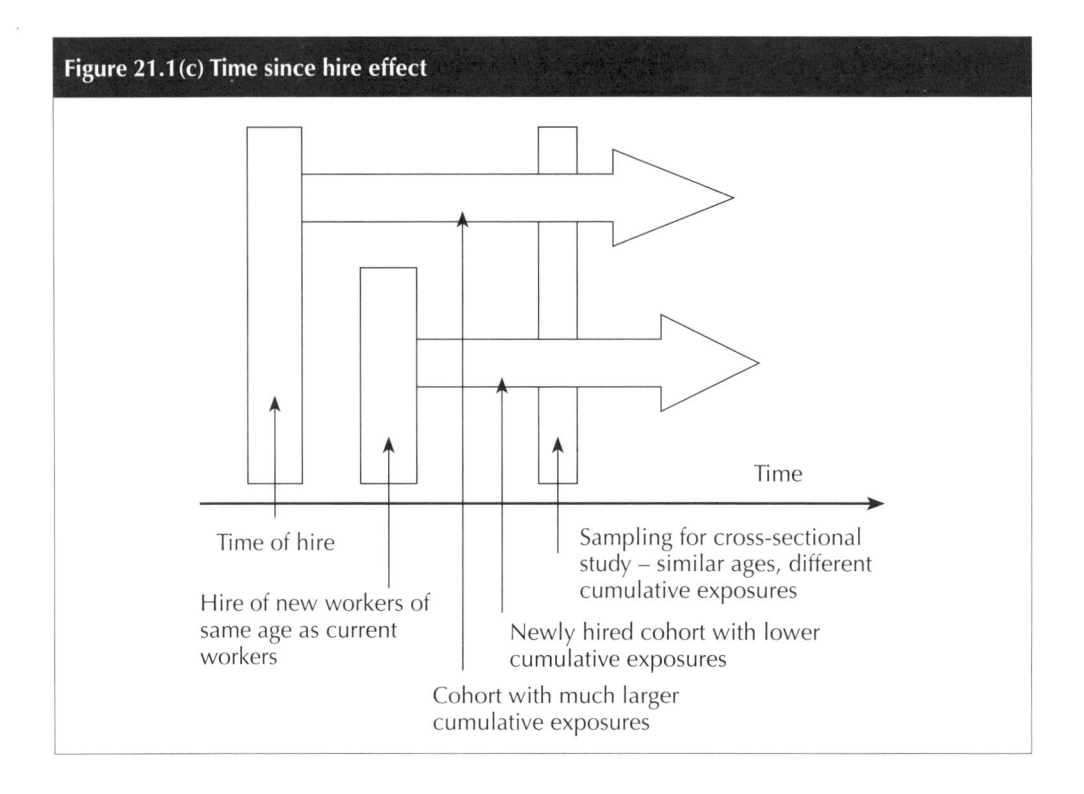

Exposure assessment

Occupational epidemiology allows the researcher to make reasonably precise assessments of exposure based on the understanding of the work processes and exposures in the study population. Quantification of exposure is an attempt to characterise the concentration of workplace toxin at the point of biological effect (human organ or cell) – the true 'dose'. We use levels of exposure in the workplace as a surrogate measure for dose.

Table 21.2 shows the process of stepwise exposure assessment. The first step in characterising exposure is the identification of the exposures and the potentially hazardous work processes. The type of exposure data that the researcher requires depends on the routes of exposure and the health outcome of interest. Acute illness episodes (e.g. asthma attacks) or biological effects occurring shortly after exposure (e.g. cross-work shift lung function changes) require short-term exposure measures such as daily averages of dust concentrations. In contrast, chronic diseases (e.g. kidney dysfunction owing to lead exposure (Ehrlich et al, 1998)) require measures of lifetime exposure. The more accurately the researcher is able to characterise exposure, the lower the likelihood of bias or exposure misclassification. With sufficient funding we may be able to conduct occupational hygiene monitoring of participants to determine current levels of exposure.

However, the reconstruction of historical exposures or the calculation of cumulative lifetime exposure is usually difficult. The first step in determining historical exposures is to identify the possible sources of data. Based on this information, the researcher defines the various processes within the industry, factory or section under observation. For this defined area, we obtain details of the different types of jobs. The varying levels of exposure in the different jobs or job categories over the period that the study

Table 21.2 Stepwise exposure assessment in occupational epidemiology

	No quantitative data available	
Increasing specificity of exposure measure ↓	Ever worked in industry	Crudest form of exposure measure in occupational epidemiology.
	Years worked in industry	
	Years worked in a specific job classified by presumed level of exposure (e.g. low, medium, high)	
	Quantitative data available	
	Industry-wide exposure data (historical data)	Generally maintained by regulatory agencies from data supplied by companies. A local example is the mining industry data maintained by the Department of Minerals and Energy.
	Factory wide exposure data – area or personal sampling (historical data)	Companies may conduct their own workplace environmental monitoring. These may be useful to the researcher, who must assess the data for quality.
	Within factory operation/ job/ exposure zone specific exposure data – area or personal sampling (current data)	Depending on the health outcomes, the researcher may require current data that are more specific to the work activity under study. The researcher will have to take the responsibility of conducting these assessments.
	Within factory operation/job/exposure zone specific exposure data – area or personal sampling (historical and current data)	Depending on health outcomes, particularly if chronic, researcher may have to make use both of historical data (collected by parties other than the researcher) and current data collected by the researcher. These datasets may have to be combined using computer modelling.
	Creation of Job Exposure Matrix (JEM)	Using current and/or historical operation/exposure zone specific data, together with knowledge of years of exposure in each operation/exposure, a JEM can be created, providing a table as shown in Figure 21.2.

participants were employed are then qualitatively or quantitatively assessed. Finally, we determine the number of years each worker has spent in each job or job category. In so doing, we begin to compile a *job-exposure matrix* (see Figure 21.2), where $X(j,t)$ is the exposure level for time period t for a particular job, exposure zone or operation j within the particular work environment under study. On the basis of this exposure matrix, the individual lifetime exposure (cumulative exposure) for each participant in the study can be calculated by $\Sigma X(j,t)$ (i.e. the sum of all individual exposures).

Typical outcomes and study designs in occupational epidemiology

Occupational epidemiology is characterised by the study of many different types of outcomes, including death (mortality studies), incident cases (case-control and cohort studies), prevalent cases (cross-sectional studies), physiological outcomes (such as lung function) or biomarker outcomes (measurement of enzyme levels or changes). Table 21.3 outlines typical outcomes in epidemiology, with their associated study design.

Figure 21.2 A job exposure matrix

Exposure zone/Job description/Operation	Time periods			
	T(1)	T(2)	T(3)	T(t)
J(1)	X(1,1)	X(1,2)	X(1,3)	X(1,t)
J(2)	X(2,1)	X(2,2)	X(2,3)	X(2,t)
J(3)	X(3,1)	X(3,2)	X(3,3)	X(3,t)
J(j)	X(j,1)	X(j,2)	X(j,3)	X(j,t)

Table 21.3 Typical outcomes and associated study designs

Outcome variable type	Study design	Exposure-outcome examples
Death	Retrospective cohort studies	Bladder cancer deaths associated with past textile dye exposures
Incident cases	Prospective cohort studies	Acute cardiac illness among carbon monoxide exposed workers
Prevalent cases	Cross-sectional surveys	Silicosis among underground goldminers
Physiological outcomes	Cross-sectional study	Hearing loss due to noise exposure
	Cohort study	Declines in lung function over time (period under study) owing to dusty work
Pathological outcomes	Autopsy studies	Emphysema in coalminers
Biomarker (biological effect) outcomes	Cross-sectional study	Blood enzyme changes among workers exposed to pesticides

Conclusion

Occupational epidemiology allows us to understand better the relationship between health effects and workplace exposures. This information, in turn, is essential to occupational medical practitioners, policy-makers, management and labour unions in their attempts to create a healthier and safer working environment for workers. The prospective occupational epidemiologist, however, needs to keep in mind the difficulties associated with conducting research in workplaces and the methodological and legal problems that typify occupational epidemiology.

Occupational epidemiology | 21

> **EXAMPLE 21.1**
>
> **Lung function changes among South African coalminers – example of healthy worker survivor effect**
>
> South Africa is the third largest producer of coal internationally, with some 100 000 workers employed in the industry. Respiratory outcomes associated with respirable coal dust exposure has not been previously described among South Africans. Researchers investigated the dose-response relationship between respirable dust exposure and lung function among current and ex-coalminers, controlling for potential confounding by smoking and history of tuberculosis. They interviewed workers (684 current and 188 ex-miners) from three coalmines in Mpumalanga province, South Africa, and obtained work histories from company records. Trained technicians performed lung function testing and did dust sampling. Regression models examined the associations of cumulative dust exposure with lung function (percentage predicted of forced expiratory volume in one second (FEV_1) and of forced vital capacity (FVC)), controlling for smoking, past history of tuberculosis and employment status.
>
> When stratifying on employment status (currently employed versus ex-employees), ex-miners had a lower mean percentage predicted lung function than current miners for each cumulative exposure category (low, medium and high categories), as shown in Figure 21.3. Among the currently employed miners, those within the high exposure category had significantly lower lung function than those in the medium exposure category, which was consistent with an exposure-related effect. However, there were no significant differences in lung function between workers in the high and low exposure categories. Multivariate regression analyses controlling for employment status, smoking history, history of tuberculosis and exposure categories indicated that ex-miners had a significantly greater exposure-related lung function loss than their currently employed counterparts.
>
> **Figure 21.3 Mean percentage predicted lung function (FEV_1) for different categories of cumulative dust exposure for current and ex-miners (with 95% confidence interval)**
>
> *Source:* Adapted from Naidoo *et al* (2002)

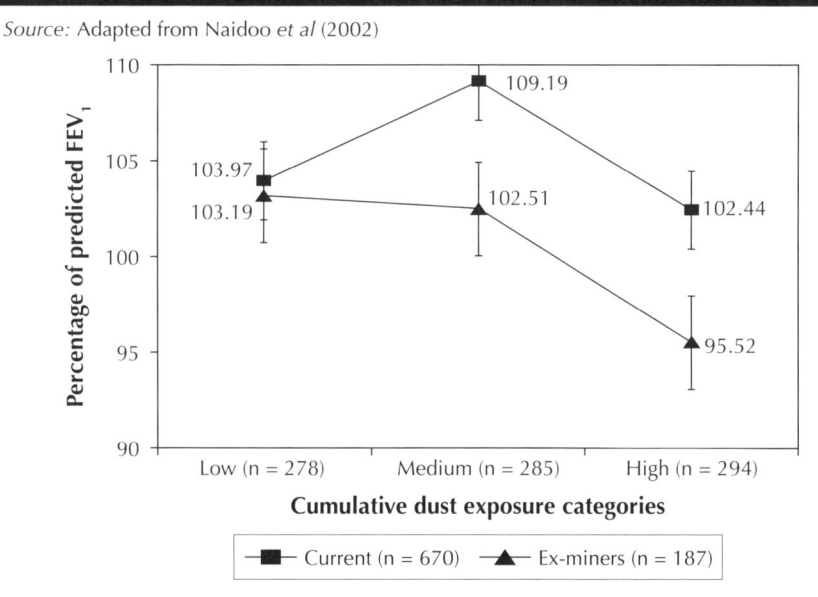

269

These differences related to employment status as well as exposure categories suggested a healthy worker survivor effect. The study concluded that the true magnitude of the dust-related loss in lung function was being underestimated in studies of active workers only, and that policies for hazard control and regulatory occupational exposure limits need to take this into consideration.

Reference:

Naidoo, RN, Robins, TG & Seixas, NS. 2002. Respiratory diseases among South African coalminers. Safety in mines research advisory committee (SIMRAC) report. *SIMHEALTH*, 607. Johannesburg: Mine Health and Safety Council.

EXAMPLE 21.2

Musculoskeletal disorders among South African steelworkers – identifying risk factors for lower back problems using standardised instruments

Lower back problems are common musculoskeletal disorders seen among industrial workers, but prevalences vary across different occupations and populations. Researchers set out to describe the prevalence of lower back problems and associated risk factors among 366 South African steelworkers, using previously field-tested guided questionnaires and a functional rating index (FRI). The FRI is used to assess the extent to which lower back problems affect daily activities. Similarly an Occupational Risk Factor Questionnaire used in previous studies was given to the participants for self-completion.

This study described the work-related risk factors associated with lower back pain problems. Twisting and bending [odds ratio (OR) = 2.8], carrying 5-15 kg objects (OR=7.2), sitting (OR=2.3), bulky manual handling (OR=5.6), kneeling and squatting (OR=4.6) and working on slippery surfaces (OR=3.6) were associated with lower back problems. Lifetime prevalence of lower back disorders in this study was 64%, compared to findings of 80% in other studies.

By using standardised instruments (see 'Useful readings' below for examples), the researchers attempted to ensure that the findings in their study were comparable to those of other studies conducted among similar populations in other parts of the world, and that any differences were not due merely to technical or instrument inconsistencies.

Reference:

Van Vuuren BJ, Becker, PJ, Van Heerden, HF, Zinzen, E & Meeusen, R. 2005. Lower back problems and occupational risk factors in the South African steel industry. *American Journal of Industrial Medicine*, 47(5):451-7.

Useful readings

National Institute for Occupational Safety and Health (NIOSH) & World Health Organization (WHO). 1987. *A joint publication on teaching epidemiology in occupational health.* 87–112. Washington: DHHS Publications..

Steenland, K. 1993. *Case studies in occupational epidemiology.* New York: Oxford University Press.

Useful web sites

Design of measurement strategies for workplace exposures. [Online]. Available: http://oem.bmjjournals.com/cgi/content/full/59/5/349. [25 February 2007].

Ethics in occupational health research. [Online]. Available: http://oem.bmjjournals.com/cgi/content/full/58/10/685. [25 February 2007].

ILO Encyclopaedia on Occupational Health and Safety: *Occupational epidemiology.* [Online]. Available: http://www.ilo.org/encyclopaedia/?d&nd=857400032&prevDoc=857000002. [25 February 2007].

National Institute for Occupational Safety and Health (NIOSH). *Respiratory questionnaires.* [Online]. Available: http://www.cdc.gov/niosh/respire.html. [25 February 2007].

NIOSH. *Quality of worklife questionnaire.* [Online]. Available: http://www.cdc.gov/niosh. [25 February 2007].

NIOSH. *Work history table.* [Online]. Available: http://www.cdc.gov/niosh/jobhist.txt. [25 February 2007].

Tools for ergonomic assessments. [Online]. Available: http://hsc.usf.edu/~tbernard/ergotools/. [25 February 2007].

US National Health and Nutrition Examination Survey (NHANES). Instruments include standardised questions about a variety of health conditions, including respiratory, cardiovascular, musculoskeletal and reproductive health. [Online]. Available: http://archive.nlm.nih.gov/proj/dxpnet/nhanes/docs/doc/nhanes3/adult/. [25 February 2007].

References used in this chapter

Checkoway, H, Kriebel, D & Pearce, N. 2004. *Research methods in occupational epidemiology.* 2nd ed. New York: Oxford University Press.

Churchyard, GJ, Ehrlich, R, teWaterNaude, JM, Pemba, L, Dekker, K, Vermeijs, M, White, N & Myers, J. 2004. Silicosis prevalence and exposure-response relations in South African goldminers. *Occupational and Environmental Medicine*, 61(10):811–16.

Ehrlich, R, Robins, T, Jordaan, E, Miller, S, Mbuli, S, Selby, P, Wynchank, S, Cantrell, A, De Broe, M, D'Haese, P, Todd, A & Landrigan, P. 1998. Lead absorption and renal dysfunction in a South African battery factory. *Occupational and Environmental Medicine*, 55(7):453–60.

Potter, PC, Crombie, I, Marian, A, Kosheva, O, Maqula, B & Schinkel, M. 2001. Latex allergy at Groote Schuur Hospital – prevalence, clinical features and outcome. *South African Medical Journal*, 91(9):760–5.

Robins, JM. 1989. The control of confounding by intermediate variables. *Statistics in Medicine*, 8:679–701.

Selikoff, IJ, Hammond, EC & Churg, J. 1964. Asbestos exposure and neoplasia. *Journal of the American Medical Association*, 188:22–6.

Wagner, JC, Sleggs, CA & Marchand, P. 1960. Diffuse pleural mesothelioma and asbestos exposure in the North Western Cape Province. *British Journal of Industrial Medicine*, 17:260–71.

Wright, WC. 1983. *Diseases of workers.* Revision with translation and notes of the original work by Ramazzini, B (1713). New York: The Classics of Medicine Library, Division of Gryphon Editions.

22

Measuring disability in surveys

Marguerite Schneider

> **OBJECTIVES OF THIS CHAPTER**
>
> The objectives of this chapter are:
> - to provide a framework for understanding and defining disability
> - to explain how to select an aspect of functioning and disability for measurement that matches the purpose of the data collection
> - to describe methodological issues in disability surveys such as choice of questions, sampling, dealing with refusals and training of interviewers.

Introduction

The measurement of disability is an emerging field of study arising from two main sources. On the one hand the efforts of the disability rights movement have highlighted the need to integrate disability issues into all planning and policies. On the other hand, the recognition from the public health field of the importance of understanding the consequences of living with a chronic condition or disability has prompted the need to collect information on functioning and disability.

In order for researchers to collect information on disability and interpret it meaningfully they need to clarify a number of elements. These include the definition and measurement of disability, the measurement tool used and the method of data collection. This chapter aims to assist the researcher in this process. The focus is on collecting disability statistics in surveys and not on clinical studies. However, we should apply the principles outlined for defining and measuring disability in surveys to clinical studies as well.

Because the definitions of disability and its measurement are currently interpreted in a range of different ways, we need to start this chapter by setting out a framework for defining disability in a way that allows us to decide on relevant measurement tools. These tools can then be applied to individual level clinical interventions, clinical studies, or surveys for establishing prevalence at population level. They can be developed for specific impairments or general disability. Impairment-specific tools focus on one impairment (e.g. spinal cord injuries), while more general tools cover a range of impairments.

The current status of disability statistics globally reveals large differences across different regions. Low and middle income countries generally have lower prevalence figures than high income countries. The United Nations Statistics Division shows variations from 0.2% (India) through to 33% (Norway) in its disability database in which data received from countries are collected (http://unstats.un.org/unsd/disability). These results are not comparable and cannot be said to be measuring the same thing.

Methodological factors influencing inter-country disability prevalence

Some methodological factors have been clearly recognised as explaining these inter-country differences in disability prevalence. These factors include:
- the type and wording of the questions used in the data collection instrument: e.g. 'are you deaf, blind or crippled?' versus 'do you have difficulty hearing, seeing or walking?'
- the definition of disability used: e.g. using 'severe' level responses only versus all levels, including mild difficulty
- the survey method: e.g. using self report versus observation or health examination
- the demographics: high income countries typically have a larger proportion of older people than low income countries, and the sharp increase in prevalence of disability in ages 60 years and above has contributed to a higher prevalence in high income countries
- the level of industrialisation, use of cars and the resulting injuries, and the availability of health care services to treat severe injuries: for example, having injury survivors with permanent impairments versus a high case fatality rate among injured people.

These are factors that operate at the *population level*. There are a number of *individual level* factors that will also play a role in whether people identify themselves as having a difficulty or not. These factors are less well understood but include aspects such as sense of self, level of independence, attitudes to disability and cultural beliefs. More research is required to understand these factors better.

Conceptualising disability

Definition of 'disability'

'Disability' is a complex phenomenon that cannot be captured in a single definition. However, the generic definition provided by the World Health Organization's International Classification of Functioning, Disability and Health, also known as the ICF (World Health Organization, 2001) is a useful starting point. The ICF defines disability as the outcome of the interaction of a health condition and the context of the person with that health condition. The context is made up of both personal factors (internal) and environmental factors (external). If the health condition, personal factors or environmental factors change, the outcome will change as well.

Interaction between ICF components

An example of the interaction between these different ICF components can be seen where, if pain is reduced in arthritis, a person's mobility and independence will be improved. Similarly, if a person with bilateral amputations using a wheelchair faces a flight of stairs, he or she will experience significant disability. The same person in a fully accessible building will experience very little disability. Disability is therefore not only about individuals, but also about the environments in which they live. It is also not a static feature of the individual but rather a changing experience. This makes it very difficult to measure in surveys. What aspect should be measured – individual factors, environmental factors, the changing relationship between them, or something else?

Impairments of body function and structure

The ICF states that the outcome of the interaction can be described at three levels. The first is the body level, where difficulties experienced are called *impairments*. Hearing loss, loss of emotional control, stuttering and loss of a limb are all examples of impairments of body function or structure.

The main focus of intervention for impairments would be accurate medical diagnostic, curative and rehabilitation services. Hence data on impairments are useful to identify service needs and are often important in clinical studies where observation and assessment of the person are possible. The identification of impairments in a self-report format is not reliable as the responses would be sensitive to factors such as access to diagnostic services and recognition of the impairment. The best way to collect information on impairments at the body level is through health examination surveys or analyses of records in the health care system. Health examination surveys are, however, generally costly and time-consuming.

Activity limitations at the person level of functioning

The second level of functioning outcome is the person level, which describes the execution of complex tasks and actions by an individual in a (mostly) conscious manner and brings together a range of different body level functions and structures. This is referred to in the ICF as the Activity component. It is measured by the construct of *capacity*, which refers to a person's ability to execute the task or activity in a standard or specified environment. A standard environment is neither facilitative nor hindering. This is typically the type of measurement undertaken in a rehabilitation clinic by rehabilitation therapists and provides an indication of the person's inherent ability to do the activity. The focus of intervention at this level will be on individually based rehabilitation (e.g. building up muscle strength to improve walking) as well as on provision of assistive technology.

Activity can be measured, for example by:
- measuring a person's capacity to hear and understand a conversation without a hearing aid in a quiet room with only one or two other people
- assessing walking capacity in an environment where the surface is smooth, non-slippery and flat and without the aid of a walking stick.

Participation restrictions at the societal level of functioning

The third level of functioning outcome is that of the societal level. This is referred to in the ICF as the Participation component and is measured by the construct of *performance*. Participation is defined as the involvement in life activities and describes what activities the person actually gets involved in within their usual environments, e.g. home, work, school, recreation and shopping. This component describes the combined effect of the inherent ability of the individual interacting with environmental factors external to that person.

For example, if we consider the walking example further, a person may have some inherent difficulty walking (i.e. mild activity limitation in walking), but is not 'involved' in walking because of the steep incline of the path just outside their dwelling (environmental barrier). The person's participation restriction is therefore moderate or severe for walking. The same person in a different environment and with the use of a walking stick might have no participation restrictions in walking. The activity limitation for walking remains the same in both instances.

Similarly, someone with a mild activity limitation in communicating because of dysarthria (impairment of facial musculature) could have very different experiences in different contexts – one with a supportive and patient listener as opposed to one with an impatient and intolerant listener. The activity limitations remain the same but the participation restrictions will vary.

The difference between activity and participation is in itself a useful measure as it provides a good indication of where the interventions should be focused – whether on the individual or the environment. Activity and participation (personal and societal levels) are aspects of disability that are relatively easy to measure using a self-report format. They require a person to describe their daily experience and rely less on access to diagnostic and other services. So they are useful for measuring disability at both the population level in surveys as well as in clinical studies to complement the measurement of impairments.

Selecting the aspect or aspects of disability to measure

When deciding how to measure disability, we first need to choose a definition, which is in turn dependent on the purpose for which the measure is being developed. There are two steps in choosing how to measure disability, both of which we should complete at the stage of protocol development. The first one is deciding which component of the disability experience should be measured. Once we have selected the component of disability at the conceptual level, decisions need to be made on how to operationalise this definition in respect of what data to collect and which categories (or combination of categories) to use as criteria for defining respondents as being disabled. This second step affects both the data collected and how they are analysed.

We must link the information on any one level of functioning (body function and structure, activity or participation) to information on the other levels of functioning as set out by the ICF in order to provide the full picture of disability in the population being studied. If we consider only impairments, we will miss the information on the impact of these on the person's everyday functioning and the role of environmental barriers and facilitators. If we ask only about activities, we will miss information on services needed to reduce impairments and on the influence of the environmental factors. If we ask only about participation, we will miss information on health care needs for impairments and rehabilitation services for activity limitations.

A historical perspective

Historically the way disability has been measured has mirrored societal understanding of and attitudes to disability. The initial statistics reported on 'deaf, blind and crippled' and reflected a view of disabled people as a marginalised, isolated group within society. The problem was seen as being within the individual and requiring medical intervention, and when this was not successful, as requiring institutionalisation. The rise of the disability movement in the 1970s resulted in disabled people pushing for policy reforms that aimed to integrate rather than isolate disabled people. The focus changed from asking not what was wrong with the person but rather what was wrong with the environment that made functioning difficult for the person. The ICF reflects a further change where both individual and environmental factors are seen as important. This has resulted in a very different manner of asking questions on disability, which is described further below.

Methodological issues in surveys of disability prevalence

Sampling

This chapter does not discuss sampling in any depth as this is covered in Chapter 8 and Appendix IV. This chapter provides some examples of how sample size issues should be considered when determining prevalence of disability in surveys. Since disability has a relatively low occurrence in the population, the sample size should be large enough to yield sufficiently high numbers of disabled people overall and within each disability type to provide accurate estimates. If there is some evidence of the prevalence of various disability types or specific impairments, this can be used to estimate the sample size required.

For example, it is estimated that there are around 6% moderately or severely disabled people in South Africa (Schneider *et al*, 1999). To measure this with great precision (e.g. with a margin of error of 0.5%), a sample of approximately 9 000 people would be needed (see Appendix IV). If the average household size is 4.5 people, a total of 2 000 households would need to be studied. However, if the objective is to measure specific types of disability or to be able to generalise about individual provinces or regions, a much larger sample size would be needed.

Within the sampling unit of the household, the individuals to be interviewed can be selected using a two stage design. The first stage involves a screening set of questions applied to the whole household. The second stage involves two possible approaches or a combination of both.

The first approach is one in which the second stage is used to confirm the responses provided to the screening questions. This will necessitate selecting all or most of the positive responses to the screening as well as a percentage (e.g. 10–20%) of those with negative responses, and administering a further assessment or set of questions to determine the 'true' disability status. The results obtained at the second stage will be used to calculate the prevalence based on the number of true and false positives and negatives obtained on the screening questions.

We would use the second approach when we want more information about people who are disabled. This would entail taking a sample of the people who responded positively on the screening questions and, for example, administering a more detailed questionnaire on life experiences. However, even in this second approach we could also take a sample of those who responded negatively on the screening questions and administer the detailed questionnaire. A combination of both second stage approaches would provide the most comprehensive use of the data – giving both estimates of prevalence as well as more detailed information on individual life experiences.

For example, disability surveys undertaken in Namibia, Zimbabwe and Malawi by Eide and Loeb (2005) used a two stage design in which the second stage involved a more detailed questionnaire for those who responded positively to the screening questions. A further example is given in Example 22.2 below.

Non-responses and interviewer training

Community surveys usually use some criteria for when it is acceptable not to interview a selected respondent, e.g. if the person is too sick or cognitively impaired, or has an impairment that precludes us from being able to administer the questionnaire in the usual mode. In disability surveys, these criteria should not be used, since by excluding such people we are excluding the very population of interest. Efforts should be made to ensure adequate support such as sign language interpreters, use of assistants, pacing the interview, and providing cue cards and other materials such as Braille for Blind people.

Interviewer training is crucial in disability surveys. It is imperative to train interviewers in facilitating the interview process. For example, hearing-impaired respondents need a quiet room with good lighting to allow for lip-reading. A number of techniques exist to manage the different impairment needs.

Data analysis and factors associated with disability

The first step in the analysis of disability data is to use a definition of disability to identify the disabled group of interest. Thereafter, analyses can be done to compare the disabled group to the non-disabled group on a number of variables such as employment status, educational attainment, level of social inclusion and need for services. Typically, the results will show the disabled group to be more socially excluded, less likely to be employed and achieving lower educational attainment than the non-disabled group.

Other analyses examine the association between chronic conditions, activity limitations and participation restrictions. Adamson et al (2004) undertook this type of analysis using a cross-sectional survey of women between the ages of 60 and 70 years in England. They found that '[l]ocomotor activity limitation was strongly associated with social participation' and that '[a]rthritis and coronary heart disease contribute importantly to locomotor activity limitation and difficulties with social participation'. Their article is a good example of asking epidemiological questions about disability.

The lack of a single definition of disability and the need to define disability according to the purpose of the data collection mean that one data set could be used for different purposes by using more than one cutoff point in the response categories. This can be done only if the data are collected using response options that go beyond a binary 'yes/no' format. Response options that reflect different degrees of difficulty (e.g. 'none', 'some', 'a lot' and 'unable to do') provide an approximation to the continuum of functioning and disability. This process is described below.

- *Using only the severe responses:* This will provide a low prevalence and will reflect the proportion of the population who are likely to need personal and technological services on a permanent basis.
- *Using only the moderate and more severe responses:* This will give a higher prevalence and will reflect the more severely disabled section of the population. This would be used for example, to estimate the proportion of the population eligible to receive free health care and disability grants.
- *Using all responses indicating some difficulty:* This will yield a higher prevalence and will include a broader section of the population. We would use this, for example, to estimate the need for services such as housing, health care and education.

Current national and international data on disability prevalence

There are two important international efforts to develop comparable data on disability across countries. One is the set of questions for censuses developed by the United Nation's Washington Group on Disability Statistics, and the other is the World Health Organization's Disability Assessment Schedule (WHO-DAS II) (see 'Useful web sites' at the end of this chapter). Both of these efforts have developed a set of questions that use the ICF as the basis. The Washington Group focuses on measuring activities in six domains of functioning using a self-report format and four response options. The purpose of the Washington Group set of questions is for use in censuses.

The WHO-DAS II has two versions – a long and a short – both of which have been validated in a number of countries. The questions are more detailed than those developed by the Washington Group and are used in surveys rather than censuses where space is limited. The WHO-DAS II questions focus on activities in a number of domains with some questions on participation and impairments. These questions use five response options.

Table 22.1 below presents these two sets of questions.

Table 22.1 Text of functioning and disability questions

Washington Group questions:
1. Do you have difficulty seeing, even if wearing glasses?
2. Do you have difficulty hearing, even if using a hearing aid?
3. Do you have difficulty walking or climbing steps?
4. Do you have difficulty remembering or concentrating?
5. Do you have difficulty with self-care, such as washing all over or dressing?
6. Using your usual language, do you have difficulty communicating (for example, understanding or being understood)?

Response options:
a. no – no difficulty
b. yes – some difficulty
c. yes – a lot of difficulty
d. cannot at all

WHO-DAS II questions:
In the last 30 days how much difficulty did you have in:
- Standing for long periods such as 30 minutes?
- Taking care of your household responsibilities?
- Learning a new task, for example, learning how to get to a new place?
- Concentrating or doing something for ten minutes?
- Washing your whole body?
- Getting dressed?
- Maintaining a friendship?

Response options:
a. none
b. mild
c. moderate
d. severe
e. extreme/cannot do

In South Africa there have been three efforts since 1996 to collect national level data on disability. The Census of 1996 (http://www.statssa.gov.za) asked a question focusing on impairments, but the term 'disability' was included. The prevalence estimate obtained was 6.7%. The Census of 2001 used a similar question but added the concept of problems in participating in daily activities. This yielded a prevalence estimate of 5%. The lower prevalence in 2001 can be explained in part by the addition of the 'participation' component to the question. The people counted were those with difficulties significant enough to cause a limitation in activities and participation restrictions. A national baseline survey on disability commissioned by the Department of Health in 1997 is discussed in detail in the example that follows.

EXAMPLE 22.1

The South African national baseline survey on disability

In 1997 the Department of Health commissioned the Community Agency for Social Enquiry to undertake a national survey on disability (Schneider et al, 1999). The survey selected a sample of 10 000 households and used a set of screening questions based on activity limitations in the domains of mobility, communication, self-care, learning, seeing, hearing, and psychological behaviour. If a member of the household was identified as having a difficulty in one or more of the domains, they were identified as being disabled. One member of the household provided proxy responses for the whole household on these screening questions.

A more detailed questionnaire was administered to people identified as being disabled or to their caregiver. The detailed questionnaire covered services needed and received, education, employment, social security, assistive devices, accessibility of the environment, inclusion within the family and feelings about being disabled or having a disabled child.

The data were standardised to the South African population based on the Census of 1996. The national prevalence of moderate to severe reported activity limitations was 5.9% (95% CI 5.7–6.1). The results were further analysed by race, age, geographical location, age of onset of the disability, sex, type of disability and severity of the overall disability (i.e. whether the person had one, two, three or more domains in which they had activity limitations). Table 22.2 presents some of the data from the study, showing the important service provision gap for most of the services listed.

Table 22.2 Proportion of all respondents reporting a service need and proportion who received the needed service

Service needed	Proportion of respondents reporting a service need (%) (n = 1703)	Proportion of respondents needing a service who reported receiving it (%) (n varies per service)
Health care	68	76
Assistive devices	44	37
Medical rehabilitation	39	39
Counselling for disabled person	28	22
Welfare services	28	22
Educational services	20	23
Counselling services for family	18	6
Traditional healer services	16	62
Vocational training	14	8

Reference:

Schneider, M, Claassens, M, Kimmie, Z, Morgan, R, Naicker, S, Roberts, A & McLaren, P. 1999. '*We also count!*' *The extent of moderate and severe reported disability and the nature of the disability experience in South Africa.* Community Agency for Social Enquiry (CASE) for Department of Health, South Africa. [Online]. Available: http://www.doh.gov.za/facts/index.html. [11 April 2007].

> **EXAMPLE 22.2**
>
> **Prevalence of childhood disability in rural KwaZulu-Natal**
>
> Couper (2002) described a prevalence survey of childhood disability (below the age of 10 years) in the Manguzi subdistrict of KwaZulu-Natal. This was a descriptive study in two stages. The first stage used 'a validated "10 question" screening tool with probes, adapted to include the under-2 year age group'. In the second stage a team of rehabilitation therapists visited the children positively identified on the screening questions and undertook a full assessment of the children to confirm the initial report. The reported rate of disability in the first phase was 8.3% (95% CI 7.1–9.5) while the confirmed rate from the second stage was 6% (95% CI 5.0–7.1).
>
> Although Couper does not provide a clear definition of what component of disability she measured, we can make the assumption from the article that it was impairments.
>
> *Reference:*
> Couper, J. 2002. Prevalence of childhood disability in rural KwaZulu-Natal. *South African Medical Journal*, 92(7):549–52.

Useful readings

Altman, BM. 2001. Disability definitions, models, classification schemes, and applications. In Albrecht, GL, Seelman, KD & Bury, M (eds). *Handbook of disability studies*. London: Sage Publications Inc.

de Kleijn-de Vrankrijker, M (ed). 2003. The international classification of functioning, disability and health (ICF): revision, content and use. *Disability and Rehabilitation Special Issue*, 25(11–12):561–682.

Useful web sites

United Nations Statistics Division: International disability prevalence data and the questions used to collect this data. [Online]. Available: http://www.unstats.un.org/unsd/disability. [25 February 2007].

Washington Group. [Online]. Available: http://www.cdc.gov/nchs/citygroup.htm. [25 February 2007].

WHO web site for the ICF: Includes the WHO-DAS II web site. [Online]. Available: http://www.who.int/classification/icf. [25 February 2007].

Referenccs used in this chapter

Adamson, J, Lawlor, DA & Ebrahim, S. 2004. Chronic diseases, locomotor activity limitation and social participation in older women: cross sectional survey of British Women's Heart and Health Study. *Age and Ageing*, 33:293–8.

Eide, A & Loeb, M. 2005. *Data and statistics on disability in developing countries*. Department of International Development Knowledge and Research Programme (DfID KaR), UK. [Online]. Available: http://www.disabilitykar.net/docs/thematic_stats.doc. [25 February 2007].

Statistics South Africa. 2003. *Census 2001: census in brief*. Report no. 03-02-03 (2001). Pretoria: Statistics South Africa. [Online]. Available: http://www.statssa.gov.za. [25 February 2007].

United Nations Statistics Division. 2004. *Briefing note on the collection and dissemination of disability statistics*. United Nations, Department of Economic and Social Affairs, Statistics Division, Demographic and Social Statistics Branch. [Online]. Available: http://unstats.un.org/unsd/demographic/sconcerns/disability/. [25 February 2007].

World Health Organization. 2001. *The international classification of functioning, disability and health (ICF)*. Geneva: World Health Organization. [Online]. Available: http://www.who.int/classification/icf. [25 February 2007].

23

Psychiatric epidemiology

Alan J Flisher

OBJECTIVES OF THIS CHAPTER

The objectives of this chapter are:
- to describe the worldwide burden of disease attributable to mental disorders
- to outline the measurement challenges in psychiatric epidemiological research, in particular those posed by culture, language, and developmental stage
- to describe the criteria that should be considered in selecting a psychiatric measurement or survey instrument
- to provide an introduction to mental health services research.

Introduction

Psychiatric epidemiology as a sub-discipline of psychiatry and epidemiology is relatively undeveloped in South Africa and other low and middle income countries. Part of the reason for this is that there was until recently under-recognition of the contribution of mental disorders to the burden of ill-health and disability. This contribution becomes apparent when considering the total number of disability-adjusted life years (DALYs) that are attributable to mental disorders (Murray & Lopez, 1996). DALYs are the years of 'healthy life' lost owing to premature death or disability (see Chapter 15). They therefore take into account the impact of both morbidity and mortality. It is particularly important to consider morbidity rather than mortality when assessing the impact of mental disorders. One exception to this is suicide, which can occur with a number of psychiatric disorders such as major depressive disorder and substance-related disorders.

In 2000 12.3% of the global burden of disease was attributable to mental disorders, and five of the ten leading causes of DALYs in the 15 to 44 year age group were psychiatric disorders (Table 23.1). A recent expert consensus panel concluded that about 17% of children and adolescents and about 25% of adults in the Western Cape suffer from mental disorders (Kleintjies et al, 2006).

Despite this evidence of the high burden of mental disorders, the overwhelming majority of people suffering from psychiatric disorders do not receive care, and many of those who do get care receive suboptimal care or are even subject to human rights abuses in treatment facilities. Only 62% of countries worldwide (and only 50% of African countries) have mental health policies (World Health Organization, 2005), and there are extreme shortages of the human and other resources that are necessary to develop and implement appropriate mental health services. Stigma continues to affect those afflicted by mental disorders, including service users, their families, and

Table 23.1. Projected leading causes of global disability-adjusted life years lost in 15–44 year olds, 2000

Source: Murray & Lopez (1996)

Rank	Disorder	% of total
1.	HIV/Aids	13.0
2.	Unipolar depressive disorder	8.6
3.	Road traffic accidents	4.9
4.	Tuberculosis	3.9
5.	Alcohol use disorders	3.0
6.	Self-inflicted injuries	2.7
7.	Iron deficiency anaemia	2.6
8.	Schizophrenia	2.6
9.	Bipolar affective disorder	2.5
10.	Violence	2.3

Measurement challenges in psychiatric epidemiological research

Psychiatric disorders differ from disorders in many other areas of epidemiology in that there is no biological gold standard that we can use to assess the presence of a disorder with sufficient specificity and sensitivity. In cancer epidemiology, for example, histological examination will in almost all cases provide a conclusion about whether malignancy is present or not. In HIV epidemiology, a blood test for presence of the virus will be definitive. In psychiatry, we generally have to rely on reports of internal states or behaviour to arrive at a diagnosis. This situation will in all likelihood change as knowledge of the biological aspects of psychiatric disorders increases, and it is possible that within a decade or two, biochemical, imaging or genetic correlates of a psychiatric disorder will be able to serve as gold standard for the diagnosis of that disorder. In the meantime, psychiatric epidemiological researchers will need to devote a lot of effort to finding or developing appropriate measurement instruments. In this section we will explore some of the considerations in developing such instruments.

Culture

Historically, instruments developed in Western Europe or North America have been applied in the developing world, including Southern Africa. This practice has been based on three assumptions: (a) universality – disorders as described in Western Europe or North America are universal; (b) invariance – the core features are identical regardless of culture or other aspects of social context; and (c) validity – the diagnostic categories of current constructs are valid (Beiser et al, 1994; Kleinman, 1988). Whether or not these assumptions are valid, there are clear advantages of this approach to psychiatric epidemiology. Specifically, it produces data that are comparable across cultures. This may contribute to uncovering the aetiology and clinical course of psychiatric disorders and to the development of effective mental health services.

The ethnographic approach to psychiatric disorders

The above approach has been criticised for imposing on other cultures Western notions of psychiatric disorder which are based on implicit assumptions of normality (Littlewood 1990). It has been argued that there is the danger of misinterpreting culture-specific behaviour as psychopathology, through assuming that certain behaviours or other manifestations of psychopathology in Western culture have the same significance in other cultures. At the very least, this approach can be criticised for ignoring the cultural and other social aspects of psychiatric disorders. An alternative approach has been proposed, which aims to use qualitative methods to understand psychopathology in the context in which it arises (see Chapter 26). Such data can be practically useful; for example, an understanding of local remedies for a psychiatric disorder can be helpful when planning interventions for people with that disorder. These *ethnographic* studies have in turn been criticised for their small scale and limited potential to answer many of the questions confronting the discipline.

What is the resolution of this situation of two apparently contradictory approaches? A consensus has emerged that the optimum solution is to exploit the advantages of both (Patel *et al*, 2006). This has practical implications when conducting psychiatric epidemiological research. For example, we should seek to understand local explanations and manifestations of psychiatric disorders to inform the development of psychiatric epidemiological instruments. This will result in instruments that are sensitive to local circumstances and which can contribute data that are comparable across cultures.

Language

A related challenge is that languages differ in how they deal with mental states such as depression, anxiety, obsessionality, anger and ruminations (Gillis *et al*, 1982). It is therefore of the utmost importance in epidemiological studies to take care in the translation process in developing a psychiatric measurement instrument.

There are generally three steps in achieving a satisfactory translation: (a) translate the concept behind each item, incorporating local idioms of distress; (b) back-translate to the original language of the instrument; and (c) compare the two translations and resolve any discrepancies. Another step that we can take is to have the translation critically examined by a group of professionals who are fluent in the original language and the language into which the instrument has been translated. Finally, the translated version can be pilot-tested with a group of people with the same characteristics as those who will be participating in the study.

Once a satisfactory translation has been achieved there are further steps that can be taken during the administration of the instrument in the pilot and actual study. These steps are listed in Table 23.2. Although much of this applies also to instruments used in studies in other branches of epidemiology, in psychiatric epidemiology we are dependent on reports of internal states and behaviour, which renders these considerations more important.

Developmental stage

Reliance on reports of internal states or behaviour when conducting psychiatric epidemiological studies presents two challenges when the target population consists of or includes children or adolescents. First, children and (to a lesser extent) adolescents may not have attained a sufficient level of cognitive or emotional maturity to identify and communicate their internal states. So if a child denies experiencing depression, this could reflect a developmental inability to label this internal state accurately. Questions should therefore be phrased in

Table 23.2 Steps that can be taken to address language issues when collecting data

Source: Adapted from Parry (1996)

- Employ interviewers who have the language of the interviewees as first language
- Ask interviewees to paraphrase questions to determine their understanding of them
- Ask interviewers to rephrase 'difficult' questions using standard alternatives
- Evaluate whether the response to items make sense based on knowledge of the language, culture and content area
- Observe the interviewee's non-verbal behaviour, taking into account cultural expressions of feelings, to ascertain whether the response to an item is as would be expected

a manner that will be understandable to children or adolescents in the target population. Alternatively, data could be obtained from adult informants, such as parents or teachers. However, adult informants may not have insight into the internal states of the child or adolescent. Conversely, youngsters may not have insight into whether their behaviour (as opposed to their internal state) is abnormal or excessive. We are most likely to obtain a valid measurement if we consider that a particular internal state or behaviour is present if either the child or adolescent or the adult informant reports that it is present (Shaffer et al, 1996).

The second challenge that arises when the target population is children or adolescents is that the significance of feelings or behaviour depends on the developmental stage of the person concerned. Normal development should form a backdrop against which mental health is assessed (Fonagy, 2002). For example, some characteristics which might indicate the presence of a disorder in an older child or adolescent (such as temper tantrums) may be normal for earlier stages of development. The converse also applies; certain sexual behaviours may be normal in older adolescents but indicate problems if manifested in younger children. So instruments that assess psychopathology in children or adolescents should take account of developmental stage.

Validity and reliability

The validity of a construct can be defined as the extent to which an empirical indicator of a concept actually represents the concept of interest. For example, if we have an instrument to assess the presence of posttraumatic stress disorder, it is valid to the extent that it accurately confers this diagnosis. Clearly, we cannot assume that an instrument for which validity has been established in Europe or North America will be valid elsewhere. In the above section, a number of suggestions were made that would have the effect of enhancing validity, such as ensuring that the development of instruments is informed by an understanding of local idioms of distress and achieving high quality translations. These and other steps that we can take to enhance validity are summarised in Table 23.3.

Reliability (also referred to as precision – see Chapter 12) refers to the degree to which an instrument produces reproducible results on repeated testing. It is important to consider reliability for two reasons: (a) if problems of lack of reliability are not addressed, it will be difficult to achieve validity; and (b) it is generally possible to correct a low reliability by structuring and standardising the assessment procedure; by improving the training of those carrying out the assessment; and by averaging repeated measurements. The most important type of reliability when adapting an instrument for use in a different context

> **Table 23.3 Steps that can be taken to enhance validity of psychiatric epidemiological instruments**
>
> *Source:* Adapted from Parry (1996) and Goldstein & Simpson (1995)

1. Take into account variations in culture, language and developmental stage.
2. Conduct pilot studies:
   - Compare results with assessments made by clinicians.
   - Compare the distributions of scores between normal and patient samples.
3. Conduct medical examinations or investigations to rule out physical disorders. Seek convergence from multiple sources of data.
4. In two stage studies (a screening survey followed by in-depth investigation of the screen positives), follow up a proportion of the screen negatives and modify estimates on the basis of the negatives who turn out to be cases.
5. Calibrate the instruments for the population under study, that is, identify the cut-off point at which sensitivity and specificity are maximised.
6. Establish the three important types of validity of an instrument in the population of interest, and make modifications where necessary. The types of validity are:
   - *Content validity:* The adequacy with which the full domain of items is elicited, for example, whether a measure of depression includes all the symptoms and signs of depression.
   - *Criterion validity:* The correspondence with a measure that is external to the measurement of the concept itself and is regarded as a 'gold standard', for example the extent to which a diagnosis obtained from the instrument corresponds to that made by consensus among experts.
   - *Construct validity:* The extent to which our measure of interest is correlated with other theoretically related concepts that are also measured, for example the extent to which a measure of self-esteem in the physical domain is correlated with a measure of general self-esteem.

from the one in which it was developed is *inter-rater* reliability, that is, the ability of two or more interviewers or raters to get the same results for the same subject. See also Chapters 9 and 12 for a general discussion of reliability and validity.

> **The ideal psychiatric measurement instrument: a summary**
>
> An ideal instrument for use in psychiatric epidemiological studies should:
> - be comprehensive in scope
> - provide the means for determining the presence or absence of psychiatric disorders in the general population
> - categorise psychiatric disorder using criteria that are in widespread use by mental health professionals
> - allow for different levels of certainty and severity of the disorder
> - have acceptable measurement properties (for example, test-retest reliability and construct validity), for the population for which it will be used
> - have a version that is suitable for use in the cultural and linguistic context of interest
> - be practically feasible to use: for example it should be brief, inexpensive and (if appropriate) equipped with computer-based scoring algorithms; and

- be able to capture data from both the child or adolescent and an appropriate adult informant (generally a parent) using parallel forms that are easily understood by both the young person and the adult informant (Bird & Gould, 1995).

Of course, there are no ideal instruments. In practice, we need to compromise on one or more of the above criteria, and take other factors into account. Tables 23.4 and 23.5 summarise some instruments in common use in respect of criteria that we should consider when selecting an instrument for studies involving adults and children and adolescents respectively. Only instruments that assess whether psychiatric disorder is present or not are included. Instruments that assess positive mental health or wellbeing, and those that confine themselves to an assessment of functional impairment, are excluded.

Table 23.4. Examples of psychiatric epidemiological instruments for adults

Source: Adapted from Parry & Swartz (1997). (Reference or web site for each instrument listed at the end of this chapter.)

	General Health Questionnaire	**Diagnostic Interview Schedule**	**Composite International Diagnostic Interview**	**Schedule for Clinical Assessment in Neuropsychiatry**
Primary application	General practice populations	Community populations	General and clinical populations	Clinical and non-clinical populations
Focus	Non-psychotic disorders	Major psychiatric disorders, excluding most personality disorders	Major psychiatric disorders, excluding most personality disorders	Neurotic or 'functional' psychotic disorders
Number of items	Varies	Extensive	288 symptom questions	Extensive
Time frame for inquiry	Past few weeks	Current/past six months	Within 2 weeks – lifetime	Present episode, last month, lifetime
Screening and/or 2nd stage	Screening mainly	Screening and 2nd stage (main use)	Screening and 2nd stage (main use)	2nd stage
Time to administer	10–20 minutes	60–90 minutes	75 minutes	60–90 minutes
Level of clinical skill advised	Trained lay interviewers; usually self-administered	Trained lay interviewers	Trained lay interviewers	Trained clinicians
Computer algorithm	No	Yes	Yes	Yes

These instruments can be used to establish the prevalence of psychiatric disorders; establish risk and protective factors for mental health problems, for example through case-control designs (Example 23.1 below); or document adverse outcomes of psychiatric problems, for example through a cohort design (Example 23.2).

Table 23.5. Examples of psychiatric epidemiological instruments for children and adolescents

Source: Adapted from Parry & Swartz (1997). (Reference or web site for each instrument listed at the end of this chapter.)

	Diagnostic Interview for Children and Adolescents	Diagnostic Interview Schedule for Children	Kiddie Schedule for Affective Disorders and Schizophrenia – Epidemiological Version
Primary application	General and clinical populations	General populations	General populations
Format	Structured	Structured	Semi-structured
Time to administer	45–60 minutes (longer if problems are present)	Child: 45–60 minutes Parent: 60–90 minutes	Child: 60–90 minutes Parent: 60–90 minutes
Age range (years)	6–17	6–17	6–18
Time frame for inquiry	Past, current	Past year/6 months	Current/past
Level of clinical skill achieved	Clinicians or trained lay interviewers	Trained lay interviewers	Clinicians
Interviewer observations	Yes	No	Yes
Computer algorithm	Yes	Yes	No

Mental health services research

The focus in the above discussion has been on the development of measures of psychiatric disorder. Studies of mental health services are also important in improving the lives of people suffering from mental disorders in the short and medium term. Figure 23.1 presents a framework that can be used to conceptualise mental health services research in the form of a 'mental health matrix', which has three geographical and three temporal dimensions (Thornicroft & Tansella, 1999).

Examples of questions that have been addressed at the country geographical level for the input, process and outcome temporal dimensions are as follows. What are the appropriate ratios of staff to population for mental health services in South Africa (input) (Lund & Flisher, 2006)? What are the appropriate admission rates and length of stay for people receiving residential mental health care (process)

(Lund & Flisher, 2001)? How have rates of suicide changed over a period of time (outcome) (Flisher et al, 2004)? Further discussion of health services research can be found in Chapter 25.

Figure 23.1 The mental health matrix

Source: Adapted from Thornicroft & Tansella (1999)

Temporal dimension ⟶

Geographical dimension	Input phase	Process phase	Outcome phase
Country or province	Expenditure on mental health services and budget allocation Mental health laws and policies Planning for training of staff	Performance/activity indicators Admission rates Bed occupancy rates Rates of involuntary service use Pathways to care Standards of care	Suicide prevalence Homelessness prevalence Imprisonment prevalence
District or catchment area	Local service budget and balance of hospital and community services Assessment of local population needs Staff numbers and mix Working relationships between services	Monitoring, service contacts and patterns of service use Audit procedures Pathways to care Continuity of care	Suicide rates Homelessness prevalence Imprisonment prevalence
Patient	Assessment of individual needs Demands made by families Demands made by patients Skills and knowledge of staff Content of treatments	Subjective quality of interventions Continuity of clinicians Frequency of appointments Pattern of care process for individual patients	Symptom reduction Impact on care givers Satisfaction with services Quality of life Disability

Note: Not all the elements of the model require epidemiological approaches, for example, mental health laws and policies. They are included in the figure for completeness.

> **EXAMPLE 23.1**

Adjustment problems among Aids orphans (case-control study)

This study examined whether adolescents orphaned as a result of Aids show elevated levels of adjustment problems compared to matched groups consisting of (a) non-orphaned adolescents from the same economically deprived communities, and (b) adolescents orphaned as a result of causes other than Aids. In addition, it investigated whether orphans' psychological adjustment was related to their perceptions of emotional connection, behavioural regulation and psychological independence or autonomy in their relationship with their carer and in their peer and neighbourhood contexts. The sample consisted of 204 10- to 19-year-old adolescents from the Eastern Cape in South Africa.

All the questionnaires were translated from English into Xhosa by translators who spoke Xhosa as a home language. The accuracy of the translated questionnaires was assured by translating them back into English, and comparing the back-translated version with the original version. Any discrepancies were resolved by negotiation between at least two of the translators. The translated measures were then piloted with a sample of 20 Xhosa-speaking adolescents orphaned by Aids living in the Cape Town metropolitan area.

Participants were recruited with the assistance of a number of local schools as well as non-governmental organisations and community based organisations who provide care and support to families affected by Aids. As the study progressed, additional participants were recruited through word of mouth ('snowballing'). Four trained and supervised Xhosa speaking interviewers who had experience in working with families affected by Aids acted as fieldworkers for the study. The interviewers administered all questionnaires verbally in the respondents' home language in a one-to-one interview format. They interviewed participants in private, in their homes or at an alternative location of their choice.

Findings indicated that Aids orphans did not experience more psychosocial problems than other orphans or non-orphaned controls. However, adolescents orphaned as a result of causes other than Aids reported more symptoms of depression and anxiety than non-orphans, and lower self-esteem than both non-orphans and Aids orphans. There were no group differences in antisocial behaviour. When both orphan groups were combined, experiences of connection, regulation and autonomy in the adolescents' relationship with their carer and experiences of connection and regulation in the peer and neighbourhood contexts, were all significantly related to one or more discrete aspects of the adolescents' wellbeing. These results support calls for increasing psychosocial support to orphans, but suggest that service providers should not distinguish adolescents orphaned as a result of Aids from other orphans or vulnerable children.

Reference:

Wild, L, Flisher, AJ & Robertson, BA. 2005. *The psychosocial adjustment of adolescents orphaned in the context of HIV/AIDS*. 15th Biennial Conference of the South African Association for Child and Adolescent Psychiatry and Allied Professions, Durban.

> **EXAMPLE 23.2**

Predictors of school dropout among Cape Town adolescents (cohort study)

The main aim of this study was to examine the predictors of diverse risk behaviours among secondary school students in Cape Town. However, the dataset was also used to examine whether use of tobacco, alcohol and illicit drugs predicted dropout among this population.

A self-report instrument was administered to 1 470 Grade 8 students in 1997. Once they had completed the questionnaire, students were asked to write the identifying number of their questionnaire on a piece of paper and place it in an envelope. They then sealed this envelope, signed across the seal and wrote their names on the outside of the envelope. To protect the anonymity of the students, the completed questionnaires were placed in separate envelopes and sealed by the students. The two sets of envelopes were handed to members of the research team separately. The students were followed up in 1999 (time 2) and 2001 (time 3). The schools were sent a list of the names of the students who had participated at the previous data collection stages. They were requested to gather these students together at a mutually agreed venue and time so that they could complete the follow-up questionnaire. The signed and still sealed envelopes were returned to each student. Once they had opened the envelopes, they were asked to transfer the identifying number onto the new questionnaire. In this way, data were linked while preserving anonymity.

At times 2 and 3, the students completed the same procedure involving envelopes to ensure linking of data. Every effort was made to ensure that as many as possible of the baseline participants completed the follow-up questionnaires at times 2 and 3. Members of the research team attempted to track students who were not present on the days of the second and/or third administrations in the following ways. They conducted repeat visits to the schools on two or three occasions to identify students who were previously absent so those students could complete the questionnaire. Where possible, those who had transferred to other schools were located, and they completed the questionnaire at that school. The research team conducted home visits for those who, despite the above two strategies, had still not completed the follow-up questionnaire. On the basis of the information obtained, the research team was able to allocate each student to one of two groups: dropped out or in school.

The proportion of students who dropped out of school between the onset of the study and its completion four years later was 54.9%. After adjusting for a range of confounders, past-month cigarette use significantly predicted dropout. However, contrary to findings from developed countries, past-month alcohol use and lifetime illicit drug use did not predict dropout. Predictors of dropout documented elsewhere may therefore not be pertinent in the developing world.

Reference:
Townsend, L, Flisher, AJ, Chikobvu, P, Lombard, C & King, G. 2004. *Relationship between substance use and high school dropout in Cape Town. South Africa.* 132nd Annual Meeting of the American Public Health Association, Washington, DC.

Useful readings

Flisher, AJ. 2007. Indicators, measures and data sources for monitoring child and adolescent mental health, risk behaviour and substance use. In Dawes, A & Bray, N (eds). *Monitoring child well-being in South Africa*. Cape Town: Human Sciences Research Council.

Parry, CDH. 1996. A review of psychiatric epidemiology in Africa: strategies for increasing validity when using instruments transculturally. *Transcultural Psychiatric Research Review*, 33:173–88.

Patel, V, Flisher, AJ & Cohen, A. 2006. Mental health. In Merson, MH, Black, R & Mills, AJ (eds). *International public health: diseases, programs, systems, and policies*. Sudbury MA: Jones and Bartlett Publishers.

Useful web sites

International Consortium in Psychiatric Epidemiology. [Online]. Available: http://www.hcp.med.harvard.edu/icpe/. [25 February 2007].

Report of the Surgeon General (USA) on mental health. [Online]. Available: http://www.mentalhealth.samhsa.gov/cmhs/surgeongeneral/. [25 February 2007].

World Health Organization mental health page. [Online]. Available: http://www.who.int/topics/mental_health/en/. [25 February 2007].

References used in this chapter

Beiser, M, Cargo, M & Woodbury, M. 1994. A comparison of psychiatric disorders in different cultures: depressive typologies in South-East Asian refugees and resident Canadians. *International Journal of Methods in Psychiatric Research*, 4:157–72.

Bird, H & Gould, M. 1995. The use of diagnostic instruments and global measures of functioning in child psychiatry epidemiological studies. In Verhulst, FC & Koot, HM (eds). *The epidemiology of child and adolescent psychopathology*. Oxford: Oxford University Press.

Fonagy, P. 2002. Outcome measurement in children and adolescents. In Ishak, WW, Burt, T & Sederer LI (eds). *Outcome measurement in psychiatry: a critical review*. Washington DC: American Psychiatric Publishing, Inc.

Flisher, AJ, Liang, H, Laubscher, R & Lombard, C. 2004. Suicide trends in South Africa 1968 – 1979. *Scandinavian Journal of Public Health*, 32:411–18.

Gillis, LS, Elk, R, Ben-Arie, O & Teggin, A. 1982. The present state examination: experiences with Xhosa-speaking psychiatric patients. *British Journal of Psychiatry*, 141:143–7.

Goldstein, JM & Simpson, JC. 1995. Validity: definitions and applications to psychiatric research. In Tsuang, M, Tohen, M & Zahner, GEP (eds). *Textbook in psychiatric epidemiology*. New York NY: Wiley-Liss.

Kleinman, A. 1988. *Rethinking psychiatry*. New York: Free Press.

Kleintjies, S, Flisher, AJ, Fick, M, Railon, A, Lund, C, Molteno, C & Robertson, BA. 2006. The prevalence of mental disorders among children, adolescents and adults in the Western Cape, South Africa. *South African Psychiatry Review*, 9:157–60.

Littlewood, R. 1990. From categories to contexts: a decade of the new cross-cultural psychiatry. *British Journal of Psychiatry*, 156:308–27.

Lund, C & Flisher, AJ. 2001. South African mental health process indicators. *Journal of Mental Health Policy and Economics*, 4:9–16.

Lund, C & Flisher, AJ. 2006. Norms for mental health services in South Africa: a systematic approach to planning. *Social Psychiatry and Psychiatric Epidemiology*, 41:587–94.

Murray, CJL & Lopez, AD (eds). 1996. *The global burden of disease: a comprehensive assessment of mortality and disability from diseases, injuries and risk factors in 1990 and projected to 2020*. Cambridge, MA: Harvard School of Public Health.

Parry, CDH & Swartz, L. 1997. Psychiatric epidemiology. In Katzenellenbogen, JM, Joubert, G & Abdool Karim, SS (eds). *Epidemiology: a manual for South Africa*. Cape Town: Oxford University Press.

Thornicroft, G & Tansella, M. 1999. *The mental health matrix*. Cambridge: Cambridge University Press.

World Health Organization. 2005. *Mental health atlas*. Rev ed. Geneva: World Health Organization.

References or web sites for instruments (Tables 23.4 and 23.5)

Composite International Diagnostic Interview: [Online]. Available: http://www.hcp.med.harvard.edu/wmhcidi/.

Diagnostic Interview for Children and Adolescents: Reich, W, Herjanic, B, Welner, Z & Gandhy, PR. 1982. Development of a structured psychiatric interview for children: agreement on diagnosis comparing child and parent interviews. *Journal of Abnormal Child Psychology*, 10:325–36.

Diagnostic Interview Schedule: [Online]. Available: http://epi.wustl.edu/DIS/DIShome. [25 February 2007].

Diagnostic Interview Schedule for Children: [Online]. Available: http://chipts.ucla.edu/assessment/pdf/assessments/disc_for_the_web.pdf. [25 February 2007].

General Health Questionnaire: Goldberg, D. 1972. *The detection of illness by questionnaire: a technique for the identification and assessment of non-psychotic psychiatric illness.* London: Oxford University Press.

Kiddie Schedule for Affective Disorders and Schizophrenia: [Online]. Available: http://www.wpic.pitt.edu/ksads/default.htm. [25 February 2007].

Schedules for Clinical Assessment in Neuropsychiatry: World Health Organization. 1992. *Schedule for clinical assessment in neuropsychiatry (SCAN).* Geneva: World Health Organization.

24

Nutritional surveys

Corinna Walsh   Gina Joubert

> **OBJECTIVES OF THIS CHAPTER**
>
> The objectives of this chapter are:
> - to define the role of nutritional epidemiology
> - to describe basic dietary assessment techniques for measuring nutrition at the population level
> - to outline methods used for processing and evaluating information obtained by dietary assessments
> - to describe the basic techniques used to assess anthropometric measurements in children and adults
> - to discuss methods used to interpret anthropometric data.

Introduction

Nutritional epidemiology describes the prevalence and distribution of malnutrition (which includes both under-nutrition and over-nutrition) as a public health problem, identifies and analyses the factors that contribute to malnutrition directly or indirectly, and provides evidence for (or against) strategies to address the problem. Diet and other lifestyle factors, such as level of physical activity and smoking, are closely associated with prevalence and risk of disease, and epidemiological studies are often undertaken to investigate these associations.

In South Africa, diseases of lifestyle such as obesity, heart disease, hypertension, stroke, type 2 diabetes and certain cancers have reached epidemic proportions in all population groups. In developing communities this is largely due to the 'nutrition transition' which is characterised by a change from traditionally healthy diets (high in fibre and low in fat) to the 'western' diet (high in saturated fat and added sugar and salt, and low in fibre) accompanied by physical inactivity (Steyn *et al*, 2006). At the same time inadequate food intake and growth faltering as well as infectious diseases such as HIV and tuberculosis continue to add significantly to the burden of disease experienced in South Africa.

Although a thorough assessment of nutritional status includes medical, social, medication and nutritional histories, physical examination, and laboratory data, nutritional epidemiology is mostly concerned with measuring nutrition at the population level, and therefore dietary and anthropometric surveys will form the focus of this chapter.

Dietary assessments in the evaluation of nutritional status

Dietary assessment estimates food consumption or nutrient intake, and is probably the most widely used indirect indicator of nutritional status. The accurate assessment of an individual's food intake is, however, the most difficult part in the evaluation of nutritional status. Various methods for collecting food consumption data exist, each with their own limitations. The most common ones are described in the next section. Table 24.1 summarises the advantages and disadvantages of the different techniques.

Two main approaches are used for dietary assessment, namely prospective and retrospective. Prospective methods involve collecting current dietary data, while retrospective methods require subjects to recall either recent or past diet.

Table 24.1 Advantages and disadvantages of dietary survey methods

Method	Advantages	Limitations
Food frequency questionnaire (FFQ)	• Ease of standardisation • Representative of usual intake • Relatively inexpensive for large sample sizes • Suitable method for research on diet-disease relationships • Reasonably accurate and valid (quantitative FFQs correlate highly with 7-day weighed records) • Relatively quick to administer	• Portion sizes can be difficult to determine accurately • Response rates may be lower if questionnaire is self-administered • Requires literacy skills if self-administered • Does not provide meal pattern data • Depends on ability of the subject to describe his or her diet • Because not all foods can be included in lists, total consumption is difficult to obtain • The burden on the respondent rises as the number of food items increases • Analysis is difficult without use of computers and special programs • Reliability is lower for individual foods than for food groups
24-hour recall	• Quick, easy and inexpensive • Subject motivation is less of a barrier, burden on the respondent is low and compliance is good • No long-term memory is required • Respondent does not alter the usual diet • Good reliability exists between trained interviewers • Suitable to use with illiterate subjects and the aged, except when memory is a severely limiting factor	• Portion sizes can be difficult to determine accurately • Data on a single-day's diet are a poor descriptor of an individual's usual nutrient intake, because of day-to-day variability • Inability to recall accurately the kinds and amounts of food eaten • Tendency for persons to over-report low intakes and to under-report high intakes of foods • Experienced interviewer required

Food record	• Portion sizes can be measured accurately • Does not depend on memory • Can provide detailed intake data • Can provide data about the respondents' eating habits, such as quantity of food eaten, how prepared, and timing of meals and snacks • Facilitates comparisons between studies using the same method, because it is widely used	• Requires highly motivated and co-operative respondents • Requires a portable scale or household measures • Items such as salad dressings and gravies are commonly omitted • Not all subjects are equally literate • Actual food intake may be influenced by the recording process • Since it is a prospective method, it takes more time to obtain data
Diet history	• A large quantity of information about eating habits can be obtained from a single interview • Assesses the subject's usual nutrient intake • Correlates well with biochemical measures • Provides the most complete and detailed description of food intake • Eliminates individual day-to-day variations	• An interview of one to two hours by a highly trained interviewer is necessary • Difficult to standardise between interviewers • Nutrient intake tends to be overestimated • A co-operative respondent with the ability to recall the usual diet is required

Basic dietary assessment techniques

Food frequency questionnaires (FFQ)

FFQs are pre-printed lists of foods that are important contributors to the population's intake of energy and nutrients. The researcher can use existing FFQ lists or compile one specifically to meet the objective of the assessment and the circumstances of the target population (e.g. to include indigenous foods that are commonly eaten). Respondents are asked to indicate the typical frequency of consumption of each food (qualitative food frequency), and/or to state, in household measures, the average amount consumed on the days when the food is consumed (quantitative food frequency). It is a retrospective review of intake frequency per day, per week or per month.

FFQs can vary in length, ranging from very short (for example, nine food items for assessing intake of a single nutrient, such as calcium intake, to assess the risk of developing osteoporosis) to very long and complex (more than 300 items for a National Food Consumption Survey designed to assess tendencies in eating patterns and usual food intake of the population). An example of a short qualitative FFQ is given in Table 24.2.

FFQs are good to use for describing intake of groups rather than individuals, and are commonly used in epidemiological research investigating the relationships between diet and disease (for example, the role that fat intake plays in the development of cancer).

Table 24.2 Short qualitative Food Frequency Questionnaire

How often are the following items consumed?
(Number of times per day, per week or per month (use only one option))

	/day	/week	/month	Columns
Sweets/chocolates				1–6
Chips (crisps)				7–12
Cake/biscuits				13–18
Cooldrinks				19–24
Coffee creamer				25–30
Coffee				31–36
Tea				37–42
Sugar				43–48
Full cream milk				49–54
Low fat/skim milk				55–60
Eggs				61–66
Peanut butter				67–72
Soya mince/legumes				73–78
Chicken/meat/ fish				01–06
Bread				07–12
Porridge				13–18
Samp/mealie rice				19–24
Margarine/oil/fat				25–30
Fruit				31–36
Vegetables				37–42
Salt/stock/soup powders				43–48
Alcohol				49–54
Water				55–60

24-hour recall

The 24-hour recall is a retrospective assessment of dietary intake, during which a trained interviewer asks the respondent to recall in detail all the food and drinks consumed during the previous 24 hours. The interviewer can obtain the 24-hour recall on single or multiple occasions. He or she should assist the respondent in estimating portion sizes of foods consumed and recalling food and drinks consumed. Multiple 24-hour recalls obtained from an individual and spaced over various seasons may provide a more reasonable estimate of the person's usual intake than one recall.

The 24-hour recall is used to determine dietary intake of large samples (>50 people), and the information is primarily used to determine trends in eating patterns. A single 24-hour recall is not recommended if we wish to determine usual or habitual intake of an individual, since it does not necessarily represent typical intake.

Daily food record or food diary

With daily food records, or a food diary, the subject prospectively records at the time of consumption the types and amounts of all foods and beverages consumed for a period ranging from one to seven days. The subject can quantify food and drink intake by estimating portion sizes using household measures (estimated food record), or by weighing the food and beverages on scales (weighed food record). Respondents must be trained to weigh and measure food correctly and to report accurately the intake of dishes that contain a variety of ingredients, such as pizza or stews. The food record is considered most accurate if the food consumed is documented immediately after consumption, or on the same day.

Multiple food records from non-consecutive, random days, including weekends and covering different seasons are necessary to arrive at useful estimates of usual intake. Food records are generally used for research in small groups (<50 people) or individuals to determine tendencies in eating patterns or usual intake.

Diet history

A diet history is used to assess an individual's usual patterns of food intake and the food selection variables that influence food intake over an extended period of time, such as the past month or year.

A trained interviewer obtains information during an interview with the subject about the number of meals the subject has eaten per day, appetite, food dislikes, the presence or absence of nausea and vomiting, use of nutritional supplements, smoking, and habits related to sleep, rest and work. Usually this is followed by a 24-hour recall or a 3-day food record to cross-check the data.

Diet histories are a comprehensive method of obtaining dietary information, together with other relevant information. They are used for research in small groups or in individuals.

Other methods for determining dietary intake

Other methods used to determine dietary intake include duplicate food collections, visual records such as photographs, and direct observation by trained interviewers (Gibson, 2005).

Factors affecting validity and reliability

When dietary assessments are undertaken, the question arises as to whether we are really measuring what people eat.

Validating dietary intake involves comparing measurements of intake obtained by a specific method with a subject's usual intake. Because it is very difficult, if not impossible, to know a person's true usual intake, investigators must turn to criterion validity (see Chapter 9). The latter can be defined as the comparison of a new instrument with another that has a greater degree of demonstrated validity. An example of a validation study would include comparing dietary intake obtained using a FFQ with dietary intake obtained by means of weighed records.

Several factors can affect the validity and reliability of a measuring instrument:
- People may consciously or unconsciously change their usual intake when attention is focused on their diet. These altered food intake patterns may be performed to simplify recording, or to impress the interviewer, thereby decreasing validity of the obtained data.
- People tend to forget what they have actually eaten.
- People have inaccurate knowledge of portion sizes.
- People over-estimate or under-estimate the amounts of food consumed.

The validity and reliability of assessments depend on the skill and training of the interviewer and the co-operation of the subject.

Methods used for processing and evaluating diet information

Adequacy of food intake is measured by comparing each individual's intake with an external reference standard. This can then be summarised as the percentage of the sample or population above or below this standard. Comparison of data with general guides of recommended food consumption, such as food groups, the food guide pyramid, or food-based dietary guidelines can be used to evaluate the adequacy of food intake.

Nutrient intake is determined using food composition tables (such as the MRC Food Composition Tables, 1991) or food composition computer database programmes (such as FoodFinder3). (See 'References used in this chapter' at the end of this chapter.)

Food composition tables usually list the amount of nutrients in 100 g of edible food and can be consulted to calculate the nutrient content of foods by hand. When food composition computer databases are used, the dietary information needs to be coded, using the specific code in the database and weight in grams of each food.

Adequacy of nutrient intake is determined by comparing the actual nutrient intakes to standards for nutrient intake, such as the Dietary Reference Intakes (DRIs) of the Institute of Medicine, USA (Table 24.3). DRI is an umbrella term for a set of reference values that indicate the amounts of nutrients needed in the diets of healthy individuals. A booklet summarising the DRIs for energy and nutrients has been compiled by the Nutrition Information Centre at the University of Stellenbosch and can be obtained from http://www.sun.ac.za/nicus. These include Estimated Average Requirements (EAR), Recommended Dietary Allowance (RDA), Adequate Intake (AI) and Tolerable Upper Intake Level (UL).

Table 24.3 Dietary Reference Intakes (DRI)	
Estimated Average Requirements (EARs)	The amount of a nutrient estimated to meet the needs of 50% of people in the same gender and life-stage group
Recommended Dietary Allowances (RDAs)	Recommendations calculated to meet the needs of nearly all healthy individuals in each gender and life-stage group
Adequate Intakes (AIs)	Intakes used as a goal when no RDA or EAR exists. An approximation of the average nutrient intake that appears to sustain a desired indicator of health
Tolerable Upper Intake Level (UL)	The *maximum* level of daily intake of a nutrient that is unlikely to pose health risks to almost all individuals in the specified group. A level that can probably be tolerated; not a recommended level

In epidemiological studies the RDA or AI of the specific nutrient is usually used. A value of $\leq 67\%$ of the RDA or AI is commonly used as the cut-off point to identify inadequate intake of a nutrient.

A dietitian, trained in dietary research methodology, can be consulted to assist the researcher to process and evaluate diet information.

Anthropometric evaluation of nutritional status

Anthropometry involves obtaining physical measurements of an individual, and relating these to standards that reflect, among other factors, the health and nutritional status of the individual. In this way malnutrition (both under-nutrition and over-nutrition) can be identified, growth can be monitored and the impact of intervention programmes can be determined. Measures of anthropometry, such as weight and fat percentage, can be used to predict risk of developing diseases of lifestyle such as obesity (see Example 24.2 at the end of this chapter).

The single most important characteristic of an anthropometric measurement is simplicity of measurement. In epidemiological studies the most commonly used measurements are height, weight, skinfold thickness and circumference measurements. All of these need to be measured using the correct techniques to ensure reliability of the results obtained (Gibson, 2005; Lee & Nieman, 2003).

Assessing the nutritional status of children

Anthropometric indicators of nutritional status

Reduced dietary intake results in reduced body size, which can be correlated with the degree of malnutrition. In children, the measurements weight, height and age are used widely, and these three measurements are used to form the indicators weight-for-age, height-for-age and weight-for-height.

Weight-for-age is the most frequently used anthropometric indicator. Weight-for-age compares the weight of a child to the weight of a 'normal' child of the same age. Its ease of measurement, low cost and suitability for screening make it particularly suitable for assessing the nutritional status of children. Furthermore, weight-for-age can alter relatively quickly as a result of seasonal food shortages, droughts, food price variations, changing availability of food, and changing health conditions. A strong association exists between weight-for-age and mortality.

The measurement of height in addition to weight is very useful. Height-for-age compares the height of a child to the height of a 'normal' child of the same age, while weight-for-height compares the weight of a child to the weight of a 'normal' child with the same height. The use of weight-for-height in addition to weight-for-age takes body size differences into consideration. This indicator is very seldom used in routine growth monitoring, but is an important measure in nutritional epidemiology, especially where birth date is not available.

Head circumference-for-age and mid-upper arm circumference-for-age can also be used as indicators of chronic protein energy under-nutrition in children (the former mainly in children under two years).

The Centers for Disease Control have published body mass index (BMI)-for-age growth charts to use as a screening tool for malnutrition in children (http://www.cdc.gov/nccdphp/growthcharts). Body mass index (BMI) accounts for differences in body composition by defining the level of fatness according to the relationship of weight to height, consequently eliminating dependence on frame size.

$$\text{BMI} = \frac{\text{Weight in kg}}{(\text{Height in m})^2}$$

Interpretation

When analysing the weights and heights of children, valid cut-off points or 'norms' need to be chosen. The National Center for Health Statistics (NCHS) tables from the USA, which present data categorised by sex and age, in percentiles or standard deviations above or below the NCHS *median*, are most commonly used (http://www.who.int/nutgrowthdb/reference/en/).

In Primary Health Care, growth charts present the NCHS weight-for-age percentiles on a chart indicating the 3rd, 50th and 97th percentile lines. By plotting the child's weight against his or her age at consecutive ages, the growth of the child can be monitored. For example, for girls aged five years the NCHS-tabulated 3rd percentile of weight-for-age is 14 kg; that is, in the reference population, only 3% of girls aged five years weighed 14 kg or less. By referring to the reference population, we can determine which children or what proportion of children are undernourished. Not only children who fall below the 3rd percentile but any child who shows a decline in weight-for-age is at risk.

Height and weight measurements below the third and fifth percentiles of the NCHS standards or below minus two standard deviations (<−2SD, also known as a *z-score* of <−2) of the NCHS median, are generally used as cut-off points to identify low weight-for-age (underweight), low height-for-age (stunting) and low weight-for-height (wasting).

A decreased height-for-age (stunting) is an indicator of chronic undernutrition, while a decreased weight-for-age (underweight) is an indication of more acute undernutrition. A reduced weight-for-height is an indicator of a recent and severe episode of undernutrition, but cannot identify children with mild undernutrition.

In children, BMI is also evaluated using percentile cut-offs that compare values for a given child with a national sample of children of the same age and sex (Table 24.4).

Table 24.4 Classification of BMI-for-age for children (kg/m^2)	
Underweight	< 5th percentile
At risk for overweight	85th to 95th percentile
Overweight	> 95th percentile

Computer software, such as Epi Info 2004 (http://www.cdc.gov/epiinfo/), is very useful in the analysis of anthropometric measurement of children. In addition, a set of training modules for health professionals to assess growth of children and adolescents can be found at http://www.cdc.gov/nccdphp/dnpa/growthcharts.htm.

Assessing the nutritional status of adults

In adults, body weight may be interpreted by various methods, including ideal weight-for-height and BMI (Table 24.5). Ideal weight-for-height can be calculated from reference standards such as the Metropolitan Life Insurance Tables, or the NCHS medians (Lee & Nieman, 2003).

Body composition

Body composition is defined as the ratio of fat mass to fat-free or lean body mass (mostly muscle and bone). These two body compartments can be indirectly assessed by anthropometric techniques, and variations in their amount and proportion can be used as indices of nutritional status (Gibson, 2005).

Body composition can be determined by a number of techniques that are mostly not practicable in epidemiological studies (Lee & Nieman, 2003) as well as by skinfold thicknesses and bioelectrical impedance.

Using a skinfold caliper the thickness of a double fold of skin and compressed fat under the skin is measured in millimetres (Figure 24.1). Accuracy of skinfold measurements decreases with an increase in body fatness.

Table 24.5 Classification of BMI in adults (kg/m²)

Source: Gibson (2005)

Underweight	< 18.5
Normal	18.5–24.9
Overweight	25.0–29.9
Obesity, class I	30.0–34.9
Obesity, class II	35.0–39.9
Extreme obesity, class III	≥ 40

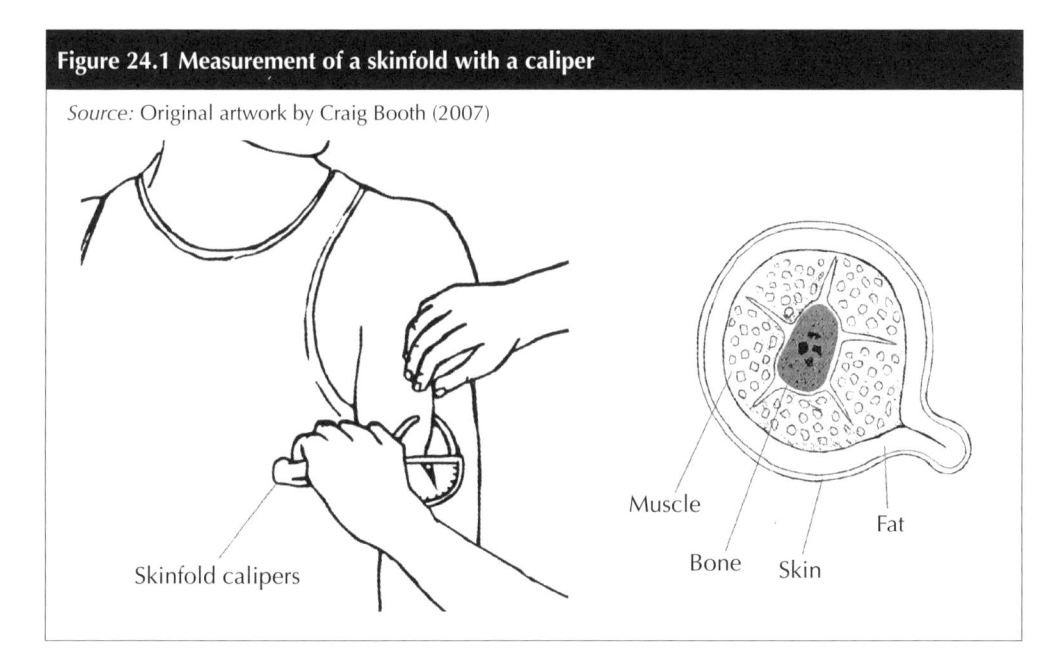

Figure 24.1 Measurement of a skinfold with a caliper

Source: Original artwork by Craig Booth (2007)

Because skinfold thicknesses vary widely among different skinfold sites within individuals, and for the same skinfold site between individuals, body composition is best assessed by measuring multiple skinfold sites, most commonly the triceps, biceps, subscapula, supra-iliac, thigh, and medial-calf. A number of formulae are available for interpretation of fat percentages from skinfold thicknesses (Gibson, 2005; Lee & Nieman, 2003).

Bioelectrical impedance analysis

Bioelectrical impedance analysis (BIA) is another method used to assess body composition. This technique is based on the principle that compared to fatty tissue, lean tissue has a higher electrical conductivity and lower impedance, relative to water, based on electrolyte content. With this method, electrodes are attached to the extremities of a patient, after which a small electrical current is passed through the electrodes to obtain electrical resistance measurements on a machine.

Reliability of measurements may be influenced by fever, electrolyte imbalance, obesity and the hydration status of the patient. Despite this, BIA is as good as, if not slightly better than, skinfold measurements in predicting percent body fat. The method is also safe and comfortable for the patient, and the measuring instrument is convenient to use, portable, quick and non-invasive, making it useful for field surveys.

Fat distribution

Determining the ratio of the waist circumference to the hip circumference (WHR) is an easy way to assess where in the human body most of a person's fat is situated (body fat distribution or body shape).

$$WHR = \frac{\text{waist circumference in cm}}{\text{hip circumference in cm}}$$

WHR provides an index of regional body fat distribution, and differentiates between android (apple-shaped) and gynoid (pear-shaped) obesity. A WHR ≥ 1.0 in men or ≥ 0.8 in women is indicative of android obesity. Android obesity has been shown to increase the risk for obesity-related diseases, including heart disease, hypertension, type 2 diabetes mellitus, certain cancers and infertility.

EXAMPLE 24.1

Energy intake and anthropometric status of Free State children aged 1 to 9 years in the National Food Consumption Survey (NFCS), 1999

As part of the NFCS undertaken in South Africa during 1999, fieldworkers collected information about the usual nutrient intake and anthropometric status of children aged 1 to 9 years. They used a cross-sectional survey of a nationally representative sample. Validated questionnaires, including a FFQ, were developed, and administered to caregivers by trained fieldworkers. Anthropometric measurements including weight and height were carried out using standard methods.

The anthropometric measurements of a total of 203 children in the Free State were included. Stunting (height-for-age < –2SD below the median), an indication of chronic under-nutrition, was the most prevalent form of under-nutrition in these children, ranging from 3.4% in children aged 7 to 9 years to 39.8% in children aged 1 to 3 years. Underweight (weight-for-age < –2SD below the median), an acute form of under-nutrition, ranged from 6.9% of children aged 7 to 9 years to 20.4% of children aged 1 to 3 years. The prevalence of wasting (weight-for-height < –2SD below the median), an indication of severe, recent under-nutrition, ranged from 1.2% in children aged from 4 to 6 years to 10.3% in children aged 7 to 9 years.

A large percentage of children consumed less that 67% of the RDA for energy, ranging from 37% of children aged 1 to 3 years to 71% of children aged 7 to 9 years.

The study identified younger children as a prime target group for nutrition intervention, including supplementary food aid and nutrition education.

Reference:

Labadarios, D. 1999. *National food consumption survey (NFCS): children aged 1-9 years.* South Africa. Directorate: Nutrition, Department of Health.

> **EXAMPLE 24.2**
>
> **Physical inactivity is the major determinant of obesity in black women in the North West Province, South Africa: the THUSA (Transition and Health during Urbanisation of South Africa) study**
>
> Associations between measures and determinants of obesity were investigated in a cross-sectional study of black women in the North West Province. A total of 1 040 women from 37 randomly selected sites in the province were stratified into five groups representing different levels of urbanisation. The association between measures of obesity, namely BMI, waist circumference, waist-to-hip ratio, triceps and subscapular skinfolds, and socioeconomic factors, dietary intakes and physical activity were analysed. The prevalence of obesity (BMI > 30kg/m^2) in the sample was 28.6%. A significant positive association between household income and measures of obesity was found. After adjustment for age, smoking, and household income, significant positive correlations were found between total energy intake, fat intake and BMI. Physical activity index (derived from a subset of 530 subjects) was negatively correlated with BMI and waist circumference.
>
> Overall, women with higher incomes and lower physical activity were at the greatest risk of increased BMI. Of all the predictive factors physical inactivity showed the strongest association with measures of obesity.
>
> *Reference:*
>
> Kruger, HS, Venter, CS, Vorster, HH & Margetts, BM. 2002. Physical inactivity is the major determinant of obesity in black women in the North West Province, South Africa: the THUSA study. Transition and health during urbanisation of South Africa. *Nutrition*, 18(5):422–7.

Useful web sites

Epi Info. 2004. [Online]. Available: http://www.cdc.gov/epiinfo/. [25 February 2007].

References used in this chapter

Centers for Disease Control. Body mass index (BMI)-for-age growth charts. [Online]. Available: http://www.cdc.gov/nccdphp/growthcharts. [25 February 2007].

FoodFinder 3. 2002. *Dietary analysis software program, version 1.0.7*. Cape Town: South African Medical Research Council.

Gibson, RS. 2005. *Principles of nutritional assessment*. 2nd ed. New York: Oxford University Press.

Langenhoven, M, Kruger, M, Gouws, E & Faber, M. 1991. *Medical Research Council (MRC) food composition tables*. 3rd ed. Parow: South African Medical Research Council.

Lee, RD and Nieman, DC. 2003. *Nutritional assessment*. 3rd ed. New York: McGraw-Hill.

NCHS. Growth standards. [Online]. Available: http://www.who.int/nutgrowthdb/reference/en/. [25 February 2007].

Nutrition Information Centre of the University of Stellenbosch (NICUS). 2003. *Dietary reference intakes (DRIs)*. [Online]. Available: http://www.sun.ac.za/nucus. [25 February 2007].

Steyn, NP, Bradshaw, D, Norman, R, Joubert, JD, Schneider, M & Steyn, K. 2006. *Dietary changes and the health transition in South Africa: implications for health policy*. Cape Town: South African Medical Research Council.

Section E

Multidisciplinary approaches complementary to epidemiology

25 Health services research
26 Qualitative methodology: an introduction
27 Economic evaluation

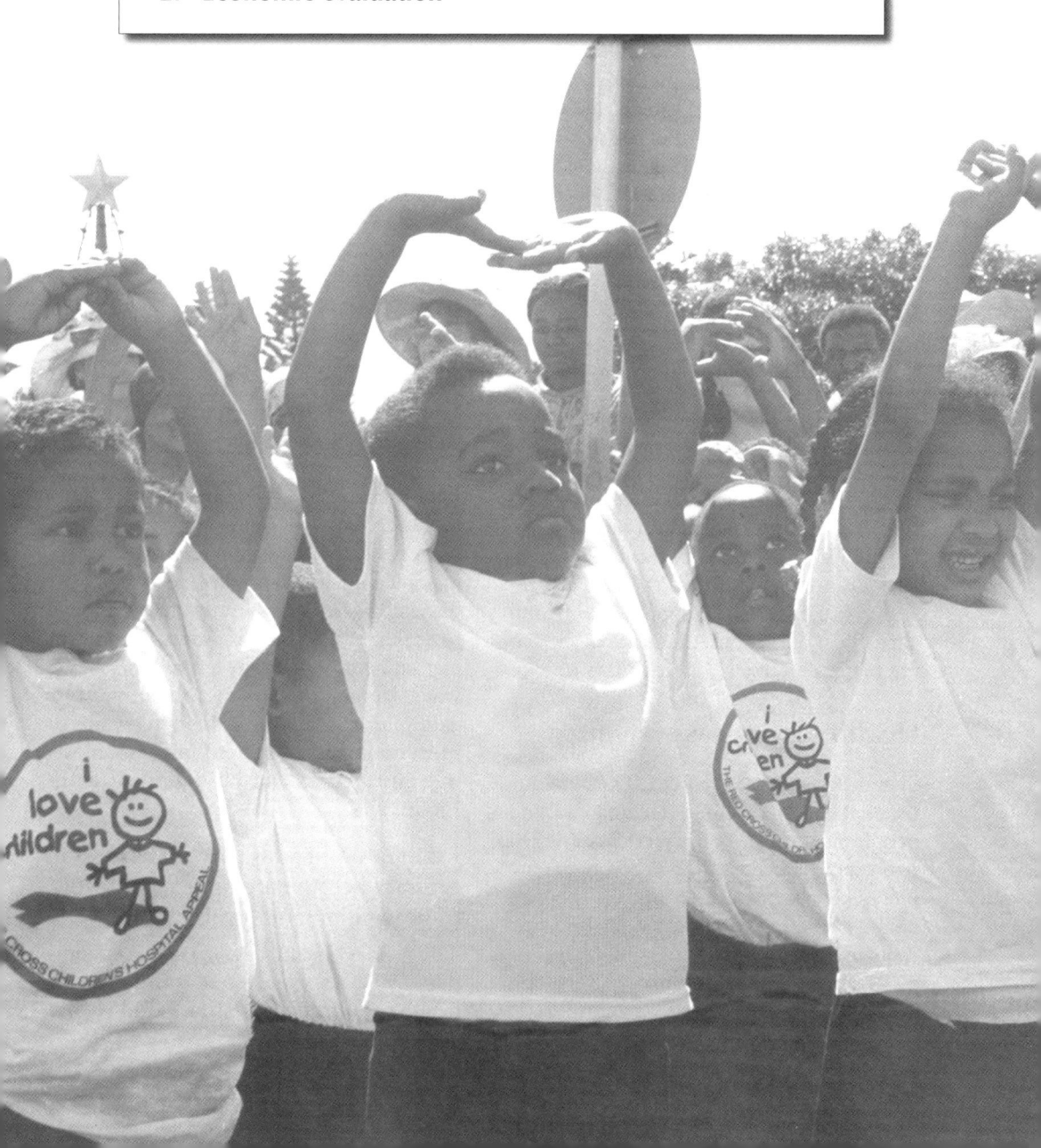

25

Health services research

Max O Bachmann

> **OBJECTIVES OF THIS CHAPTER**
>
> The objectives of this chapter are:
> - to provide a framework for analysing health systems
> - to provide an overview of research methods used in health services research
> - to describe measurable dimensions of the quality of health care
> - to show how different epidemiological study designs can be used to describe and analyse health care
> - to show how epidemiological studies can be used to evaluate disease prognosis and the effectiveness of interventions.

Introduction

Health services can be studied using various methods and perspectives. The appropriate method depends on the type of question we want to answer. This chapter starts with some useful frameworks and terminology for thinking about health services. It then uses examples to show how different research methods can be applied to health care. Most of these methods are discussed at greater length elsewhere in this book.

Health services as systems

Health services are complex. They include the organisations, facilities, technologies and people that provide or use services designed to promote good health and prevent or cure illness. A systems framework can help to analyse anything complicated, by breaking it down into three kinds of component:
- structure (inputs: resources, users, and organisations)
- process (what happens: actions, services provided and used)
- outcome (effects: changes in health, behaviour, knowledge).

Everything else can be called the environment. Dynamic systems are systems with feedback loops, for example, where changes in population health profiles require changes in health care, or where evaluation leads to health service changes. Any health system can be bounded and described in various ways, depending on the objective. For example, the health system relevant to prevention and treatment of tuberculosis in South Africa can be described as in Figure 25.1.

Examples of health care systems: the primary health care approach, levels of prevention and levels of care

The primary health care approach encompasses the key features of good primary health care as defined by the World Health

Figure 25.1 The health system and tuberculosis care

Environment
- Politics (government)
- Economics
- Risk factors (HIV, poverty, nutrition, housing)

Structures (inputs) →	Processes →	Outcomes
Infected people	Clinic visits	Death
Clinics and hospitals	Hospital admissions	Cure
Health professionals	Tests	Quality of life
Health departments	Treatments (provision and adherence)	Employment status
Drugs, laboratories, X rays		Infectious people (not fully treated)

Feedback: Monitoring and evaluation; disease transmission

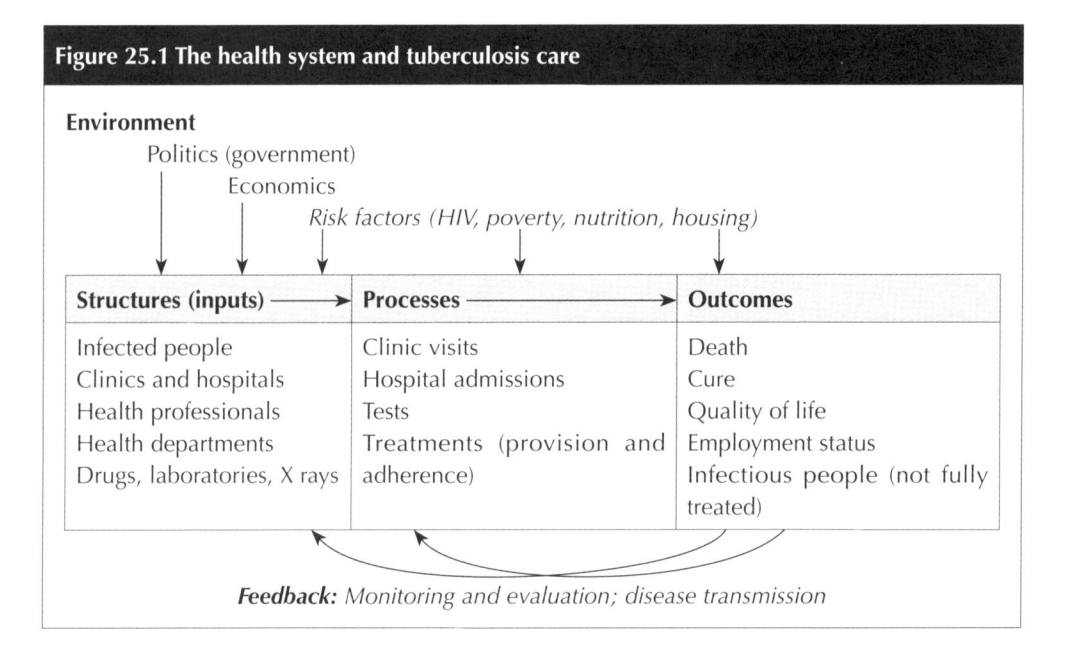

Organization (WHO) in the Alma Ata Declaration. This definition is often confused with two other useful frameworks for analysing health services – probably because they all use the word 'primary'. The first framework is holistic, the second is based on objectives for prevention, and the third is based on the structure and pathways of health services. Each has its uses.

The primary health care approach

This has been defined as '[e]ssential health care based on practical, scientifically sound and socially acceptable methods and technology made universally accessible to individuals and families in the community by means acceptable to them and at a cost that the community and the country can afford to maintain at every stage of their development in a spirit of self-reliance and self-determination' (World Health Organization, 1978).

Levels of prevention (see Chapter 2)

- *Primordial prevention:* Preventing the development of unhealthy or injurious social, environmental or lifestyle patterns.
- *Primary prevention:* Preventing a health problem before it even starts (e.g. immunisation or health education).
- *Secondary prevention:* Preventing a problem from getting worse (e.g. preventing opportunistic infections in people with HIV, screening for and treating early cervical cancer).
- *Tertiary prevention:* Preventing the problem from causing impairment, disability and handicap (e.g. rehabilitation).

Levels of care

- *Primary care:* The point of first contact with the health service (e.g. a clinic).
- *Secondary care:* The first level of care to refer to (e.g. a regional hospital).
- *Tertiary care:* A higher level of specialisation and referral (e.g. a regional transplant unit).

How do different levels of prevention or care relate to each other? An integrated system has good communication and co-ordination between its different parts, offering 'seamless' care without gaps or overlaps. A fragmented system has the opposite. *Vertical integration* is about linkages between different levels of care. For example, how are clinic services linked to hospital services? There may be ambulances, referral protocols or data sharing. *Horizontal integration* is about linkages at the same level of care. For example, in clinics, how are general curative services co-ordinated with chronic disease and child health clinics? Types of care that often need emergency referrals – like obstetrics – need good vertical integration. They may also need horizontal integration, for example, with child health services after delivery of the baby. Chronic disease management and health promotion mostly need good horizontal integration, because of co-morbidities and opportunities for prevention.

People need different kinds of primary care at different times which need to be co-ordinated. Analysis of service integration and fragmentation therefore makes up an important part of health services research. This requires a complex systems approach to evaluation research.

Typical questions in health services research

Health services research tries to solve problems so as to improve services and outcomes. To answer different types of questions, we need different kinds of research evidence, from different studies. The research design in turn determines the kind of evidence that results. For example, for the problem of multi-drug resistant tuberculosis the following kinds of evidence would be relevant (Table 25.1), and would need to come from descriptive studies, analytical studies or trials.

Table 25.1 Typical questions and research designs in health services research applied to tuberculosis drug resistance in a TB programme

Question	Research design	Examples of evidence
1. What is the problem, and how bad is it?	Qualitative or descriptive	Prevalence of resistance to TB drugs TB treatment programme quality (case holding, adherence) Staff and patient perceptions (barriers)
2. What causes it?	Analytical	Patient, community and health service factors associated with increased TB drug resistance
3. What solves it, and how well does it do so?	Controlled trials	Reduced TB drug resistance, attributable to programme to improve adherence

Evaluating health service quality

The quality of health care can be analysed along different dimensions. Four key concepts cover most of the quality of care, and each needs a different type of evidence for evaluation. Other aspects of quality such as accessibility and acceptability can be thought of in terms of these four concepts. For example, accessibility is an aspect of equity, and acceptability overlaps with humanity.

Effectiveness: Does the service do what it is intended to do? Does it improve health? Or does it cause changes that we can assume will improve health and prevent disease? If so, how well does it do so? How large is the effect? Sometimes we distinguish between 'efficacy', which means effectiveness under ideal circumstances, and 'effectiveness' in realistic situations. The best method for evaluating efficacy and effectiveness is with randomised trials. If these are not feasible, other epidemiological designs may provide useful evidence, as discussed below.

Efficiency: This refers to maximising outcomes for a given amount of resources. A fuller discussion of efficiency is provided in Chapter 27.

Equity: Is there equal care for equal need? 'Need' means capacity to benefit. Equity can be about different ways in which different people with the same disease are treated. For example, some people with Aids get antiretroviral drugs but others, who could benefit as much, do not. Or it can be about differences in care between people with different diseases, or living in different areas. For example, how much of our limited health resources should be used to care for people with Aids and how much for people with other diseases, such as diabetes? Should people with good incomes be entitled to buy better health care than those who have no income? If so, how much better? These examples show that equity, or fairness, can be a matter of opinion. But some opinions are more logical and evidence-based than others. If we can define what we mean by equity, and develop a valid and reliable way of measuring it, then research showing inequity can be powerful in shifting priorities.

For example, a lot of South African research has shown that poorer and rural areas have the largest burden of illness, and that these illnesses could be cost-effectively prevented or treated, but that these areas have the fewest primary care resources. This is inequitable – and also inefficient. This knowledge has led to and supported policies to improve primary care in such areas. Note that *equality* is different from equity, because equality does not consider need. To evaluate equity we measure the provision, accessibility, use or outcomes of health care, and how they are distributed in relation to different people's needs. Epidemiological designs are often appropriate for such measurement.

Humanity: The emotional and social well being of users and providers of care is an important health outcome. Is the health care humane? Are people treated with respect? Are they satisfied with their care? Do they get what they expect? If not, what is the problem? What do they expect or want? What do patients think about their care, and what do nurses think? The answers to these questions are subjective. Qualitative research methods are a good way to answer them. Quantitative research methods such as patient satisfaction, utilisation, or market research surveys may also be appropriate, if we know what we mean and can measure it. If not, we may need to start with qualitative research to clarify our concepts (see Chapter 26).

These four dimensions of quality are inter-related. Effectiveness is a prerequisite for the others. If a service does not work, it cannot be cost-effective and is not needed, so efficiency and equity are irrelevant. However, effectiveness and efficiency may depend on equity and humanity. For example, it is said that the South African health system, including public and private sectors, is relatively ineffective and inefficient because it is so inequitable. Improving equity may increase both effectiveness and efficiency through improving primary care for poorer populations. As another example, if people are treated disrespectfully they may not use primary care services appropriately, which could impair health and waste costly care later. Inhumane care is therefore ineffective and inefficient. Efficiency may, however, conflict with equity. For example, it is more expensive to provide equitable emergency services to remote areas than to urban areas. Studies that evaluate several dimensions of quality at the same time can show such inter-relationships.

Different research methods used in health services research

Researchers try to understand health care using different research methods and theories. These are briefly introduced in this section (see 'Useful readings' at the end of this chapter for more detail.)

Epidemiology, the focus of this book, investigates the determinants and distribution of health outcomes, and is a large part of health services research. *Clinical epidemiology* applies epidemiological principles to health care, for example to evaluate the effectiveness of treatments, the accuracy of diagnoses, or inequities in health care. It can be descriptive, for example, describing the natural history of disease or inequitable use of health care. Clinical epidemiology can also use analytical designs to investigate the causes of things that happen in health care. For example, why do patients use hospital services inappropriately, or why do some hospitals have higher death rates? Clinical epidemiology is described in more detail from page 311 onwards.

Health economics investigates how efficiently scarce resources are used to improve health. Economic evaluation combines evidence about effectiveness and costs (see Chapter 27). Health economists also study subjects such as health care financing, decision analysis, valuation of health outcomes and equity.

Organisational research is a multidisciplinary field that uses various qualitative and quantitative social science methods. Organisational sociology and anthropology emphasise cultures and interactions of groups of people, such as providers and users of health care. Organisational economics studies the boundaries and configuration of health service organisations and their co-ordination mechanisms. These characteristics depend in turn on economic factors such as economies of scale, scope and specialisation. They also depend on aspects of information such as uncertainty, information technology, and differences in information held by different people ('game theory').

Qualitative research is drawn from social science methodologies. It aims for deeper understanding of people's feelings, beliefs and values, especially by interpreting behaviour and use of words (see Chapter 26). It is especially useful for researching the humanity of health care, and is also valuable in investigating how and why existing services are ineffective, inefficient or inequitable.

Policy analysis originates in political science, described as the study of government. This includes government services. It emphasises the effects of power, interests and ideologies of different organisations and groups on the formulation and implementation of polices. It can be applied to government health policies, for example to health care financing or Aids treatment in South Africa. It can also be applied to private firms and non-governmental and international organisations. It uses quantitative and qualitative methods to analyse official statistics, statements and documents, media reports and interviews. Historical research can shed light on new situations. For example, the history of public responses to previous epidemics helps us to understand political responses to HIV/Aids.

Operations research is a specific methodology based on analysis of industrial production processes, including health services. It uses mathematical models which are simplified representations of reality. These make it possible to put together different types of evidence such as on the incidence, prevalence and prognosis of disease, and the effectiveness and resource requirements of different treatments, and to explore interactions between these variables that are too complex to see intuitively. These techniques help to plan health services and to allocate resources. Typical health service applications of operations research include analysis of patient flows and queues, inventory control, design of resource and service mix, and decision analysis. Simulation modelling is used to represent random variations over time and in populations such as the numbers of patients needing emergency care in a city.

Evaluation of programmes and projects

Health services are often organised, or thought of, as programmes or projects. A programme is a set of related measures or activities with a long-term aim. For example, a national tuberculosis control programme includes the structures and processes listed in Figure 25.1, and aims to improve the listed outcomes. The quality of each part of a programme can be evaluated in detail. Alternatively, the quality of a whole programme can be described using frameworks such as levels of care, levels of prevention, and health systems.

A project is a set of activities intended to produce a specific output, which has a definite beginning and end, such as building a hospital or carrying out an immunisation campaign. This is typically based on a plan that sets deadlines for each step to be completed. The critical path is the sequence of steps that must be completed before subsequent steps can be taken. For example, we need to complete the walls before we can paint them and build the roof. So, while carrying out the project, it is important to monitor whether each step is completed in time. If there are unexpected delays, plans need to be modified. Computer software can make it easier to plan and monitor complex projects. Once a project is completed, its effects can be evaluated using the methods described elsewhere in this chapter.

It may be useful formally to take into account the beliefs or preferences of *stakeholders*. Stakeholders are the people involved in programmes or projects, such as members of the public, patients, professionals, managers or politicians. They can be surveyed using questionnaires. Or their views can be explored more deeply using in-depth, key informant or focus group interviews, or other qualitative or policy analytical methods. If we are evaluating a programme or project as an outside consultant, we usually need to discuss with our clients beforehand what they want, and to report our findings as our evaluation goes ahead. This helps to ensure that our research is relevant and useful. It is important that project and programme evaluations are completed on time, so that they can support decisions when they are needed. If time is lacking, it can be helpful to interview rapidly a wide range of stakeholders and to summarise what they say in a short report but without using formal qualitative research methods.

Epidemiological studies of health care

Experimental studies of the effectiveness of health service interventions

Randomised controlled trials, also known as experimental studies, provide the most valid estimates of effectiveness and the strongest evidence of causation. This is because randomisation can minimise selection bias and confounding. The design of randomised controlled trials, and of quasi-experimental and before-after trials, is described in Chapter 7. A trial is a study in which the researcher intervenes, in contrast to an observational study. Trials can be randomised or non-randomised.

In principle, randomised trials can be used to evaluate the effectiveness of any kind of intervention, or to compare any two or more different ways of providing health care. Despite the availability of this methodology, there is still no good evidence about many types of care. There is much more evidence about the effectiveness of drugs than there is about the effectiveness of other health technologies or programmes. This is because governments require randomised trial evidence that new drugs are effective before they may be sold. It is also relatively simple to allocate individual patients randomly to get one drug or another. Since governments do not demand that other kinds of treatment, or diagnostic technologies, are supported by randomised trials, we know much less about their effectiveness. Partly this is because randomised trials of these kinds of care may be unacceptable to patients, professionals or others who have strong preferences. For example, patients may have strong preferences about getting medical or surgical treatment, or being treated at home or in hospital, and so be unwilling to support or participate in a comparison of different types of care. But often the reasons for not doing randomised trials are based on misconceptions, lack of imagination, or lack of resources. We need more randomised trial evidence to be able to provide effective services, which are a prerequisite for efficiency and equity. When a randomised trial is logistically or ethically not possible, well designed observational studies can provide useful information.

One experimental design – the *cluster randomised trial* – is not discussed in detail elsewhere in this book, so we do so here. This design is especially useful for evaluating complex health service interventions that could affect whole groups of people at the same time. For example, a new educational method to train clinic nurses could affect the health of large numbers of each nurse's patients. Providing sex education in schools could positively influence the sexual behaviour of many students in each school. With a cluster randomised trial, whole groups of participants are assigned together to different trial arms. For example, clinics may be allocated, together with all of their eligible patients, to different trial arms. Entire schools can be assigned either to get sex education or not. The aim is to have balanced (similar) groups, so we need to have enough clusters to randomise.

Why use cluster randomisation?

There are three main reasons for using cluster randomisation.
- It is logical if the intervention is aimed at clinics and all their staff (even if outcomes are measured in individual patients). If enough clinics are randomised, we can be confident that the clinics, their staff, and their patients in each of the trial arms are balanced at the start. As a result, any difference in outcomes afterwards must be due to the intervention, or to chance.
- Physical separation of participants in different trial arms can avoid contamination. *Contamination* means the unintentional exposure of participants belonging to one trial arm to the intervention intended for the other arm. For example, in a trial of health education, control arm participants may receive information that was intended only for the intervention arm and this could affect their behaviour. Contamination, like non-adherence, may lead to underestimation of the effects of the intervention. The risk of contamination may not be a sufficient problem in itself to justify this design – it depends on the type of intervention. For example, it would make more sense to use a cluster randomised design if we were evaluating health promotion using local radio, but less sense if we were evaluating health education given privately to individual patients.
- Cluster randomisation can be convenient, because we need not randomise each patient during the trial - we need only randomise each clinic beforehand. Outcomes can be analysed at patient level or at cluster level (comparing the average outcomes in each clinic), depending on our level of inference. That is, do we want to know what this intervention means for patients or for services?

The main disadvantage of cluster randomised trials is that they tend to reduce statistical power and precision. The reason is that members of the same cluster are often more similar to each other than to members of other clusters. This is called *intra-cluster correlation*. For example, the health of patients attending clinics in wealthier areas may be very different from that of patients attending clinics in poorer areas. If patients within each clinic are similar to each other, then each extra patient effectively provides less information. This is especially so if intra-cluster correlation is strong, or if there are few clusters, even if each cluster is large. Sample size calculations and statistical analyses therefore need to take intra-cluster correlation into account (for which assistance of a statistician will be needed).

Another disadvantage of cluster randomised trials is that, if we are randomising only a few units, it is more likely that the trial arms will differ owing to chance. Cluster randomisation should be used only for very good reasons. Otherwise, it is better to randomise individuals.

Observational studies of health care

Observational studies – including cohort, case-control, cross-sectional and ecologic designs – can also provide evidence about the effectiveness of health care.

Descriptive epidemiological studies can be used for a number of purposes:
- to estimate the need for health care (that is, the prevalence and severity of disease that would benefit from such care)
- to quantify inequity in health care (that is, unequal supply or use of health care in relation to need)
- to quantify indicators of health care quality (such as delays in receiving care, patient satisfaction and inappropriate health care utilisation).

Analytical epidemiological designs can be used to try to determine and quantify the predictive factors in health care outcomes, distribution or usage. For example:
- Case-control studies can be used to investigate why patients with mild illnesses go to hospital rather than to nearby clinics, or why some patients do not adhere to treatment. In the former example, the cases are those who use the hospital and the controls those who use the local clinic for the same illness.
- Cohort studies of patients can identify patient and health service characteristics associated with better or worse prognoses, or can compare costs of different types of health care utilisation over time.
- Ecological studies could test whether countries with better primary care provision have better health outcomes than wealthier countries that spend more on health care but have less primary care.

The validity of these studies, as always, depends on the quality of their data and the ability to control bias and confounding. Observational studies of effectiveness can be useful if randomised trials are practically or ethically unacceptable. For example, it would be unethical with present knowledge to allocate trial patients randomly to get either placebo or triple antiretroviral treatment. So there is no direct randomised trial evidence about the effectiveness of triple antiretroviral treatment. We can estimate the results using evidence from cohort studies, as well as indirect comparisons of different trials. Observational studies can consequently evaluate the effectiveness of treatment in realistic situations, instead of under trial conditions. They can also follow large populations for long periods, which might not be feasible or ethical for randomised trials.

Problems inherent in observational studies of health care effectiveness

Compared to randomised trials, observational studies are at much greater risk of confounding and selection bias. These must be avoided by good study design if possible, and adjusted for as far as data allow. Selection bias can be an insurmountable problem in health care evaluation, because treatments are usually selected according to the severity of disease, and it is rarely possible to measure and adjust for disease severity perfectly. Both treatments and their outcomes are often associated with patients' health status in the beginning, which confounds the treatment effect. For example, we can estimate the effectiveness of antiretroviral treatment by comparing the survival of a cohort of HIV-infected patients who do or do not get antiretrovirals. But patients with more severe disease are more likely to get antiretrovirals, so we need to adjust for measures of disease severity, such as Aids stage, CD4 count and body mass index. Even so, we are unlikely to have perfect information on disease severity or other confounders. *Regression models* are usually the most efficient way to adjust for several confounding variables. Discussion of these is beyond the scope of this book.

Studies of diagnosis and screening

Effective health care depends on accurate diagnoses. The validity of diagnostic information, such as test results, can be evaluated in terms of *sensitivity*, *specificity*, and *predictive values* (see Figure 9.4, Chapter 9). This entails comparing test results with a reference standard, such as the most accurate test possible.

Sensitivity is the proportion of people who truly have the disease who correctly test positive. Sensitive tests are most useful for ruling out disease, as in screening, where we would want to be confident that disease is unlikely if the test is negative.

Specificity is the proportion of people who truly do not have the disease who correctly test negative. Specific tests are most useful for confirming disease, for example as a second line confirmatory test, where we would want to be confident that the disease is present if the test is positive.

The positive predictive value is the probability that someone truly has the disease if the test is positive. The negative predictive value is the probability that someone truly does not have the disease if the test is negative. Unlike sensitivity and specificity, predictive values depend on disease prevalence. For example, the less prevalent the disease is, the lower the positive predictive value will be.

Screening aims to identify early disease that can be effectively treated, usually in people who do not yet have symptoms. It can be organised as large scale programmes that invite patients without symptoms to be tested (e.g. cervical and breast cancer screening, and HIV voluntary counselling and testing), or it can be opportunistic (e.g. testing for hypertension among adult patients who go to a clinic for any reason).

Seven pertinent questions to justify a screening programme

To justify a *screening programme*, we need good reasons and strong evidence to answer at least seven questions:
1. Is this an important public health problem?
2. Do we know the natural history of the disease, with and without treatment?
3. Is there an effective treatment?

4. Is the screening test valid and reliable?
5. Is there capacity to confirm and treat everyone diagnosed?
6. Is there good evidence that such screening programmes have been effective?
7. Will the programme be effective and cost-effective enough compared to other priorities?

We can evaluate the effectiveness of screening by using randomised trials. However, these trials usually need to be large and lengthy to be able to show effects, and so they are scarce. Where randomised trial evidence is lacking, mathematical modelling can be used to put together evidence on disease incidence and prevalence, diagnostic validity, and treatment effectiveness.

Observational studies can also be used to evaluate the effectiveness of screening but may suffer from various biases. For example, survival could seem longer just because the diagnosis was made earlier, and not because earlier diagnosis and treatment were effective. This is called *lead time bias*. The bias known as *length time bias* occurs when the type of disease detected by screening differs from the type detected without screening. Therefore people with less aggressive disease with a longer asymptomatic period are more likely to be detected by screening than those with more aggressive disease, who are more likely to present with symptoms to the health service. This bias may also make it appear as if screening improves prognosis or prolongs life. Finally, *volunteer bias* occurs when people who present themselves for screening have a different risk of disease from those who do not.

Studies of prognosis

Patients with specific diseases usually want to know what will happen to them in future, that is, their prognosis. This may be especially important when cure is not possible, for example with chronic and fatal diseases. Cohort studies provide the best evidence of prognosis. Otherwise, without longitudinal data, we need to model prognosis using cross-sectional data. Prognosis can be expressed in various ways. For example, we can express the prognosis for patients with HIV/Aids as the probability of being alive after five years, as the median time to death, or as the incidence rate of severe infections and hospital admissions.

Survival analyses, based on time-to-event data, are especially useful when studying prognosis. They estimate the risk of the event occurring at any instant among those who have not yet experienced the event. This kind of risk is called a hazard. *Cox proportional hazard* regression models are used to identify the prognostic factors that are independently associated with time to event or survival. Their results can be used to predict prognoses for individual patients by entering their characteristics into the model. For example, WHO Aids staging criteria divide patients into prognostic groups according to their clinical features and are based on survival analyses of cohort data. A more advanced text should be consulted for further information on this topic.

Conclusion

From a public health or epidemiological perspective, since health services can be considered as an exposure or determinant of population health, they can be analysed using the basic epidemiological toolbox. Evidence from health care evaluations is essential for people providing health care to patients, whether planning and organising services or managing individual patients. Randomised trials of treatments and studies evaluating diagnostic methods are essential for clinicians to know how best to diagnose and treat their patients. Prognostic studies can provide information that patients want to know (but are rarely told).

However, knowledge about specific tests and treatments does not tell us much about why health care works well or badly. Organisational structures, complex interventions, and economic and political environments can have large effects too. Systems, problem-based and multidisciplinary approaches can help to capture the complexity of a health service, while still allowing us to focus on those elements of health services that are most relevant to the research question.

> **EXAMPLE 25.1**

Developing and evaluating a practical approach to lung health in South Africa

This study evaluated an educational intervention based on a diagnostic and treatment guideline, with outreach of trainers to clinic nurses. Forty Free State province clinics were randomly allocated either to get the intervention or not. Randomisation was stratified by district, because tuberculosis outcomes varied between districts, and because the researchers expected that the intervention could be more effective in some districts than in others. After training had started in the intervention clinics, outcomes were measured and analysed at patient level.

In each clinic, about 50 adults with cough or difficulty in breathing were interviewed after a clinic visit and again three months later. By the time of follow-up, the odds that patients in intervention clinics were newly diagnosed with tuberculosis was 72% higher, and the odds that they received preventative asthma treatment was 90% higher, than in control arm patients. Statistical analyses were adjusted for intra-clinic correlation of outcomes. The study showed that a relatively inexpensive educational intervention improved primary respiratory care over a period of months.

Evaluating the effectiveness of the final product was just part of the research programme. While the training package was still being developed, qualitative group and individual interviews were used to help understand what primary care clinicians thought of the original WHO guideline, what the greatest barriers to following the guideline were, and how it should be changed. Qualitative research was also used during the training of trainers and in clinic settings, to understand what was happening during the training process. It showed what parts of the educational package people liked and carried out, and what they could or would not do.

A cost effectiveness analysis was also carried out alongside the randomised trial. This estimated the costs to each patient, and to the health service, of illness, health care, and the training package. Combined with the trial results, this provided an estimate of the extra cost per extra patient who benefited. A fourth set of studies was carried out in a Cape Town health centre, to evaluate the diagnostic accuracy of the guideline as used by a nurse compared to a specialist diagnosis. This combination of qualitative research, randomised trial, observational epidemiology and economic evaluation can provide powerful evidence about a relatively complex health service intervention.

Reference:

Fairall, L, Zwarenstein, M, Bateman, ED, Bachmann, MO, Lombard, C, Majara, B, Joubert, G, English, R, Bheekie, A, Mayers, P, Peters, A & Chapman, R. 2005. Educational outreach to nurses improves tuberculosis case detection and primary care of respiratory illness: a pragmatic cluster randomised controlled trial. *British Medical Journal*, 331:750–4.

> **EXAMPLE 25.2**

Analysing tuberculosis care and control

In a recently published project, several studies analysed the steadily worsening tuberculosis epidemic in South Africa so as to find its causes and to recommend changes. This multi-disciplinary programme included methods and perspectives from microbiology, history, sociology, organisational research, economics, communication studies and other interdisciplinary fields. Some studies used published sources to describe how South Africa's political and economic history affected tuberculosis and health services, before and after the end of apartheid. Other studies used qualitative information from patients, clinicians and health service managers. This information was gathered using individual and group interviews and direct observation. Further studies analysed interactions between the tuberculosis and HIV epidemics, health services, and the growing problem of antibiotic resistance. Health service resources were critically examined. Evidence from previous economic evaluations of tuberculosis programmes was reviewed. Principles of good health education strategies were outlined alongside a critical analysis of actual health education programmes. These diverse studies together provide a rich picture of health service problems and possible solutions and emphasise the multidisciplinary nature of health services research.

Reference:

Van Rensburg, D, Meulemans, H & Rigouts, L (eds). 2005. Tuberculosis. *Acta Academica*, Suppl 1: whole issue.

Useful readings

Fulop, N, Allen, P, Clarke, A & Black, N (eds). 2001. *Studying the organisation and delivery of health services. Research methods.* London: Routledge.

Health Systems Trust. *South African health review.* Durban: HST. [Online]. Available: http:// www.hst.org.za. [25 February 2007]. [Published annually.]

Hunink, M, Glasziou, P, Siegel, J, Weeks, J, Pliskin, J, Elstein, A & Weinstein, M. 2001. *Decision making in health and medicine. Integrating evidence and values.* Cambridge: Cambridge University Press.

Muir Gray, JA. 2001. *Evidence-based health care: how to make health policy and management decisions.* 2nd ed. Oxford: Churchill Livingstone.

Pencheon, D, Guest, D, Meltzer, D & Muir Gray, JA (eds). 2001. *Oxford handbook of public health practice.* Oxford: Oxford University Press.

Van Rensburg, HCJ (ed). 2004. *Health and health care in South Africa.* Pretoria: Van Schaik.

Useful web sites

British Medical Journal. [Online]. Available: http://bmj.bmjjournals.com/series/. [25 February 2007].

Health Systems Trust. [Online]. Available: http://www.hst.org.za. [25 February 2007].

National Health Service Research and Development. *Health technology assessment.* [Online]. Available: http://www.ncchta.org/. [25 February 2007].

Reference used in this chapter

World Health Organization. 1978. *Primary health care. Health for all series, no 1.* Geneva: World Health Organization.

26

Qualitative methodology: an introduction

Donald Skinner

> **OBJECTIVES OF THIS CHAPTER**
>
> The objectives of this chapter are:
> - to describe the uses and value of qualitative research in health research
> - to provide a framework for qualitative research methodology, namely the philosophy and narrative base of the data
> - introduce the methods of qualitative research and their diversity
> - to provide an understanding of the analytical process in qualitative research.

Introduction

The answers to many of the most pressing questions about human health care are influenced by the attitudes and perceptions of both caregivers and users of health services. Sometimes people behave in ways or hold views which are difficult to understand. For instance, some people stubbornly refuse to take their medication, no matter what. If we try to understand their motivation, they may tell us a number of things that we did not think were important, but are important to them.

Qualitative research methods are a useful and valuable addition to an epidemiologist's collection of skills. They encompass a broad range of research and fieldwork methods, as is the case with quantitative research. Epidemiology has traditionally focused on the use of quantitative data, which allows for focused projects and the testing of pre-set hypotheses. Qualitative methods provide research opportunities which extend the type of information which can be collected.

These methods allow researchers to understand how the subjects of research perceive their situation and their role within this context. It is out of these perceptions and social influences that behaviour, including health-related behaviour, is born. Qualitative research can help us find out why these behaviours occur or why people hold these views. As in quantitative research, a range of formal research methodologies exist. These allow researchers to get and interpret in-depth information on their subjects, generally by talking to them or observing them. Qualitative data consists mainly of descriptions of people or places, or of conversations. Such information cannot easily be handled by statistical procedures, and these procedures are generally inappropriate. At present qualitative research still remains an underdeveloped field in public health, but with the importance of trying to understand what determines behaviour in the context of diseases such as HIV/Aids and conditions such as obesity, its influence is rising.

Philosophical approach

Underlying the qualitative approach is a philosophy concerning how behaviours and social processes are determined. This philosophy argues that explaining the social world merely in terms of overt behaviour misses the most vital element, namely that each behaviour or action carries meaning which needs to be explored. People and contexts are seen as being shaped by the norms and conventions of the society in which they are found. All these norms, conventions and social institutions find their final form in cultural and belief systems. The personal and social meaning that people use to structure their lives cannot just be treated as a statistical variable, but needs to be explored if the researcher hopes to answer many basic research questions (Babbie & Mouton, 2001).

This philosophy implies an interpretive or subjective approach with the focus being on how the respondents experience and understand the particular situation.

Uses of qualitative research

Qualitative research can be used in multiple contexts with the four major instances outlined below.
1. Qualitative research may be used in the early phase of a study to explore an area before starting with a survey, to clarify the basic conditions that are present or to establish hypotheses for future research.
2. Qualitative research can be used along with other types of research in order to get an additional perspective on the problem. It can provide the meaning behind a significant connection made by a quantitative survey.
3. It is often the only methodology used when the aim is to get an in-depth sense of what people think of a particular object or event.
4. The in-depth interaction between the researcher and the participant makes this approach particularly appropriate when used as part of a process to establish some form of action or campaign in a community, and for intervention-based research.

Methods of data collection

In qualitative research objectives are formulated broadly and not framed around variables defined in measurable (quantitative) dimensions or in terms of specific hypotheses. The emphasis is on investigating the variables in their complexity and in context. Overviews of the three most commonly used methods of qualitative data collection are provided below. The manner in which the research method is used has to be adapted to the situation and the demands of the research question.

Depth interviews

The depth interview is probably the most common form of qualitative data collection. It generally takes the form of a discussion between the interviewer and interviewee on the research topic. The interview is commonly recorded on a tape recorder with permission from the interviewee. The interviewer has to direct the discussion to some extent so that the required information can be obtained, but respondents are allowed to talk and cover the area in their own terms and from their own perspective (Terre Blanche & Durrheim, 1999). This method is generally used when detailed information is needed from individuals. The major advantage is that it gives the respondent the opportunity for personal explanation and detailed responses. In addition, the individual focus allows the interviewer to draw out the information in more detail while the respondent is talking and thinking about the subject. Examples of its use would be to assess the illness experience of a person with cancer, or to find out how patients with sexually transmitted infections (STIs) feel about the idea of using condoms.

Considerable preparation must take place before starting fieldwork. The researcher needs to be clear about the purpose of the research, have a good knowledge of the setting in which the research takes place and have read widely in the area to be researched. Interviewers may also have to prepare themselves emotionally as they often have to deal with difficult and emotive issues.

Most commonly, the interviewer will enter the field with a list of points to be covered in the interview. These points give direction, but ideally should not inhibit the interviewer from discussing other points if they seem important during the course of the interview. No sequence is imposed, and each point can be the beginning of a particular discussion. The greater the level of structure provided, the less spontaneity the interviewee is allowed.

An appointment should be organised well in advance at a mutually acceptable place, so that time is allocated and the respondent can prepare. The fieldworker who organises the meeting should explain the nature of the research. A person's unwillingness to be interviewed must be respected, and reservations should be discussed if possible.

The atmosphere should be cordial and open. An interview should preferably not last more than an hour. It can be carried on later if more time is required. The initial phase of the interview is very important, as this is when trust is established or lost. Openness and frankness about the nature of the research will help to gain trust at this point. The researcher should confirm that the person is agreeable to having the interview taped, reaffirm the nature of the research, and re-establish consent. Privacy and quiet are very important.

The interviewer asks an open question, and then by the use of summarising techniques and questions of clarification, draws out the meaning, understanding and beliefs that the interviewee places on the issues under question. Summarising involves reflecting back to the interviewee what was said in such a way as to provide an immediate check on the interviewer's understanding, and to allow the interviewee to develop his or her thoughts on the question further. Clarification questions serve to get explanations on issues raised by the interviewee about which the researcher is unclear.

The interviewer needs to conclude the interview with great discretion and care. Any emotions and hopes that the interview raises should be respected and talked through as appropriate. At the end of the interview, the respondent must be told where the research will be going from this point, should be reassured about confidentiality, and where possible the offer of later feedback should be made.

Focus group interviews

The focus group method involves a number of people meeting in a group in which the participants talk to one another under the guidance of a facilitator. The purpose is to gain insight into the attitudes, perceptions and opinions of participants on a pre-arranged topic (Silverman, 2004). Focus groups can produce results that may directly represent how people are feeling as they attempt to re-create the social situation. People are often stimulated by the discussion, and reveal facts and opinions that they might not otherwise have chosen to reveal. It may also give group members the chance to clarify their attitudes and beliefs.

Focus groups can be used flexibly, for example, to evaluate health projects and educational attempts, and to obtain perceptions of what the major needs in a community are. Focus groups can help to build community involvement in the research or the intervention being evaluated or planned. The major disadvantage of this method is possible peer pressure within the group, which may prevent the members from saying what they believe.

Ideally, a group should number between six and ten members, plus a facilitator and observer or recorder. Membership of the group should be fairly homogeneous. If the subject is sensitive, care needs to be taken in mixing groups. For example, if the subject is sexuality, one should consider interviewing men and women separately.

The site selected for the discussion should be private and comfortable, free from disturbance and at a convenient spot for the members of the group. The optimal time span for a group discussion is between 60 and 90 minutes, but the demands of the study and respondents need to be taken into account. It may also be possible to organise more than one meeting of the group.

As with the depth interviews, the facilitator should work from a pre-established list of points or schedule, which can be used to ensure that all important points are covered. The facilitator should not allow the schedule to limit discussion.

Setting up and conducting the focus group interview

Prior to starting the group interview, it is important for the facilitator to open the discussion by welcoming the group and getting everybody introduced, providing an overview of the topic, outlining the ground rules of the discussion, getting permission for the use of the tape recorder, and explaining the role of the observer or recorder. The facilitator should be aware of the following:

- Potential group members need to be reminded of the meeting by the facilitator (or some other intermediary person) in advance, to minimise the problem of cancellations and no-shows.
- The group must remain focused and discussions on side issues should be limited.
- Difficult personalities such as dominant people, those who ramble, and argumentative members need to be monitored and controlled so that they do not disrupt the group. It is important to get a balance of participation between the different members.
- The facilitator needs to guard against his or her powerful role biasing the group.
- The facilitator will at times have to use probes, such as direct questions, to elicit additional information of interest. Probes should not be overused, as this will inhibit discussion.

At the end of the discussion, group members should be thanked for their participation and told what will happen to the information that was gathered in the group. For every group discussion, there should be an audiotape recording. In addition, the recorder should keep detailed notes on the body language and social processes in the group, as well as brief notes on what was said.

Participant observation

Participant observation requires researchers to involve themselves directly in the lives and worlds of those being studied and experience their reality to gain a greater understanding of the context. The method is based on the assumption that understanding of the inner perspectives of subjects can be achieved only by actively participating in the subjects' world and gaining insight by means of observation. This makes it potentially the most powerful tool for developing an understanding of the experience and meanings attached to behaviours and social norms. The classical form of the research involves the researchers living or working with the research subjects over a period of months. Its major disadvantage is its time-consuming nature (Silverman, 2004).

The method is not commonly used in health research, but it does have potentially important applications, including observations of the flow of patients through a clinic (health services setting), an assessment of how well safety regulations are adhered to and how the workers feel about these (occupational health setting). In investigations of infectious diseases (such as Aids), it may identify indicators of risky patterns of sexual behaviour. The data collection covers a range of activities, including observing, listening, asking questions, and recording, which can be done either covertly or overtly. The combination of methods is often termed *ethnographic research* to indicate the additional depth of information gained even over other qualitative approaches.

The process of gaining access is vitally important, as it determines in many ways how responsive the community or group is likely to be to the researcher, as the researcher needs to be free to move around easily and participate in the activities of the community or group, while preferably remaining relatively inconspicuous. The researcher should explain the nature of the research to the research subjects as far as possible, especially how the information will be used. Where possible, the researcher should negotiate access not only with those in authority, but also with individuals at different levels.

Once in the field, the researcher has to decide to what extent he or she should participate in the activities of the community. Some researchers merely act as observers and try to maintain a distance from the activities of the community, while others seek to get involved as much as possible. This is both a practical and an ethical decision.

While it will be impossible to record everything that happens, it is vital that very detailed data recording takes place. This can be done in a range of ways; most commonly the researcher will use field notes, audio taping, and video taping. Field notes should consist of relatively concrete, complete, accurate, and detailed descriptions of social processes and their contexts. As the subjects being observed may be threatened by the note-taking, only brief notes should be made as unobtrusively as possible and the fuller version should be done at a later stage from memory. It is important to avoid any impressions of evaluating the respondents, as this will compromise results.

Finally, when leaving the field, the researcher must be aware of the powerful social connections made in this type of research, and the effect that the research process has had on the community. Full and proper goodbyes need to be said and details of the future research plans given. The researcher needs to be clear about when to leave the field by setting either a date or a point defined by the quantity of data obtained.

Participant observation also works well in combination with other fieldwork approaches. For example, it has been used in conjunction with individual depth and focus group interviews in research on the situation of orphaned and vulnerable children and an assessment of services for prevention of mother-to-child transmission of HIV infection. In these studies, observations of conditions inside the homes of the children, including the nature of the housing, amenities inside the house and interactions between family members during an interview, often provided as much information as the interview itself, and assisted the interpretation of the data. Likewise observations made in clinics offering prevention of mother-to-child transmission (PMTCT) services in an area of the Eastern Cape showed clearly the problems of lack of necessary resources and the real difficulties of travelling to the clinic (see Examples 26.1 and 26.2).

Other qualitative methods

There are a number of other qualitative methods which are available to the researcher but are less commonly used. These are often variations on the above approaches. It is important to note here that qualitative methods can be very flexible, allowing for adaptation to a range of contexts.

Researchers often keep research diaries to supplement the data collected. Research diaries utilise valuable information picked up while the researcher is in the research setting. The use of documentary evidence includes the analysis of photographs, tapes, life histories, and old documents. Other more experiential methods include activities such as role-play, projective techniques and visualisation exercises.

While the methods of data collection discussed in this chapter are often used individually, they may also be used in combination. The different methods are used to assess different types of information and to back up findings found in one of the other research methods.

Two useful applications of qualitative methods were applied in a review of policy for the Department of Education. In the first a number of experts in policy analysis were each asked to produce a ten-page review of a set of policies. These accounts were then analysed using a qualitative analytical approach to produce a single account of these policies.

A second application looked at the levels of implementation of policy in the Department. Senior managers in the Department attended a three-hour workshop to observe implementation. Following that discussion a report was produced which became the subject of a second workshop, after which the final report was produced, representing a valid account of the implementation of policy (Simbayi *et al*, 2005).

Methodological issues in qualitative research

Sampling

The usual epidemiological practice of formal random sampling with concern for adequate sample size is inappropriate in qualitative studies. The depth of the data gathered is the primary goal, rather than statistical inference. Within qualitative methods, greater emphasis is placed on *purposive sampling*. This is a sampling method in which the researcher deliberately chooses respondents or settings in order to ensure that the sample covers the full range of possible characteristics of interest. The researcher aims to obtain a sample that represents all important subgroups of the population. This includes sampling deviant or extreme cases, typical cases, critical cases, politically important or sensitive cases, and sampling to maximise the variation. The researcher hopes to cover the diversity of the target group, as well as what is typical, in this way. Haphazardly selecting people for convenience is discouraged, as the results can be heavily biased.

The constraints of available time and funding often determine sample size. Two potential ways of defining sample size in the field are firstly to continue until the researcher has enough information to answer the initial research questions, or until no more or very little new information is being gained from successive interviews. The second method is to use the initial interviews to establish hypotheses and use successive interviews to validate or adjust these hypotheses. Interviews will continue until the hypotheses require no further adaptations in respect of the new information being gathered, and the researcher feels that the information collected adequately explains what is being researched.

Analysis of qualitative data

A range of approaches to analysis have been developed (Miles & Huberman, 1984; Strauss, 1987; Glaser, 1998). It is important that the researcher does not blindly follow others' practices, but adapts the analytical procedures to the demands of the situation and the data. While there are no fixed rules for the analysis of qualitative data, there are some key processes that need to be noted (Silverman, 2001).

The general term often used for the analytical process is *content analysis*, which means that the data are explored in detail for common themes and these are then established into units of meaning or codes. Although costly and time-consuming, taped material should be transcribed (typed or written out) as the written word is the basic medium for analysis. The task of transcribing should not be underestimated and requires someone with skill and a budget to pay them. Every single word that is said by both the interviewer and the interviewee has to be written down. From early on in the data collection process, analysis should begin so that the key areas can be drawn out to inform the data collection process.

Coding consists of searching the data for common themes which can be established as categories into which ideas and information can be collected (see Figure 26.1). Over time, this coding should move from the original crude codes to becoming more complex. At this point, codes should start to overlap, so more complex codes may need to be developed and sub-dimensions of these codes created. For example, if the general code concerns attitudes towards the use of condoms, the sub-dimensions could be that they are unerotic, that they are embarrassing to use, or that they are difficult to obtain.

Figure 26.1 An example of qualitative data analysis

Text	Themes
I think in a big sense some of the older people have to provide for the younger people as I said … my idea is that the elder people were always the respected ones and they were provided for, the younger people provided for the older people when they retired or they helped them and so on. Now it's not working that way, now the older people have to work and have to provide for the grandchildren. So in that instance it's changed. And as I said, many of my age group the people have to help their friends, or have to tend to their friends who are sick and who are dying. It's just not you can just be friends and ondersteun, I don't know what the word is, support one another in the various ways that you always did with personal problems or with family problems or what like that. It's becoming more a caring situation, the younger people have to care for their friends and care for their children because they can't do it for themselves.	Care systems, support structures Traditional systems Impact of the epidemic Care systems, support structures Change in culture, community context Care burdens Levels of support required Community care Caring for children

As the data collection continues and the codes become more complex, there is a need to start summarising and to begin making some sense of the data. The use of theoretical memos is **important** and should begin early on. These are brief notes of potential hypotheses or observations that can be made while coding and examining the data. All notes should be filed away to be used as a resource later on when doing the final interpretation of the data. During the project, the notes will become more complex and closer to the final interpretations that will need to be made. From all of the above, the key issues and important factors need to be drawn out and the final interpretations stated. It is important to relate the final interpretations to existing findings and information about the subject to obtain greater depth and understanding.

Researchers may use a number of techniques to verify and interpret results. One useful method is to set up initial hypotheses and then to search the transcripts for contradictions. If any such results are found, then the hypotheses may need to be adapted to take them into account. These techniques increase confidence in the qualitative results. Validity can be further enhanced by comparing results between interviewers, by getting a number of people to analyse the same sections of the same material, or by relating the results to the theory on which the research was based. On a more sophisticated level the *triangulation method* compares the results using any number of different methods to see if they complement each other (Silverman, 2001).

Training

This chapter is a brief overview of qualitative methods and cannot be considered a training guide. The references at the end of this chapter will give some additional guidelines on theory and techniques, but do need to be backed up with experiential learning and support. Initial training can often be done via a short set of workshops presented by someone who is skilled in this area. Short courses on qualitative methods are offered by most research training institutions. Additional suggestions for training include the establishment of study groups within institutions to learn about the methods. Another would be to work alongside more senior and experienced researchers. It is only in the process of working with others that the techniques can really be known and mastered. Key to this is the fact that the researcher as a person is the research instrument for qualitative methods. Just as the questionnaire is the instrument in a survey, the researcher is the means by which information is collected in qualitative techniques. For this reason, we need to do a lot of hard work in getting ourselves ready for the task, even though many skills are simply extensions of existing social skills.

Table 26.1 outlines the main advantages and disadvantages of qualitative research.

Table 26.1 Advantages and disadvantages of qualitative methods

Advantages of qualitative methods
- Since qualitative research is done within people's contexts, it can produce results that directly represent how people feel. During this process, the researcher will also get a closer feeling of the general social functioning of the person or the community.
- The results obtained are often more accessible than questionnaire research, as they are descriptions of real situations rather than statistical measures or diagrams, which are often beyond readers' experience.
- In new areas of research, qualitative methods can be useful for the production of new ideas. They can also provide information for other studies.
- If new information appears during the research process, there is space within the research structure to explore it.

- A common research problem is that respondents may produce responses that they feel are socially appropriate rather than what they genuinely believe. Their responses may also seek to hide behaviours that they believe may be negatively judged (e.g. discriminatory actions). In qualitative research, a skilled researcher will be able to use the greater flexibility of the qualitative method to get around these problems by developing a relationship with the respondent in the fieldwork situation and by using probes and picking up non-verbal cues.

Disadvantages of qualitative methods
- Researcher subjectivity and bias can be serious problems in the analysis of the information.
- The process of transcribing and analysing data can be time-consuming and costly.
- It may not be easy to generalise the conclusion owing to the small sample size and the non-random sampling technique often used.

> **EXAMPLE 26.1**

Depth interviews to evaluate services for prevention of mother-to-child transmission (PMTCT) of HIV infection in a rural area

As part of an assessment of PMTCT services in a rural area of the Eastern Cape for the purpose of developing tools to deal with the service backlog, fieldworkers conducted a number of qualitative interviews. The sample included nursing and other medical staff at the health services, the pregnant women using the clinics, and their partners and mothers or mothers in law. The interviews were able to identify core problems that the women faced in using these services, for example, distance and transport problems in getting to the clinic, deficiencies in the health services, personal fears of the women and their families in relation to HIV/Aids, and some community and cultural restrictions on accessing the PMTCT services. The fieldworkers established a system of trust and a relationship with the staff in which they made it evident that both fieldworkers and staff were trying to achieve the same goals. As a result, interventions could be identified and later implemented to assist the extension of the PMTCT services in this deep rural and largely inaccessible area.

Reference:
Skinner, D, Mfecane, S, Gumede, T, Henda, N & Davids, A. 2005. Barriers to accessing PMTCT services in a rural area of South Africa. *African Journal of AIDS Research*, 4(2):115–23.

> **EXAMPLE 26.2**

Development of a shared definition of orphaned and vulnerable children

This piece of research was the first part of a large project aimed at developing interventions for orphaned and vulnerable children. A common definition was sought across six communities in Botswana, South Africa and Zimbabwe where the study was to be done, so as to form a common understanding of who the target recipients for the intervention were. The emphasis of the interventions was to draw on community strengths and systems, so it was important that community members participated at this point. Two focus groups were held in each community, representing community-elected and traditional leadership, key professionals and service providers, direct caregivers of orphaned and vulnerable children, and the children themselves. Each of the three countries analysed their own data to produce a country-specific definition. These were combined into a single definition to set out a framework for the rest of the project, which has included depth interviews, focus groups and observational research, survey research, and intervention development, implementation and evaluation.

Reference:

Skinner, D, Tsheko, N, Mtero-Munyati, S, Segwabe, M, Chibatamoto, P, Mfecane, S, Chandiwana, B, Nkomo, N & Tlou, S. 2006. Towards a definition of orphaned and vulnerable children. *AIDS and Behaviour*, 10(6): 619–26.

Useful readings

Glaser, B. 1998. *Doing grounded theory. Issues and discussions*. Mill Valley, CA: The Sociology Press.

Searle, C, Gobo, G, Gubrium, J & Silverman, D. 2004. *Qualitative research practice*. London: Sage.

Silverman, D. 2001. *Interpreting qualitative data: methods for analysing talk, text and interaction*. London: Sage.

Silverman, D. 2005. *Doing qualitative research: a practical handbook*. Thousand Oaks, CA: Sage.

Useful web sites

Forum: Qualitative social research. [Online]. Available: http://www.qualitative-research.net/fqs/fqs-eng.htm. [26 February 2007].

QSR International. [Online]. Available: http://forums.qsrinternational.com/. [26 February 2007].

The Qualitative Report. [Online]. Available: http://www.nova.edu/ssss/QR/web.html. [26 February 2007].

References used in this chapter

Babbie, ER & Mouton, J. 2001. *The practice of social research*. Cape Town: Oxford University Press.

Glaser, B. 1998. *Doing grounded theory. Issues and discussions*. Mill Valley, CA: The Sociology Press.

Miles, MB & Huberman, AM. 1984. *Qualitative data analysis: a sourcebook of new methods*. Beverly Hills: Sage Publications.

Silverman, D. 2001. *Interpreting qualitative data: methods for analysing talk, text and interaction*. London: Sage.

Silverman, D. 2004. *Qualitative research: theory, method and practice*. Thousand Oaks, CA: Sage.

Simbayi, L, Skinner, D, Letlape, L & Zuma, K. 2005. *Workplace policies in public education*. Pretoria: HSRC.

Strauss, AL. 1987. *Qualitative analysis for social scientists*. Cambridge: Cambridge University Press.

Terre Blanche, M & Durrheim, K (eds). 1999. *Research in practice: applied methods for the social sciences*. Cape Town: University of Cape Town Press.

27

Economic evaluation

Susan Cleary   Marianela Castillo-Riquelme

> **OBJECTIVES OF THIS CHAPTER**
>
> The objectives of this chapter are:
> - to define health economics and the place of economic evaluation within the discipline
> - to describe specific techniques for economic evaluation such as cost-effectiveness and cost-utility analyses
> - to introduce methods for measuring costs and outcomes.

Introduction

Health economics is the discipline that studies the allocation of scarce resources among competing health care needs. Because of this scarcity, all societies are faced with decisions about what health care to provide, how much to provide and what not to provide. Within health economics, economic evaluation is a set of techniques that can be used to measure the costs and benefits of alternative health care interventions such as, for example, different ways of treating a particular disease.

While economic evaluation has the potential to assist in resource allocation in a country's health care system, it cannot be of benefit unless detailed studies are actually conducted. For this reason, health care providers (governments, international funding agencies and medical insurance companies) are requiring that results from economic evaluations inform decisions about whether new medical interventions should become health care benefits.

The first part of this chapter reviews basic concepts in economic evaluation including opportunity cost, outcomes, efficiency and equity. After this, we describe the four types of economic evaluation, their key characteristics and methods for calculating costs and benefits. We review how the results of economic evaluations can be interpreted by decision-makers and reflect on limitations of the methods used. Finally we present two studies that have looked at the costs and benefits of different treatment interventions in South Africa.

Basic concepts in economic evaluation

Opportunity cost and economic cost

Opportunity cost is defined as the benefit sacrificed when using resources for one purpose rather than another. For example, if a nurse were recruited to a clinic to perform child immunisations rather than antenatal care, the opportunity cost of her work in immunisations would be the number of antenatal patients she could have seen otherwise. This concept of trading off one course of action against another is the key to understanding economic evaluation. It is not simply about avoiding costs, but rather about getting the most benefit from each resource. A related concept is the economic cost. This should not be confused with prices or patient fees. In a public health system, patient fees are often subsidised and so the fee is lower than the cost, while in private health care the fee would normally be higher than the cost. We therefore define an *economic cost* as the value of the resources used to produce an output such as an outpatient visit.

Outcomes (or effectiveness)

Economic evaluation in health works from the principle that we are prepared to incur costs so that we can get health care benefits. There are many different types of health care benefits – we will use the word *outcomes* to refer to these collectively. For example, the outcome of providing antiretroviral treatment to HIV-positive people as opposed to doing nothing could be measured as its effectiveness in delaying death. This type of outcome would be derived from epidemiological studies. Other outcomes of antiretroviral treatment could be improvements in quality of life and economic production gains. Outcome measurement is one of the most difficult aspects of economic evaluation, but it is crucial to the priority-setting process. Without outcome measurement, we cannot assess whether resources are being channelled into beneficial activities.

Efficiency

In economic evaluation, efficiency is defined as maximising outcomes for a given amount of resources. There are two main types: *allocative* and *technical* efficiency.

Allocative efficiency is about doing the right thing – if we want to maximise health, where should resources be allocated? Should new resources be directed to primary health care (PHC) or to hospital care? Should breast cancer screening receive priority over child immunisations? Assuming resources are allocated to child immunisations, *technical efficiency* assesses how to do it the right way: how can the programme be delivered so as to immunise the most children at least cost?

Equity

Many public health care systems have policies aimed at equity, which reflect recognition that health care should be fairly available to all members of society irrespective of ability to pay. There are two dimensions of equity. *Horizontal equity* is concerned with providing equal access to health care to those with equal needs. *Vertical equity*, on the other hand, is concerned with how people with different health care needs should be treated differently, or unequally. It may result in 'discriminating' in favour of those with greater needs by providing them with more health care.

Equity-efficiency trade-off

While both efficiency and equity are important goals for a health care system, it is sometimes necessary to sacrifice efficiency in order to achieve a fairer distribution of health care benefits. For example, providing primary health care in rural areas could be less efficient than in urban areas because of the need to pay rural allowances to attract clinical staff. This trade-off between equity and efficiency is an important consideration for policy-makers.

Characteristics and types of economic evaluation

In economic evaluation, studies can be conducted from a *societal perspective* (i.e. including costs and outcomes affecting all members of society) or from a *provider perspective*, including costs and outcome that are incurred by the health care provider. Also, while it is possible for a partial economic evaluation to consider a single

E   Multidisciplinary approaches complementary to epidemiology

Table 27.1 Types of economic evaluation and their key characteristics

Type of economic evaluation	Type of outcome	Type of efficiency	Main advantages of the method	Example of study question
Cost-minimisation analysis	Not needed (the same for all options)	Technical efficiency	Simple, does not require measurement of outcomes	What is the lowest cost method of immunising 2 000 children against measles?
Cost-effectiveness analysis	Natural or disease-specific (e.g. reductions in cholesterol levels, infections averted, deaths prevented)	Technical efficiency	Measurement of outcomes may be less biased as natural or disease-specific data often readily available	What is the most efficient approach to reducing malaria infections: indoor residual spraying or mosquito nets?
Cost-utility analysis	Generic (i.e. comparable across a wide variety of interventions)	Allocative efficiency	Can compare different interventions and diseases	Would health gains be maximised by prioritising HIV/Aids treatment or malaria prevention?
Cost-benefit analysis	Money	Allocative efficiency	Because outcomes are in monetary terms, can determine whether the benefits outweigh the costs	Do the monetary benefits of HIV prevention outweigh the costs?

intervention, a full economic evaluation examines the competing costs and outcomes of two or more interventions. For example, a study examining the costs and effects of running a voluntary counselling and testing (VCT) service would be a partial economic evaluation. A full economic evaluation would compare VCT services to other competing strategies for HIV/Aids prevention, such as the treatment of sexually transmitted diseases, in order to see which approach would have the largest impact on HIV prevention within a given budget.

There are four types of economic evaluation: *cost-minimisation analysis, cost-effectiveness analysis, cost-utility analysis*, and *cost-benefit analysis*. The key difference between them is the way that outcomes are measured. In general, the more complex the approach to outcome measurement, the broader the assessment of efficiency becomes. Table 27.1 provides examples of each.

A *cost-minimisation analysis* is the appropriate study design if alternative interventions have the same outcomes and the objective is to find the least costly intervention. This method has limited practical applicability because it is rare for interventions to have the same outcomes.

Cost-effectiveness analysis, probably the most popular form of economic evaluation, uses natural or disease specific outcomes. An advantage of this approach is that there is less bias in the way that outcomes are measured, but a disadvantage is that comparability across interventions for different diseases or health programmes is limited.

Cost-utility analysis transforms disease-specific measures into generic outcomes by combining quality of life and life expectancy into one outcome measure. This allows comparability across different diseases and interventions in the health care sector (see the later section on outcomes for details). The disadvantage is that assumptions and modelling might be required to achieve this transformation.

Cost-benefit analysis goes one step further and converts outcomes into monetary values in order to provide further comparability between health care interventions and other sectors of the economy.

A diagram of the economic evaluation research process is presented in Figure 27.1.

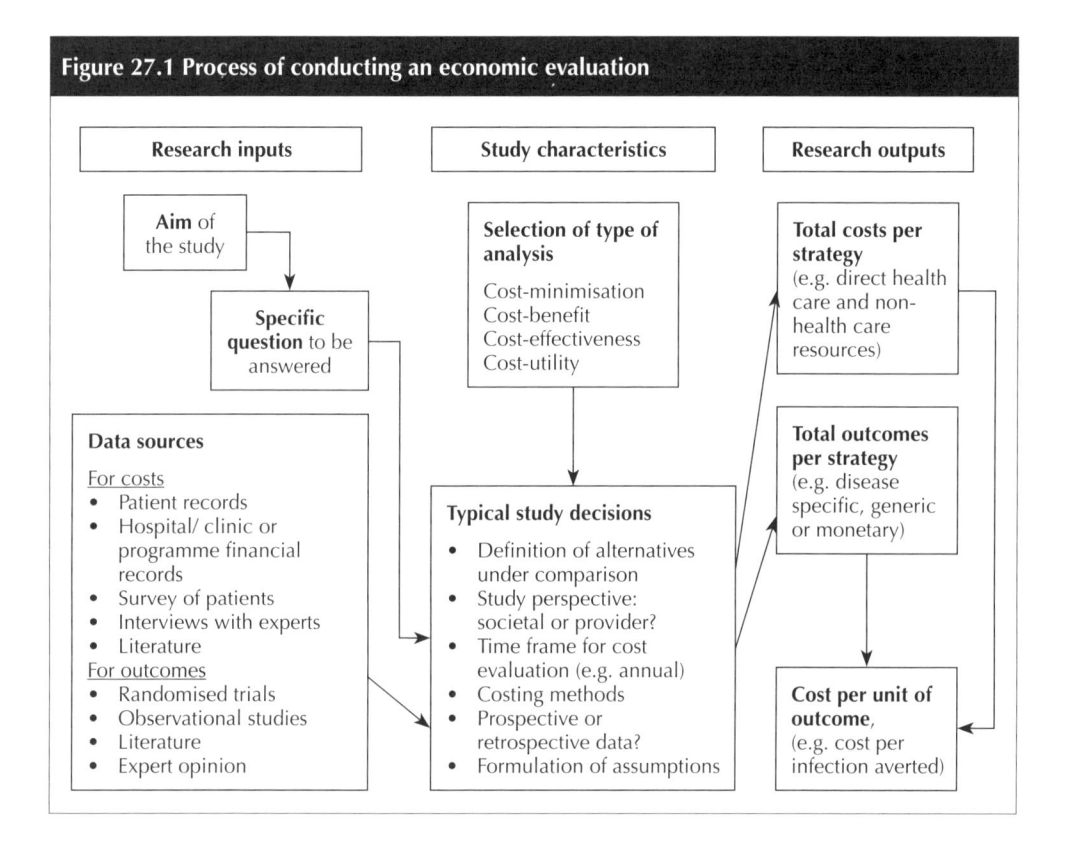

Figure 27.1 Process of conducting an economic evaluation

Research inputs
- Aim of the study
- Specific question to be answered
- Data sources
  - For costs
    - Patient records
    - Hospital/clinic or programme financial records
    - Survey of patients
    - Interviews with experts
    - Literature
  - For outcomes
    - Randomised trials
    - Observational studies
    - Literature
    - Expert opinion

Study characteristics
- Selection of type of analysis
  - Cost-minimisation
  - Cost-benefit
  - Cost-effectiveness
  - Cost-utility
- Typical study decisions
  - Definition of alternatives under comparison
  - Study perspective: societal or provider?
  - Time frame for cost evaluation (e.g. annual)
  - Costing methods
  - Prospective or retrospective data?
  - Formulation of assumptions

Research outputs
- Total costs per strategy (e.g. direct health care and non-health care resources)
- Total outcomes per strategy (e.g. disease specific, generic or monetary)
- Cost per unit of outcome, (e.g. cost per infection averted)

Scope of costs and outcomes

Figure 27.2 presents the scope of costs and outcomes that could be associated with an intervention. Outcome A – improving health status and/or delaying mortality – is normally derived from epidemiological studies. An intervention might also create non-health benefits such as *production gains or losses* associated with improved or impaired ability to work (B). For certain interventions, there could be a variety of intangible elements that occur during the process of receiving care (C). For example, fearing the outcome of an HIV-test might imply *process disutility* (e.g. severe anxiety) but confirmation of negative HIV-status might bring *process utility* (e.g. relief from anxiety), despite there being no impact on health status.

Direct costs can be defined as the value of goods, services, and other resources consumed in providing or accessing an intervention. These are depicted in Figure 27.2 as D to G. The delivery of treatment consumes health care resources including medicines, laboratory investigations and health professional time (D). Non-health care resources include the patient's transport costs to and from the health facility (E). In addition, a considerable burden of care, with associated costs, might be placed on the households of an ill person (F). Finally, the time costs of the patient might be considered, including travelling time, waiting time and time receiving treatment at a health facility or in hospital (G).

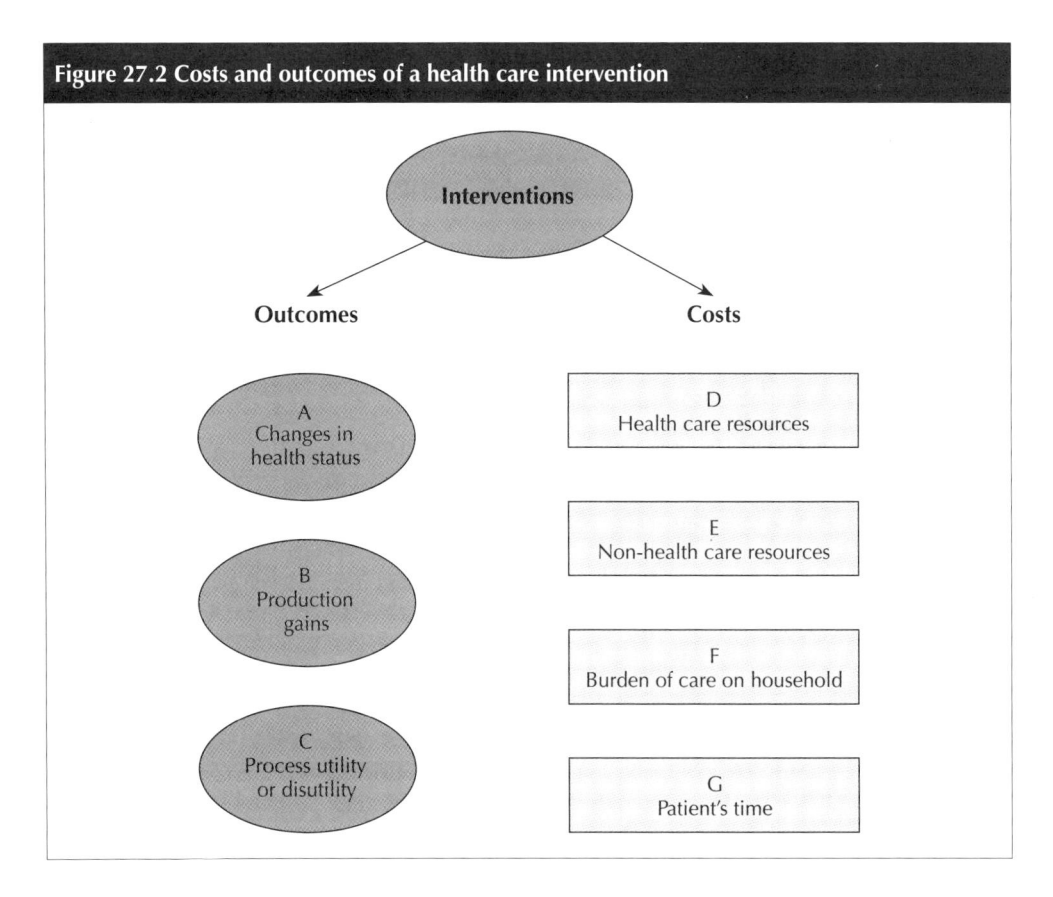

Figure 27.2 Costs and outcomes of a health care intervention

Interventions
→ Outcomes
→ Costs

Outcomes:
- A: Changes in health status
- B: Production gains
- C: Process utility or disutility

Costs:
- D: Health care resources
- E: Non-health care resources
- F: Burden of care on household
- G: Patient's time

Measuring costs

When calculating the costs of health care services it is common to relate these to a unit of output, such as a visit to a community health centre or a day in hospital. These costs per unit of output are termed *unit costs*, and include all relevant *recurrent* and *capital* costs. Recurrent costs are staff salaries, medicines and laboratory investigations. Capital costs include resources whose lifespan is greater than one year, such as equipment, furniture and buildings.

Capital costs are calculated by establishing the replacement value of each item, estimating the approximate working life of the item and using this information to estimate an annual cost. In this way, a share of the value of the capital item can be included in the unit cost.

There are two basic methods of allocating resource use to units of output: the *ingredients approach* (also called micro-costing) and the *step-down method* (gross costing). The former involves identifying the ingredients involved in delivering a service – such as medicines, laboratory investigations, and imaging. Step-down methods, on the other hand, can be used to allocate shared resources that are not directly linked to patient use, including most capital costs and certain recurrent costs such as water, electricity and non-clinical staff such as cleaners. There are many ways of allocating shared costs using step-down methods. The key is to use a method that makes sense in the setting – for example, cleaning costs might be allocated to hospital wards on the basis of the percentage of hospital space occupied by the ward, and then equally to all patients in the ward.

An example of recurrent and capital costs is provided in Table 27.2. The unit cost per visit has been calculated by dividing annual costs by annual visits, using step-down allocation.

Once unit costs have been calculated, these should be linked to the utilisation of services by patients. For example, if the research objective were to calculate the cost per patient completing tuberculosis (TB) treatment, we would need to calculate the quantities of different services used by tuberculosis patients (such as health facility visits for diagnosis and for treatment observation). The total cost per tuberculosis case treated would then be calculated by multiplying the use of these services by the relevant unit cost.

Table 27.2 Example of unit costs for an outpatient clinic

Inputs	Annual cost (Rand)
Capital	
Vehicles	10 000
Equipment	14 000
Building	30 000
Staff training	1 000
Subtotal	**55 000**
Recurrent	
Personnel	150 000
Medicines	50 000
Overheads	45 000
Subtotal	**245 000**
Total	**300 000**
Outputs	**Annual visits**
	5 000
Unit cost per visit	**60**

If a societal or patient perspective has been taken, it is also necessary to quantify non-health care resource costs (such as transport and waiting time). These data are often collected during patient exit interviews. Interested readers are referred to 'Useful readings' at the end of this chapter for additional information on calculating costs.

Measuring outcomes

In *cost-effectiveness analysis*, intermediate outcomes are used such as 'cases cured', and 'children immunised'. *Final* outcomes, such as life years gained, can also be used. These can be derived from a parallel epidemiological study or from secondary data.

Another type of outcome is found in *cost-benefit analysis* where intermediate, final or generic outcomes are transformed into monetary terms. This can be done by assessing the economic production gains that can be achieved through health improvements or by asking members of the public how much they would be willing to pay for these improvements.

QALYs and DALYs

In *cost-utility analysis*, outcomes are measured as *Quality Adjusted Life Years* (QALYs) or *Disability Adjusted Life Years* (DALYs). In essence, these try to put mortality and morbidity on the same measuring rod in order to provide a broader measure of health gain and to allow comparison across different healthcare interventions.

QALYs consist of years of life-expectancy adjusted by a *'health related quality of life'* (HRQoL) factor. One year of life in perfect health would be equivalent to one QALY, while a year in less than perfect health would be less than one QALY.

In contrast, DALYs consist of years of life lost added to years of life lived with disability – a DALY is therefore a 'negative' (see Chapter 15 for more on the DALY). Desired outcomes would thus be QALYs gained in contrast to DALYs averted.

While the life-expectancy component of the QALY (or DALY) might be derived from epidemiological studies, HRQoL (or disability) is measured by administering a questionnaire to patients receiving the intervention. The questionnaire is designed to capture different aspects of health such as functional, physical and emotional status. Once measurement has been completed, health states are *valued* against one another. Although QALYs or DALYs have gained popularity as measure of outcome, there are many unresolved issues including how valuation should be done and whose values should be used.

Decision-making 'rules'

This section describes how the results of economic evaluation can be interpreted. Under what conditions would interventions be implemented and when would they not? In cost-minimisation analysis, the least costly intervention should be implemented. In cost-benefit analysis, implementation would be recommended if benefits (in monetary terms) were higher than costs. Decision rules for cost-effectiveness and cost-utility analyses are more complicated.

First, one calculates results in terms of an *incremental cost-effectiveness* or *utility ratio* (ICER), as follows:

$$\text{ICER} = \frac{(TC_1 - TC_2)}{(O_1 - O_2)}$$

where:

TC_1 = total costs of new intervention
TC_2 = total costs of comparator (e.g. existing intervention/status quo/doing nothing)

O_1 = total outcomes of new intervention

O_2 = total outcomes of comparator

The ICER gives an indication of the increased (decreased) cost required, and the increased (decreased) outcomes that could be obtained from implementing a new intervention versus a comparator. To assist interpretation, the ICER can be plotted on a cost-effectiveness or utility plane with four quadrants (Figure 27.3). The comparator is plotted at the origin, which means that the horizontal axis is the difference in outcomes between the interventions (e.g. QALYs gained or additional children immunised) while the vertical axis shows the difference in total costs.

If the ICER falls in quadrants II or IV, then decision rules are straightforward. For II, the new intervention has better outcomes and lower costs and should be implemented. In the case of IV, the new intervention has higher costs and lower outcomes, and should not be implemented. If the ICER falls in quadrants I or III, a trade-off is required. In the case of III, the new intervention is less costly, but also has lower outcomes, and the decision-maker will have to trade off cost savings against reduced outcomes. In the case of I, the new treatment is both more costly and has higher outcomes. Now the decision-maker would need to decide whether the additional costs are worth the additional outcomes. To operationalise this trade-off, some countries have created a *maximum acceptable ICER* (represented by the dotted line in Figure 27.3). For example, if R50 000 were the maximum value assigned by a decision-maker to a QALY, then any intervention with an ICER greater than R50 000 per QALY (to the left of the dotted line in quadrant I) would not be accepted. Equity and feasibility would also be taken into account when making a final decision.

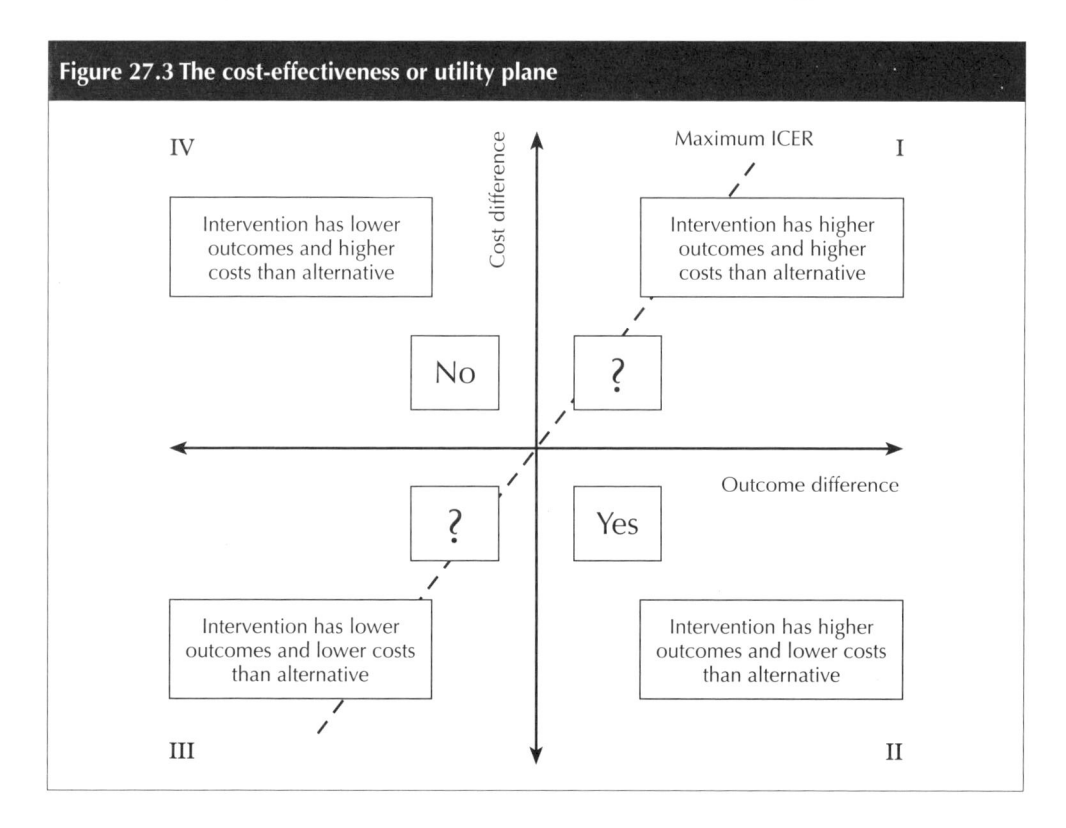

Figure 27.3 The cost-effectiveness or utility plane

IV — Intervention has lower outcomes and higher costs than alternative

I — Intervention has higher outcomes and higher costs than alternative — Maximum ICER

No | ?

? | Yes

III — Intervention has lower outcomes and lower costs than alternative

II — Intervention has higher outcomes and lower costs than alternative

Cost difference (vertical axis); Outcome difference (horizontal axis)

Other issues in economic evaluation and potential limitations

Dealing with uncertainty

Many of the estimates used in economic evaluation are uncertain and context-dependent. For example, where cost-effectiveness estimates are derived from a large randomised controlled trial in a hospital, these would not necessarily be applicable to general practice. *Sensitivity analysis* is a powerful technique that varies one or more of the input values or assumptions in order to see whether the results are sensitive to such changes.

Discounting

Frequently, costs and outcomes in an economic evaluation are *discounted*. The logic of this practice is grounded in the principle of *time preference*, which states that people prefer to postpone payments but to receive benefits as soon as possible. For example, paying R1 000 today is less preferable than paying R1 000 in two years' time, even after inflation adjustments. In economic evaluation, this time preference is applied to both costs and benefits – such that any costs and outcomes that happen in the future are reduced by a discount rate. A rate of 3% is often used in published studies.

Limitations of economic evaluation

There are various limitations which might restrict the use of economic evaluation techniques, especially in developing countries. Economic evaluation is resource and researcher intensive. Epidemiological studies are expensive to conduct and the research capacity is scarce; for example, there are few health economists available. Poor recording and lack of information systems mean that routine health service data are either unavailable or inaccurate. In addition, because local peer-reviewed publications are scarce, secondary data are unavailable. Rapidly changing medical technology means that studies are applicable only to the context (time and place) in which they were conducted. For example, the cost-effectiveness of rapid diagnostic testing for malaria will depend on the prevalence of malaria and local prices for the test.

Other limitations include methodological controversies about measuring and valuing costs and outcomes. Inaccuracy in these measures can jeopardise the validity, acceptability and comparability of results. Finally, the potential contribution of economic evaluation to policy decisions is constrained by the capacity of policy-makers to understand and accept these methods, which can prove difficult to follow given the technicalities involved.

Despite these limitations, economic evaluation offers objective methods for gathering information on the costs and outcomes of health care interventions. Decisions about what and how much health care to provide are frequently based on 'gut feelings' and political expediency. Often we continue to provide interventions because a decision has been taken in the past, even though the intervention has become relatively inefficient. Economic evaluations are becoming more widespread, accepted and even demanded among the main stakeholders in health care, including the pharmaceutical industry, ministries of health, international donors and healthcare providers.

Examples of studies linking economic evaluation and epidemiology are provided below.

EXAMPLE 27.1

Cost-effectiveness of starting antiretroviral treatment at different points in HIV-infection

In South Africa, HIV-positive adults qualify for antiretroviral treatment (ART) if they have an Aids diagnosis or a CD4 lymphocyte (CD4) count lower than 200 cells/µl. Evidence suggests that it may be more effective to start therapy earlier, although there may be additional cost implications.

This study examined the cost-effectiveness of starting highly active antiretroviral therapy in three CD4 categories: >350 cells/µl, 200-350 cells/µl or <200 cells/µl. ART strategies were also compared against the treatment of and prophylaxis for opportunistic and HIV-related infections in the absence of ART. Intermediate outcomes (e.g. increases or decreases in CD4 count) and final outcomes (deaths) were derived from a previous study of a cohort of HIV positive patients not receiving ART and from a clinical trial of ART. These data were extrapolated where necessary to calculate life-expectancy. Secondary HRQoL data were used to calculate QALYs.

The study took a provider perspective. Unit costs included all health care resources, categorised into inpatient care, outpatient visits and antiretroviral drugs. The utilisation of these units by patients at different stages of illness and CD4 count categories informed the calculation of lifetime costs. Results included estimates of life-expectancy, QALYs and lifetime costs.

The lowest ICER was obtained for initiating highly active antiretroviral therapy with CD4 < 200 cells/µl. Earlier initiation was more effective but more costly. Policy-makers would thus need to choose whether the better outcomes of earlier therapy were worth the additional costs, taking into account the constraints of limited resources and the need to provide equitable access to such treatment.

Reference:

Badri, M, Cleary, S, Maartens, G, Pitt, J, Bekker, L-G, Orrell, C & Wood, R. 2006. When to initiate HAART in sub-Saharan Africa? A South African cost-effectiveness study. *Antiviral Therapy*, 11:63–72.

EXAMPLE 27.2

Cost-effectiveness of cervical cancer screening in developing countries

Screening has been a priority intervention in the prevention of cervical cancer. However, the conventional cytology method with multiple visits to the facility has proved impractical in developing countries. In this study different cervical cancer screening strategies were evaluated in six developing countries (including South Africa). Computer-based models were used to simulate the natural history of human papilloma virus (HPV)-induced cervical neoplasia ('pre-cancer' cells) under 25 different screening strategies. The strategies were formulated as a combination of (a) number of clinic visits per screening: 1, 2 or 3; (b) frequency of screening: 1, 2 or 3 times per lifetime; (c) age groups targeted; and (d) type of screening test used. Screening tests evaluated were visual inspection of the cervix, cytologic examination of cervical cells and DNA testing for HPV in cervical cells.

Lifetime costs were calculated for each approach. Outcomes were defined as lifetime reduction of the risk of invasive cervical cancer with associated years of life saved. Costing included direct medical costs (staff, supplies, equipment and specimen transport), patient time costs (travelling and getting care), transport costs and costs specific to each screening strategy. Results were expressed as cost per year of life saved.

The results suggested a reduction in lifetime risk of invasive cervical cancer between 25% and 36% per country. In all countries the most *effective* strategy was 'screening at one clinic visit, using HPV DNA testing, at 3 intervals per lifetime (at 35, 40 and 45 years of age)'. The most cost-effective strategy (except for South Africa) was 'screening at one clinic visit, using visual inspection at one point in the lifetime (at 35 years of age)'. The cost per year of life saved ranged from $10 (in India) to $134 (in Kenya). In South Africa, the most cost-effective strategy was HPV DNA testing with same-day treatment at a cost of $467 per year of life saved. This was because the costs of the three different methods of diagnosis were fairly similar in South Africa, with the consequence that the most accurate screening method (HPV DNA) was the most cost-effective.

Reference:

Goldie, S, Gaffikin, L, Goldahaber-Fiebert, J, Goedillo-Tobar, A, Levin, C, Mahé, C & Wright, T. 2005. Cost-effectiveness of cervical-cancer screening in developing countries. *New England Journal of Medicine*, 353(20):2158–68.

Useful readings

Creese, A & Parker, D (eds). 1994. *Cost analysis in primary health care: a training manual for programme managers*. Geneva: World Health Organization.

Drummond, MF, O'Brien, B, Stoddart, GL & Torrance, G (eds). 1997. *Methods for the economic evaluation of health care programs vol 2*. Oxford: Oxford University Press.

Useful web sites

British Medical Journal series. *Economic notes*. [Online]. Available: http://bmj.bmjjournals.com/series/. [26 February 2007].

World Health Organization: WHO-CHOICE. *Choosing interventions that are cost effective*. [Online]. Available: http://www.who.int/choice/en/. [26 February 2007].

Appendix I: Standardisation (adjustment) of rates

Gina Joubert

If one needs to compare morbidity or mortality rates of two or more populations, a variable (for example, age or sex) which is related to the outcome of interest can distort the comparison if the populations differ with respect to the distribution of that variable. One therefore needs to standardise or adjust rates before they can be compared. This appendix outlines standardisation with respect to age distribution – a similar approach would be used to standardise for sex or for age and sex. Standardisation is also dealt with in Chapter 15, as it is often used in mortality studies.

Standardisation can be direct or indirect, depending on the type of information that is available for the populations (see Table A1.1).

To perform *direct age-standardisation*, the researcher needs age-specific rates for each population, as well as a standard or reference age distribution. A step by step example is provided in Table A1.2. For each population the standardised rate is calculated by (a) multiplying each age-specific rate by the number of persons in that age category in the standard population, (b) adding these numbers, and (c) dividing by the number of people in the standard population. (The same results can be derived by multiplying each age-specific rate by the *proportion* of the standard population which falls into that age category, and then adding these weighted age-specific rates.) Directly standardised rates are therefore obtained by mathematical manipulation of category-specific rates (in this case age-specific rates). These standardised rates are *hypothetical* summary rates for purposes of comparison.

The researcher can choose as standard distribution the age distribution of either of the populations of interest, their joint distribution, or some other standard such as the World Standard (Ahmad *et al*, 2001). As standardised rates depend on which standard is chosen, various standards can lead to varying conclusions.

Researchers often pay too little attention to the informative category-specific rates by focusing only on the standardised rates. No single summary rate can reflect the richness of category-specific rates, but if there are many categories it may be difficult to make useful deductions based just on category-specific rates.

Indirect age standardisation is used when age-specific rates are not available for one or more of the populations of interest. For this standardisation method, the researcher uses the crude number of cases in each of the populations (the 'observed' number), the age distribution of each of the populations, and the age-specific rates of a standard population (which could be one of the populations being compared, if the information is available). See Table A1.2 for a step-by-step example. By (a) multiplying each age-specific rate of the standard population by the number of people in the matching age category of the population of interest and then (b) adding these, one obtains the 'expected' number of cases in that population. By (c) dividing the observed by the expected number of cases, a *standardised morbidity (or mortality) ratio* (SMR) can be calculated for the population.

The various standardised rates for the data provided in Table A1.2 are summarised in Table A1.3.

A word of caution about indirect standardisation: we use the category distribution (in our example, age distribution) of each population to calculate each population's expected number of cases. The distributions may differ vastly, and this method has therefore also been called the 'changing base' method. When one compares SMRs, one is actually comparing measures based on differing standards. By contrast, direct standardisation (or the 'fixed base' method) involves the comparison of measures based on the same standard, and therefore represents the essence of standardisation.

It can be seen from Table A1.3 that the value of a relative index depends on the method used to calculate it. While the direction of the relationship will remain the same, the magnitude depends on what population was selected as standard. It is crucial to report details of the standard population and the method of standardisation when reporting standardised rates.

Standardisation can also be used if the researcher has done a study on a sample in which the proportion of the *sample* in each stratum (for example age category) does not correspond to the proportion of the target population in

339

each stratum (that is, one does not have a proportional stratified sample). For example, strata of equal size may be included in a sample (say, 100 subjects in each age and sex category) where this distribution does not reflect the population composition. Crude (unadjusted) prevalences or rates found in such samples could be very distorted because of the unrepresentative age distribution. One has to adjust the stratum-specific rates to obtain the overall rate in the population. Table A1.4 provides an example.

Table A1.1 Information needed for age standardisation

Direct standardisation	age-specific rates of each population of interest
	age distribution of a standard population
Indirect standardisation	total number of cases (deaths or illness) in each population of interest
	age distribution of each population of interest
	age-specific rates of a standard population

Table A1.2 Age standardisation to compare mortality rates in two populations

Population A

Age category (years)	Population size	Proportion of population in age group	Number of deaths in age group	Mortality rate (per 1 000)
< 25	18 000	0.45	90	5
25 to 49	10 000	0.25	50	5
50 to 69	6 000	0.15	210	35
70+	6 000	0.15	270	45
Total	40 000	1.00	620	15.5

Population B

Age category (years)	Population size	Proportion of population in age group	Number of deaths in age group	Mortality rate (per 1 000)
< 25	5 000	0.25	5	1
25 to 49	5 000	0.25	10	2
50 to 69	5 000	0.25	150	30
70	5 000	0.25	200	40
Total	20 000	1.00	365	18.25

The crude mortality rate in Population A is 620/40 000 = 15.5 per 1 000, and in Population B 365/20 000 = 18.25 per 1 000. However, the age-specific mortality rates are consistently higher in Population A than in Population B. From the population figures it is clear that Population A is a much 'younger' population than Population B. Younger people tend to have lower mortality rates than older people.

To remove the effect of the difference in age-distribution from the comparison of the mortality rates, we can directly age-standardise the rates. We can use the *joint* age distribution of the two populations as our standard population by adding together the numbers in each age category.

Population A plus population B

Age category (years)	Population size (A + B)	Proportion of population in age group
< 25	23 000	0.383
25 to 49	15 000	0.25
50 to 69	11 000	0.183
70+	11 000	0.183
Total	60 000	1.000

The directly age-standardised rate (per 1 000), using the above proportions, for Population A is: $(0.383 \times 5) + (0.25 \times 5) + (0.183 \times 35) + (0.183 \times 45) = 17.8$ per 1 000.

This can also be calculated, using numbers rather than proportions, as $[(23\,000 \times 5) + (15\,000 \times 5) + (11\,000 \times 35) + (11\,000 \times 45)]/60\,000 = 17.8$ per 1 000.

The directly age-standardised rate (per 1 000) for Population B is $(0.383 \times 1) + (0.25 \times 2) + (0.183 \times 30) + (0.183 \times 40) = 13.7$ per 1 000.

The *comparative mortality factor* (CMF) is the ratio of the 'directly' standardised rate of the one population divided by that of the other population. The CMF when comparing group A to Group B is 132% (17.8/13.7). The CMF could be reported as an index around 1; in this case it would be 1.30.

To illustrate *indirect standardisation*, let us assume that in Population A we know only how many deaths there were in total (620), but that we do *not* know how many occurred in each age category. We do, however, have the age distribution of Population A. For Population B let us assume we have all the information as provided above. We can therefore use Population B as our standard population, applying its age-specific mortality rates to the age distribution of Population A. The standardised mortality ratio for Population A is calculated as follows:

Expected number of deaths: $(1/1\,000 \times 18\,000) + (2/1\,000 \times 10\,000) + (30/1\,000 \times 6\,000) + (40/1\,000 \times 6\,000) = 18 + 20 + 180 + 240 = 458$.

Observed number of deaths = 620.

SMR = observed / expected = 620/458 = 1.35

In Population B the SMR = 1, since the expected number of deaths using the group's own category-specific mortality rates would equal its observed number of deaths. The reference SMR is frequently expressed as 100, in which case Population A's SMR would be expressed as 135.

Table A1.3 Comparison of crude and standardised mortality rates

	Crude mortality rate (per 1 000)	Directly standardised mortality rate* (per 1 000)	Comparative mortality factor* (CMF)	Indirectly standardised mortality rate (SMR)
Population A	15.5	17.8	130	135
Population B	18.25	13.7	100	100

*Using the pooled population as standard age distribution.

Table A1.4 Age-adjusting a sample to the population age structure

In a study to determine the prevalence of diabetes mellitus, hypertension and related factors in inhabitants of QwaQwa, Free State province, the aim was to select randomly 100 respondents in each sex and age group below (Mollentze, 2003). The resulting sample was much older than the population of QwaQwa as indicated by the *proportions* in each age group by sex below.

	Sample proportions		Population proportions	
Age (years)	Males	Females	Males	Females
25–34	0.20	0.25	0.36	0.33
35–44	0.24	0.19	0.25	0.22
45–54	0.10	0.17	0.16	0.14
55–64	0.16	0.18	0.10	0.15
65+	0.30	0.21	0.13	0.16

The crude female prevalence of diabetes mellitus overall was 6.7%. The age-specific prevalences of diabetes mellitus in females were:

Age (years)	Prevalence
25–34	0.7%
35–44	3.7%
45–54	7.1%
55–64	14.0%
65+	9.9%

Using the population weights for females and the age-specific prevalences, the age-adjusted prevalence is $(0.7 \times 0.33) + (3.7 \times 0.22) + (7.1 \times 0.14) + (14 \times 0.15) + (9.9 \times 0.16) = 5.7\%$, i.e. lower than the crude rate.

References used in this appendix

Ahmad, OB, Boschi-Pinto, C, Lopez, AD, Murray, CJL, Lozano, R & Inoue, M. 2001. Age standardization of rates: a new WHO standard. *GPE discussion paper series, no 31*. Geneva: EIP/GPE/EBD WHO. [Online]. Available: http://www3.who.int/whosis/discussion_papers/pdf/paper31.pdf. [11 April 2007].

Mollentze, WF. 2003. *Diabetes mellitus, hypertension and related factors in black subjects residing in QwaQwa and Bloemfontein*. Unpublished PhD thesis. Bloemfontein: University of the Free State.

Appendix II: Random number table

Source: Fleiss et al (2003)

08939	53632	41345	65379	20165	32576	13967	90616	17995	92422
92578	23668	08801	39792	59541	99117	58830	60923	36068	68101
83994	91054	90377	22776	23263	34593	98191	77811	83144	98563
43080	71414	40760	01831	44145	48387	93018	22618	98547	87716
39372	46789	26381	37186	85684	79426	05395	17538	56671	82181
83046	58644	04452	98912	53406	30224	00687	32099	86414	29590
99808	32539	96961	88917	60847	64826	41332	64557	15354	11111
28478	70870	68912	75644	33648	21097	23745	52593	01849	37760
09916	19651	28659	95093	12626	19919	05879	56003	83100	94572
19537	66067	20569	28808	87722	67059	12851	73573	25776	92500
23013	05574	26320	07754	09642	88068	41626	57139	68199	94938
55838	80585	80967	60540	34528	62310	63106	17843	39104	74036
92279	87344	93556	75233	09394	79265	91047	32891	77925	71530
27850	23332	89336	26026	52130	78544	02090	05645	15060	39550
01760	54605	11794	79312	69728	04554	99775	57959	47981	68954
81889	70751	87501	88247	41966	57574	67745	88304	20118	25964
74722	14654	15425	60665	25162	04987	03467	75915	24282	62456
56196	75068	44643	92240	51651	79743	13598	63901	61020	91003
96842	62021	00543	45073	65545	87612	35765	26079	34589	72821
25619	98328	59393	71401	93871	20611	78830	87477	15390	05044
91746	05084	04781	82933	54564	80986	94843	40178	87483	63288
92384	84706	76778	98313	98875	08427	60687	88272	83448	06237
86390	62208	95735	14535	25591	22730	06059	31786	36181	31016
60458	83606	57510	92609	38061	94881	26736	06489	98303	31419
03783	39922	05489	73630	92379	91602	18193	84741	44704	05558
31011	36035	37113	98362	56149	51634	04468	62096	32361	35301
20555	05621	48728	41776	12101	96615	70781	55151	93876	66892
56466	36766	12400	43510	49456	05140	85736	68155	37306	10438
26875	67304	61950	65962	38223	35676	70043	99178	64677	95457
90648	84770	92791	93814	27760	22232	83545	01183	55188	20482
26197	72840	01264	52019	00739	36259	10905	39097	36437	66743
72522	34445	53975	13840	97262	59007	78685	41044	38103	59216
12370	41270	36290	46307	51230	90614	82613	80148	37371	02895
81028	60112	31415	47478	02131	85480	93699	92876	13958	47867
61573	38634	77650	18189	10283	97999	95442	90657	84963	93863
98511	46300	91199	30492	62159	98525	31710	03540	35844	83200
76606	10834	75548	55779	54744	26450	66001	57949	53685	00567
20237	16311	15733	47599	43998	35594	17577	85113	52487	48900
21022	86025	26951	87480	82317	06580	98627	32536	07573	52612
47512	11564	41777	46581	03492	01722	78900	57901	37307	02727
80598	59041	28861	41793	91007	69907	00376	73086	35132	53014
01892	34226	88327	21926	36607	22307	04376	25491	13563	51955
89657	70349	15176	57916	10911	44218	67108	04678	24097	02476

Reference used in this appendix

Fleiss, JL, Levin, B & Paik, MC. 2003. *Statistical methods for rates and proportions*. 3rd ed. Hoboken, NJ: John Wiley & Sons, Inc.

Appendix III: Writing a report

Rodney Ehrlich

Research should be written up as soon as possible after project completion. In research involving human subjects or their records, it should be considered an ethical requirement to provide a written communication, whether it be to stakeholders, funders or members of the peer scientific community. Even a study which had flaws in its methods should be written up so that other researchers can learn from the researcher's experiences. Depending on whether one is writing up the research as a dissertation, a journal article or a report for a funding agency, one needs to make sure one knows what the requirements of the institution, journal or agency are. Some general principles are outlined below.

Principles of writing up research

1. *Define the readership and their requirements.* In the case of dissertations, one's readers are one's small group of examiners. In the case of journals, one needs to consider whether the journal has a general readership of health professionals or a readership more narrowly focused on disciplinary or methodological questions.
2. *Try to be as concise as possible and observe any word limit set.* Excessive length is a more frequent problem than excessive brevity. Writing everything one needs to say within a word limit is an art which comes with practice.
3. *Allow enough time.* Write-ups are frequently done under pressure of time, for example to hand in a dissertation, or complete a report before a contract comes to an end. Steps in the write-up that are particularly at risk of being compromised by time pressure are writing the Discussion, cutting the length to meet word limits, careful proofreading, and achieving the required layout.
4. *Strive for a coherent, logical narrative.* Research write-ups are not chronicles of everything that was done or happened. Rather, while remaining honest to the data, one needs to decide on what one wants to convey. The more focused the research protocol, with a limited number of primary objectives, the easier it will be to write up the results. With the addition of the Results and Discussion sections, the protocol should form the basis of the report write-up.
5. *The objectives are the hub of the write-up.* These determine every aspect of the research: what the problem statement is, what literature one reviews, what methods one uses, which results one presents and what one discusses. Every aspect of the write-up should be tested against its relevance to the objectives. If it is not relevant to the objectives, it should be omitted.
6. *Use appropriate scholarly language.* One should use clear and direct language that is suitable for the readership. For example, one should avoid emotional language and exclamation marks.

Table A3.1 provides a guide in summary form to each of the components of a research write-up. These follow the logic of the protocol (see Chapter 4).

Table A3.1 Steps in a write-up: tips and pitfalls

Step	Tips and pitfalls
Title	This should be informative but also designed to catch the attention of readers, particularly in journals.
Acknowledgements	These should cover everyone who contributed to the study, including those granting permission for access, funders, and research staff not listed as authors.
Declaration	Dissertation rules may require a statement that it is one's own work. Journals increasingly require statements regarding conflict of interest and funding.
Abstract	This should be a brief structured summary: for example, background, objectives, study design, population/setting, methods, results, conclusions.

Problem background/ Introduction	A write-up should not start with a detailed literature review. The Introduction should rather explain why the study was done, for example, the size or urgency of the health problem, the gap in knowledge, or a specific opportunity that arose for research. It should progress from the general to the particular and should lead logically to the objectives of the study. The Introduction could also include a description of the structure of the thesis or the argument to be proposed.
Objectives or hypotheses	These should be expressed in as precise and measurable terms as possible. Sometimes they are divided into primary and subsidiary objectives. (Subsidiary objectives should not merely be a list of the stages of the study, but should be able to stand on their own as answering some question.) Objectives could be expressed as hypotheses.
Literature review (for dissertations)	The literature should be precisely guided by the objectives. Reviews are usually of what is known about the question being posed, but may also be directed to methodological questions. They should be based on relevant, recent information from reputable sources. The review should be critical rather than merely being a summary, that is, it should attempt to evaluate the quality of other studies and of the evidence as a whole. (See Chapter 6 on systematic reviews.)
Methods	These should provide details of the setting of the study, study design, the population and sampling strategy, sample size calculation, measurement instruments used and their known validity or attempts to validate them. Pilot study activities and particularly how these contributed to quality improvement should be reported here. Ethical issues should be stated here with a description of formal ethics approval and permission granted for access to study subjects. Statistical analyses conducted should be outlined – one must ensure that one has used the correct statistical methods for the data.
Results (including Tables and Figures)	This section should always start with the response rate. The tables and figures should follow logically, for example, from baseline characteristics through bivariate comparisons to multivariate modelling. Each objective should be clearly covered. The text should not simply repeat the contents of tables and figures but rather direct the reader to the main findings and point out important, interesting or surprising results. Good tables take a long time to get right and a lot of thought should go into their presentation. Tables and figures need logical numbering, explanatory titles, and footnotes explaining abbreviations.
Discussion	This section should start with a summary of the main or surprising findings. This should be followed by an honest appraisal of the limitations of the study method, including sample size constraints, measurement error and possible biases. The implications of each limitation for the study findings should be examined and a conclusion drawn as to whether the findings are still likely to be valid. The study findings should then be related to the literature – their concordance with other studies and possible reasons for discordance. Conclusions can be drawn about the ability to generalise (depending on how particular the study circumstances were) and implications for knowledge and or action. (A negative or inconclusive study should be stated as such.) If appropriate, recommendations can be made for future action or research.
References	All those genuinely used and cited should be included in dissertations. Journals may set limits on the number allowed.
Appendices	In dissertations it is common practice to include the questionnaire or data capture instrument as well as consent form. Highly technical descriptions in an article designed for a non-technical readership, for example of a laboratory assay, could be placed here.

Appendix IV: Sample size calculation

Abdul-Rauf Sayed

Before a sample is drawn it is essential to know how many individuals will be needed for a study. Calculating the correct sample size is important because a sample that is too large may waste time and limited resources. On the other hand, a sample that is too small may lead to inconclusive or imprecise results. A result is inconclusive if the sample size of the study is too small to declare an observed effect statistically significant. A result is imprecise if the small sample size results in wide confidence limits for the population characteristic being estimated. The statistical methods appropriate for sample size calculation will depend on the research question, the study design and the types of outcome measures, specifically whether they involve categorical or numerical data. Furthermore, the formulae also differ depending on whether one is interested in *estimation* or *hypothesis testing* (see Chapter 11).

The following quantities have to be specified when calculating a sample size for estimating a single proportion with a specified precision, as in a survey. (This section should be read with Chapter 11.) This is an example of estimation.

a) *The anticipated population proportion* (p), for example the expected prevalence of the disease in the population to be surveyed. This estimate has to be based on a prior idea of what one will find, for example, from the literature or a pilot study.
b) *The confidence interval.* One has to choose the level of confidence at which one wants to state that the true population proportion is within certain specified limits. The commonly used confidence level is 95%.
c) *The acceptable margin of error* on either side of the proportion, that is, the desired precision, denoted by d. Precision is a measure of the uncertainty associated with a single measurement arising from random error (see Chapters 11 and 12). The required precision will determine the width of the confidence interval. What is 'acceptable' or 'desirable' depends on the use to which one will put the results.

The following quantities have to be specified when calculating a sample size for testing a difference between two population parameters (for example, incidences or means). This is an example of hypothesis testing.

a) *Level of significance*: The level of significance (denoted by α) is the probability of rejecting the null hypothesis when it is assumed to be true (Type I error). Conventionally, one sets α at 0.05, meaning that there are about 5 chances in 100 of rejecting a true hypothesis.
b) *Power of the test*, denoted by $(1-\beta)$: The probability of correctly rejecting the null hypothesis when it is false (1 - Type II error). Conventionally, one sets the power at 80%, the probability that a test will produce a significant difference at a given significance level if there is in fact a difference.
c) *The anticipated outcomes in the group(s)*, for example incidence in each group or the mean and standard deviation in each group. Note again that one needs these estimates *before* doing the calculation.

If, when comparing group means or incidences, one is interested in estimation, one should also specify:

- *The size of the effect or the magnitude of the difference to be detected.* This 'difference worth finding' should be decided on clinical or public health grounds. For example, in a case-control study, if the size of the increased risk to be detected is specified as two-fold (odds ratio = 2) the sample size would need to be much larger than to detect a four-fold risk (odds ratio = 4).

Other important factors that must be taken into consideration before calculating sample sizes are the following:

- If one is estimating more than one outcome, one should calculate the sample size for the rarest outcome, or the outcome with the smallest mean. A larger sample size is needed to detect small differences or a low prevalence, for example.
- The calculated sample size should be large enough to allow for non-response or loss to follow-up.
- Simple random sampling is assumed in sample size calculations. In cluster sampling a larger sample size is required because of

the 'design effect', an indication of the variation owing to clustering. The design effect is the ratio of the variance when cluster sampling is used to the variance when simple random sampling is used.
- Sample size is often limited by budget and time restrictions. However, one needs to estimate the *power* of the study (see above) under various assumptions and decide between what is desirable and what is logistically feasible.
- In a case-control study, if the number of cases is limited, the precision of the study can be improved by increasing the number of controls per case.

Detailed discussions of optimal sample size calculations for clustered and other epidemiological study designs can be found in Kirkwood & Sterne (2003) and Lemeshow et al (1990).

Some examples of calculation of sample size by different methods are given below.

Example 1: Calculating sample size manually, focusing on hypothesis testing

The sample size formula for a two-sample test of equality of means with significance level $\alpha = 0.05$ and 80% power is:

$$n = \frac{(\sigma_1^2 + \sigma_2^2)(1.96 + 0.84)^2}{(\mu_1 - \mu_2)^2}$$

where the anticipated mean and variance (variance = standard deviation squared) of the two samples are μ_1, σ_1^2 and μ_2, σ_2^2 respectively, 1.96 is the cut-off value of the Normal distribution (see Chapter 11) and n represents the sample size in each group. So if the expected means are 15 and 18 and the variances 25 and 26 respectively, n in each group will be 44.

Example 2: Determining sample size from a published table

The minimum sample size for estimating a population proportion when assuming random sampling from a large population can be calculated using the following formula:

$$n = \frac{p(1-p)z^2}{d^2}$$

where p is the anticipated population proportion, d is the precision required on either side of the proportion, and z refers to the cutoff value of the Normal distribution (= 1.96). Table A4.1 shows the required sample sizes for varying proportions and precision levels derived from the formula above.

Example 3: Calculating sample size using a software programme

Several statistical software packages compute sample size. *Epi Info* is a downloadable public domain software programme designed to provide for easy database construction, data entry and analysis. It includes sample size calculations for categorical data.

EpiCalc 2000 is a public domain statistical calculator that analyses tabulated data from

Table A4.1 Sample size required for different levels of precision and anticipated proportion

Precision (d)	Anticipated proportion (p)				
	0.10	0.20	0.30	0.40	0.50
0.01	3 457	6 147	8 067	9 220	9 604
0.02	864	1 537	2 017	2 305	2 401
0.03	384	683	896	1024	1 067
0.04	216	384	504	576	600
0.05	138	246	323	369	384
0.1	35	61	81	92	96

public health or epidemiological contexts and includes sample size calculations for studies with categorical and numerical response measures. The program can be downloaded from the web site.

For example, a cross-sectional study may be used to investigate whether two groups have different proportions of a disease. Assuming the anticipated population proportions are 30% in the exposed group and 20% in the non-exposed group, the *EpiCalc 2000* screen below (Figure A4.1) shows that the required sample size with significance level $\alpha = 0.05$ and 80% power is 292 in each group.

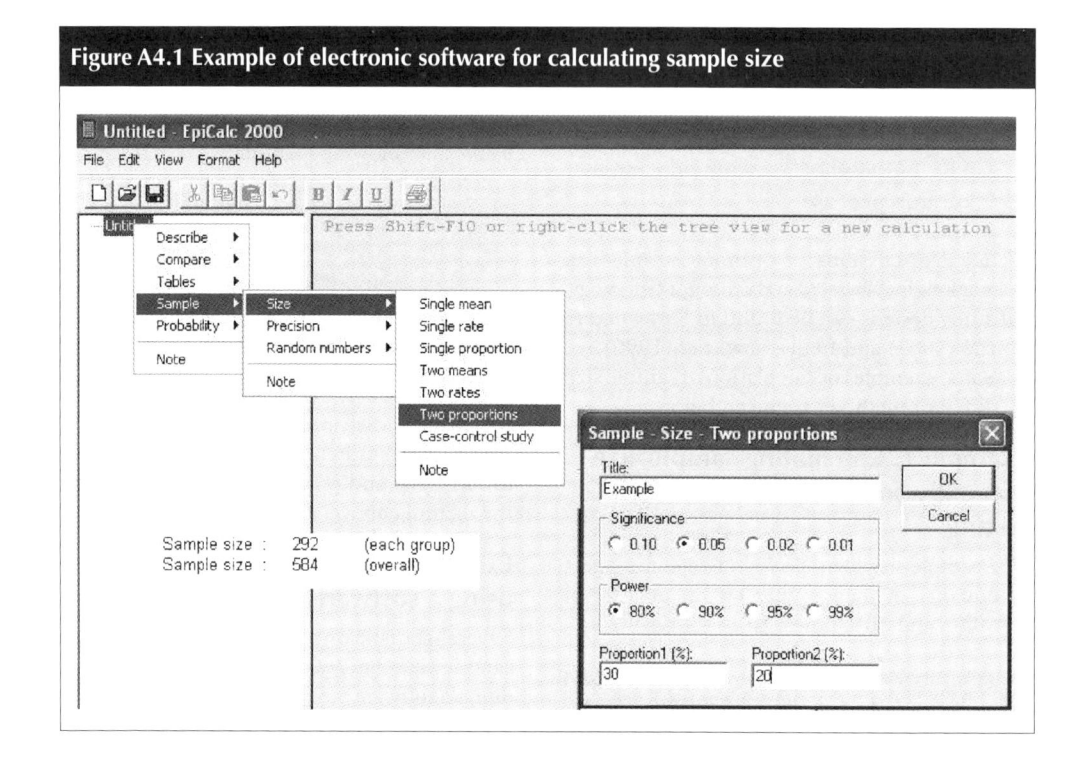

Figure A4.1 Example of electronic software for calculating sample size

Useful readings

Kirkwood, BR & Sterne, JAC. 2003. *Essential medical statistics*. 2nd ed. Oxford: Blackwell Science.

Lemeshow, S, Hosmer, DW, Klar, J & Lwanga, S. 1990. *Adequacy of sample size in health studies*. New York: Wiley. [Published on behalf of the World Health Organization.]

Useful web sites

EpiCalc 2000. [Online]. Available: http://www.brixtonhealth.com/epicalc.html. [26 February 2007].

Epi Info. [Online]. Available: http://www.cdc.gov/epiinfo/. [26 February 2007].

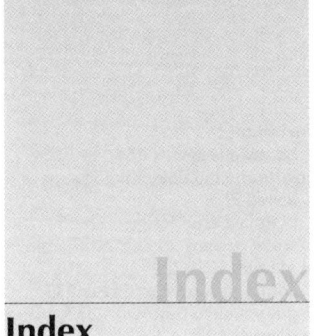

Index

Page numbers in bold refer to figures and tables.

A

acute lower respiratory infections 257–258
Adequate Intake (AI) 298
adolescents 198, 283–284, 290
advocacy 36–37
agent of disease 222
age standardisation 201–202, **340**
age-specific fertility rate 27
Aids, *see* HIV, HIV/Aids
alcohol
  abuse 256
  dependence 86
allocative efficiency 329
Alma Ata Declaration 307
analogy in causation 16
analysis, choosing appropriate 147–154
analytical epidemiology 6
analytical study, objective of 62
  designs 78–88
Annecke, Siegfried 7
antiretroviral treatment (ART) 41, 175, 337
applied epidemiology 2
applied research 3
arithmetic mean 137
attributable risk in the exposed 150
autonomy (respect for persons) 32

B

bar graph **135**
basic reproductive number 223, 224
basic research 3
before-after studies 92
Belmont Report 31–32, 34
beneficence (ethics) 32–33
betablocker therapy 73, **73**
bias 16, 52–54, 160–163, 315
Bill of Rights 36
Binomial distribution 143
bioethics 30–31
biological plausibility 16
biological sciences 5
biomedical ethics 31–34
biostatistics 126–127
birth data (sources) 175
Birth to Twenty study 257
bivariate (scatter) plot 133–134, **134, 153**
blinding/masking of participants 89–90, 164

block chart **136**
blood lead levels **256**, 256–257
body composition 300–301
body mass index (BMI) 299–300, **300, 301**
box plot 131–133, **133**
bull's-eye diagrams 117–118
burden of disease 200–201, 208–209

C

CAGE Questionnaire 86
CANSA 50
cancer 8, 163, 254, 261, 302, 337–338
  breast 163
  of cervix 78, 168, **206, 207**
capacity 35
  context of 274
  development 40–41
  informed consent 35
capital costs 332
cardiovascular disease 18
case
  definition 231–232
  primary and secondary 233
  reports 225, 254–255
case-control studies 79, 161, 164, 226, 257, 313
  calculations **84**
  design **82**
  example 84
  limitations 85
  matching 83–84
  random measurement error **159**
  selection 83
  strengths 84–85
case-detection (incidence) rate 180, 182
categorical variables 135, 136, 158
causal relationships 15–16, 263
causation 12–16
  biochemical marker 15
  genetic marker 15
  infectious diseases 222
  levels 15
  modified triangle/triad 222
causes
  immediate 203
  notion of 13
  underlying 203
  'upstream' versus 'downstream' 15
census data 24, 25
Census Enumerator Areas (EAs) 190
Centers for Disease Control (CDC) 177, 299
Centre for Epidemiological Research in Southern Africa (CERSA) 9
cervical cancer 8, 78, 168, 206, 337–338
chi-squared (χ^2) test 147
cholera **176**, 229
chronic diseases 29, 182, 272
  social networks 218–219
circulatory diseases 207

circumcision, male 247–249
  high-risk groups **248**
  and HIV **249**
clinical disease phase 17
clinical epidemiology 310
closed questions 110
cluster randomised trials 91, 92, 312–313
cluster random sampling 98–99
Cochrane Collaboration **69**
coding of data 113, **115**, 324
coefficient of variation (CV) 138
coherence (causal relationships) 16
cohort studies 79, 150, 161, **162**, 168, 206, 226, 257, 313
  calculations 80
  design of 80
  example 80–81
  limitations 82
  prospective 81
  retrospective (historical) 81
  strengths 81
  types 81
Commission on Health Research for Development 5
communicable disease, *see* infectious disease
community
  access to 190
  assessment 39
  education 40
  materials development 40
  orientated primary care 8
  participation 37–39, **40**
  randomised intervention trial 89
  South African model 39–41
  surveys 188–189
Community Advisory Board (CAB) 39
comparative mortality factor (CMF) 202
component causes 13, 14, **14**
condoms 247
confidence intervals 144–145
confidentiality 35–36
confounding bias 165–167, **165, 166**
consecutive sampling 100–101
consistency (causal relationships) 16
CONSORT initiative 141
content
  analysis 324
  validity 120
continuous variables 158
control(s)
  best friend 83
  group 82
  hospital 83
  measures 179, 239
  neighbourhood 83
coronary artery disease 14, **14**
correlation 142, 151–153
  coefficient 151, **152**
correlational study 87
cost-benefit analysis 331, 334
cost-effectiveness
  analysis 330, 334
  or utility plane **335**

349

Index

cost-minimisation analysis 330
cost-utility analysis 331
Council for International Organisations of Medical Sciences (CIOMS) 34, 37
Cox proportional hazard regression model 315
criterion-related validity 120
  sensitivity and specificity **121**
critical thinking 56
cross-classification 113
cross-sectional studies 79, 161, 225, 255–257
  calculations **86**
  design 85–86, **86**
  example 86
  limitations 87
  strengths 87
crude birth and death rates 27
crude (overall) rate 23
cumulative incidence 22
cumulative nature of science 67
cytological screening (Pap smears) 206

D

data
  analysis 113–114, 129, **324**
  capture sheet **114**
  checking 127–129
  management and analysis 50
  methods of collection 108
  missing 117, 182
  quality of 116
  routine collection systems **185**
  routinely available **173–174**
  types of distribution **131**
data collection 53, 117, 120–122, 195
  methods 108, 319–323
death data (sources) 175
Declaration of Helsinki 34
deductive methods 3
demographic indicators **28**
demographic process 27
demographic transition 29
demography 24–29
denominator 21, 22, 182
Department of Health 9, 36, 78, 183
depth interviews 319–320, 326
descriptive epidemiology 6
descriptive (narrative) synthesis 72
descriptive studies 62, 225, 313
descriptive v analytical studies 78
developmental stage 283–284
diabetes 13–14, 256, 302
diagnosis, studies of 314–315
diagnostic/detection bias 163
diarrhoea 206–207, 219, 252
  outbreak 238
  population pyramid 232
diet
  history 297
  information 298
dietary assessment techniques 295–297
  validity and reliability 297

dietary intake 297, 298
Dietary Reference Intakes (DRIs) **298**
dietary survey methods **294–295**
diphtheria 176, 183
direct age standardisation 339
direct costs 331–332
directly observed therapy (DOT) 91
disability 272, 279–280
  activity limitations 274
  data analysis 277
  functioning **278**
  measurement of 273–275
  national baseline survey 278, 279
  participation restrictions 274–275
  prevalence 277–278
  surveys of prevalence 276–277
disability adjusted life years (DALYs) 205, 281, 334
Disability Assessment Schedule (WHO-DAS II) 277–278
disclosure (informed consent) 35
discounting (costs and outcomes) 336
disease
  consequences and treatment 17
  identification 254
  natural history of 17–18, 178
  outcome of 17
  surveillance 176–182, **177**
distribution-free methods 147
District Health Information System (DHIS) 175
DNA fingerprinting 235
dogma, received 72
dose response 15–16, 263
drug abuse 256
DTP vaccination 179
dummy (mock) tables 50
  demographic characteristics **50**

E

Ebola virus 223
ecological studies 87, 226, 255, 313
  data from **88**
  limitations 88
  strengths 87–88
economic cost 328–329
economic evaluation
  basic concepts 328–329
  characteristics and types 329–331, **330**
  costs and outcomes 331–334
  decision-making 'rules' 334–335
  evaluation and limitations 336–338
  limitations 336
  process of conducting **331**
  uncertainty 336
effect modification 167–168
effectiveness
  economic evaluation 329
  health service 308–309
efficiency
  economic evaluation 329
  health service 309
endemic disease 223, 226, 229

environment
  hazardous agents 253
environmental epidemiology 251–252
  planning and design 252–257
  study designs 254–257
epidemics 178, 229
  common source outbreak **233**
  point source outbreak **233**
epidemiological transition 29
epidemiological triangle/triad **222**
epidemiology
  analyses commonly used 148–149
  definition 6
  ethics guidelines 34–35
  notion of 'cause' 13
  prevention 17–18
  in South Africa 7–10
  terminology 229–230
equity–efficiency trade-off 329
equity of health service 309, 329
error 142, 155
essential national health research (ENHR) 6
Estimated Average Requirements (EAR) 298
estimates **143**, **145**
estimation 147
ethical considerations 52
ethics 30–31, 120–121
  guidelines 34–35
ethnicity 217–218
ethnographic research 322
Expanded Programme on Immunisation (EPI) 179, 183–184, 237
experimental epidemiology 6
experimental evidence 16
experimental studies 88–93
exploratory data analysis 129–138
exposure 79, 151
  analysis 253
  to asbestos 261–262
  assessment 253–254, 266–267
  to contaminants 251
  hazardous 254
  smoke 257
  sulphur fire 252
exposure-response relationships 263
extraneous factor (confounder) 151

F

face validity 120
Falsificationists 3
fatal injuries (surveillance) 186
fat distribution 302
fertility rates 27
field supervision 122, 195–196
fieldwork
  planning 193–194
  report 196
fieldworkers 193–194
final outcomes 334
Fisher's exact test (chi-squared (χ^2) test) 147, 148
focus group interviews 320–321

350

Index

follow-up
  loss of 161, **162**
  study 79
food
  diary 296–297
  intake 298
  poisoning 240
food frequency questionnaires (FFQs) 295, **296**

G

Gay Related Immunodeficiency Disease (GRID) 242
Gear, James 8
general fertility rate 27
geographic distribution of illness 178
Geographic Information Systems (GIS) 235
geographic variations 205–206
Gluckman, Henry 8
graphical display 130–135, 139, **152**
  for confounding bias 165
  honesty in **139**
gross costing 332
growth charts 300

H

haemangiosarcoma of liver 262
Haemophilus influenzae 176, 183
haphazard/convenience sampling 100
Harvard v Vancouver citations 74
hazard and risk 315
hazardous environmental agents 253
health
  economics 310
  indicators 184–185
  information system 172–175
  practices 179
  resource inequalities 9
  workers 39, 160
Health Act (1977) 175
health care intervention **332**
'Health for All' strategies 8, 9
Health Metric Network (HMN) 172
health services
  evaluating projects 311
  evaluating quality 308–309
  epidemiological studies 311–313
  examples 306–308
  observational studies 313–315
  questions 308
  research methods 310–311
Health Systems Trust 50
healthy worker
  selection effect 264, **265**
  survivor effect 264–265, **265**
  time since hire effect 264, 265, **266**
heart disease 302
hepatitis B virus (HBV) **176**, 183, 223, 225
Hill, Bradford 15, 16
Hippocratic Oath 33
histogram (graphical display) 133

HIV 78, 92, 242–245
  blood transfusions
  co-infection 182
  epidemic **245**
  infection 6–7, 168
  prevalence **181**
  prevention 246
  risk factors 245–246
  seroprevalence 223
  transmission 243–244
  vaccine trial **40**
HIV/Aids 5, 28, 29, 177, 223, 242
  denialists 10
  education 92–93
  information systems 175
  mortality rate 203
  orphans 289
  prevention 330
HIV Prevention Trials Network (HPTN) 39
horizontal equity 329
horizontal integration 308
hormone replacement therapy (HRT) 163
hospital
  controls 83
  data 175
host (infectious disease) 222
households 24, 189, 190, 192–193, 256
humanity 309
human papilloma virus (HPV) 168
human rights
  abuses 36
  advocates 37
Human Sciences Research Council (HSRC) 5, 36
hypertension 9, 256, 302
hypothesis 179, 235–237
  research 62
  testing 145–146, 237–238

I

immunisation 9
  see also vaccination
impairment of body function 274
incidence 78, 160, 245
  infectious disease 223
  and prevalence **20**, 23, **23**
  rate 22
  tuberculosis 180
incident cases 19, 79
inconsistent validity 120
incremental cost-effectiveness ratio (ICER) 334–335
incubation period 225, 233
indirect age standardisation 339
inductive methods 3
infant mortality rate (IMR) 21, 202, 207, 255
  water sources **255**
infectious agents 179
infectious diseases 14, 221–222
  occurrence and transmission 223–224
  study designs 225–227
  surveillance 223

infertility 302
influenza epidemic 7
information
  bias 163–165
  case-control study **164**
  overload 67
  routine health systems 185–186
informed consent 35
ingredients approach 332–333
Initial National Burden of Disease Study 208
injury surveillance 183
Inquests Act (1959) 183
Institute of Family and Community Health 8
instrument variation 119
interaction (variables) 168
intermediate outcomes 334
International Classification of Diseases (ICD-10) 203
International Classification of Functioning, Disability and Health (ICF) 273–275
International Ethical Guidelines for Biomedical Research Involving Human Subjects 34
International Guidelines for Ethical Review of Epidemiological Studies 34–35
inter-observer variation 119
interquartile range 132, 138
intervention
  behaviour change 257
  health services 311–313
  studies 18, 88–89, 257–258, 263–264
  see also experimental studies
interviewers 122, 194–195
  training 276–277
interviews 319–321
intra-cluster correlation 313
intra-observer variation 119
ischaemic heart disease 14

J

Jali, Amelia 7
Jali, Edward 7
job-exposure matrix 267, **268**
justice (ethics) 33

K

KABP surveys 188–189
Kappa statistic **120**
Kark, Emily 7
Kark, Sidney 7, 8
Khomanani Campaign 190, 196–197
  intergenerational sex **197**

L

language 283
  collecting data 284
  in mental state 283
latent period (infectiousness) 225
lead time bias 315
leading question 109
legal considerations (informed consent) 52

351

Legionnaire's disease 240
length time bias 315
life expectancy 28
Lind, James 2
Lister, F Spencer 7
literature reviews 66–68
　traditional **68**
　writing up 74–76
loaded question 109
logistics 49–50, 193–194
Lognormal distribution 143
lung
　cancer and smoking 15
　function changes 269–270
　health 316
　predicted function **269**

M

McLaren, Margie 9
malaria 7, 222
management sciences 5
map of houses **96**
Maputo Conference 9
masking, *see* blinding
matched case-controlled pairs 84
mean differences 91
measles 183, 227
　immunity **224**
　vaccine **179, 226**
measurement
　costs 332–334
　error 117–119, 157–159, 163–164
　instruments 106
　outcomes 334
　scale of 127
　sciences 5
measures
　of aassociation 148–150
　central location 137–138
　variability (spread) 138
median 131
media relations 40
mediation 167–168
mediators/intermediate variables 168
Medical Officer of Health (MOH) 4
Medical Research Council (MRC) 10, 36, 256
MEDLINE 70, 71
meningococcal disease cases **176, 180,** 226
mental disorders 281–282
　see also psychiatric disorders
mental health
　matrix **288**
　services research 287–288
mesothelioma 261
meta-analysis 72–73
methodology 49
　qualitative research 318–327
micro-costing 332
migration 28–29, 246
mines/mining 7, 251
　coalmining 269
　goldmining 263

misclassification
　differential 163–168
　non-differential 158–160
mode 137–138
mortality 27–28, 200
　age- and sex-specific 201
　age-specific **201**
　age standardisation **340**
　crude and standardised rates **341**
　premature 208
　rates 201–205
multiple linear regression 154
multiple logistic regression 154
multivariate analysis 153–154
musculoskeletal disorders 270
Mycobacterium tuberculosis 13, 213, 221

N

National Antenatal HIV and Syphilis Seroprevalence Survey 78
National Cancer Registry (NCR) 78, 183
National Committee for the Confidential Enquiry into Maternal Deaths 183
National Health Act (2003) 36, 175
National Health Research Ethics Council (NHREC) 36
National Health Service Commission 8
National Injury Mortality Surveillance System (NIMSS) 183
National Institute for Communicable Diseases (NICD) 175–176, 235
National Library of Medicine (NLM) 70
National Medical and Dental Association 9
necessary cause 13–14
neighbourhood controls 83
Nightingale, Florence 2
non-communicable diseases 13–14, 18
non-governmental organisations (NGOs) 5, 39
non-maleficence (ethics) 32–33
non-parametric method 142–143
non-random sampling 100–101
non-responses 276–277
Normal (Gaussian) distribution 142, **144**
notifiable diseases 176, 178, 230
　in South Africa **176, 178**
notification
　HIV infection 223
　maternal death 183
　pesticide poisoning 186
　statutory system 175
number needed to treat (NNT) 91
numerator 21, 22
numerical variables 130–134, 136
Nuremberg Code 31
nutrient intake 298

nutritional status 8
　adults 300
　anthropometric evaluation 299
　children 299
　dietary assessments 293–297
　nutrition survey 7, 293–294

O

obesity 13, 302–303
objectives of research 55–63
　death rate of children 63
　implementation 63
　safe sex 64
observational studies
　health care 313–314
　race 218
　versus experimental studies 77
observations, listing of **129**
observer variation 119
occupational epidemiology 260–262
　exposure assessment **267**
　methodological issues **262**
　outcomes and study designs 267–268
occupational hazards 9, 261–264
odds
　of exposure 150
　prevalence ratio 150
　ratio 82, 142, 150, 160
open-ended questions 109–110
operations research 310–311
opportunity cost 328–329
OPV vaccination 179
organisational research 310
outbreaks of disease 229
　common source **233**
　investigation **230,** 230–239
　person to person **234**
　point source **233**
　propagated 234
　questionnaires **237**
outcomes 79, 267–268, 329
　associated study designs 268
outliers 234

P

parameter 142
parametric versus non-parametric methods 147
partial correlation coefficient 152
participant observation 321–322
Pearson correlation coefficient 152
peer review 3
performance 274
pesticides 254
phthisis 7
philosophical approach (qualitative research) 319
philosophy of science 3
PICO method 69–70
pilot study 50
placebo 89
plagiarism 74
　rules for avoiding **74**
Plasmodium falciparum 222
pneumococcal vaccine 7

Pneumocystis carinii 230
pneumonia 7, 8, 252
Poisson distribution 143
policy analysis 310
poliomyelitis 8, **179**, 183
pollution 252, **253**
Popper, Karl 3
population
   age structure **342**
   attributable proportion 150–151
   composition 25
   estimates 143
   five-year age group by sex **25–26**
   level 15
   pyramids 25
   sample 143
   under-five mortality rate 28
postal questionnaire 107
potential years of life lost (PYLL) 204–205
poverty and health 212–213, 222
precision 155, 157–160
   and validity **156**
preclinical/pre-symptomatic phase 17
predictive factors 12
predictive validity 120
predictive values 314
prevalence 23, 78, 160
   data surveillance 181
   differences 86
   of disease 85
   infectious disease 223
   odds ratio 150
   ratio 86, 150
prevalent cases 19–20, **20**
prevention
   levels of 16–17, **19**, 307
   of disease 264
Prevention of Mother-to-Child Transmission (PMTCT) 175, 322
primary health care (PHC) 307, 329
   approach 307–308
   facility data 175
   Pholela 7–8
primary prevention 18, 307
   versus secondary prevention 20
Primary Sampling Units (PSUs) 190
primordial prevention 18, 307
probability
   distribution 142
process
   disutility 331
   utility 331
problem
   analysis diagrams 58, 59
   exploration process 60, 61–62
   research 55–56
production gains or losses 331
prognosis 315
prophylaxis 9
proportion 20–23
   precision and anticipated **347**
proportional hazards model 154

Proportional Mortality Ratio (PMR) 204
proportional stratified sampling 98
prospective method 294
protocol, *see* study protocol
provider perspective 329–330
psychiatric disorders 283–287
psychiatric epidemiology 281–282
   disability-adjusted life years **282**
   ethnographic approach 283
   instruments 284–290
   instruments for adults **286**
   measurement challenges 282–287
   validity and reliability 284–285
   validity of instruments **285**
public health 4
   ethics 31, 34–35
   principles of ethics **34**
   professionals 5
   research 5–6
   scope of 4
   seven-step framework 34
PubMed® 71–72
purposive sampling 101

Q

qualitative data analysis 324
qualitative research 310, 318–327
   advantages and disadvantages 325–326
   analysis of data 323–325
   methodological issues 323–326
   methods 325
Quality Adjusted Life Years (QALYs) 334, 335
quality control 195–196
quartiles (sample values) 132
quasi-experimental study designs 92–93
questionnaires 107, 195
   identification information 112
   layout and design 112
   piloting/pre-testing 116
   steps in development 107, 109–116
   technology 113, 115
   visual presentation 112
questions 109–110
   organisation and structure 110–111
   sequence 111
quota sampling 100

R

race as variable 216–218, **218**
random allocation sequence 89
randomisation 89
randomised controlled trial (RCT) 89–92, 227
   calculations **91**
   design **90**
   two-arm individual 89
random measurement error 157–158, **159**
random number
   grid **192**
   table **343**

random sampling 89, 95
   error 157
range (variability) 138
rate(s) 20–23, 79
   comparison of 23–24
   components of 21, **21**
   crude and specific 23
   difference 150
   key **21–22**
   ratio 150, 160
ratios 20–23
recall bias 163, **164**, 262
Recommended Dietary Allowance (RDA) 298
records, review of 106–107
recurrent costs 332
reference level 151
regression 142, 153
relative risk 150, 227
reliability
   inter-rater 285
   measurement 117, 119
   and validity **118**
   versus validity 155–156
reporting of results 52, 344–345
research 3, 46
   access to 67
   country-specific 5–6
   ethics 10
   global 5–6
   process **46**
   proposal, *see* study protocol
   regulation 36
   team 46–47
   voluntary nature 35
   write-up **344–345**
researcher, emotional state of 53, **53**
research ethics committees (RECs) 36
research participants, protection of 40
resources 50–51
respect for persons 32
respondents 117
   purposive choice 189
   random choice 189
response rate 102, **345**
retrospective method 294
review questions 69–70
Revised National Essential Data Set for Primary Health Care **184**
rheumatic heart disease 9
rickettsial diseases 8
right to privacy 36
risk 79, 91
   differences 79, 91, 149
   factors 12, 14, 17, 78
   ratios 79, 91, 160
rubella 183, 225

S

sample 94–95, 339
   data 135–138
   design effect 103
   electronic software **348**
   estimates 103
   size 102–103, 149, 346–348

Index

sampling 190–191, 276, 323
  bias 101–102, 160
  error 142
  example 104–105
  frame 95
  multi-stage stratified design 190
scatter plot **152**
Schools of Public Health 9
science, cumulative nature of **67**
screening programmes 17, 314–315
search strategy in PubMed® 71
secondary care 307
secondary prevention 18, 307
selection bias 53, 83, 89, 160
  information bias and confounding **168**
self-administered questionnaire 107
sensitivity analysis 158, 314, 336
sentinel surveillance 183
serogroup patterns 180
service need survey **279**
Severe Acute Respiratory Syndrome (SARS) 225
sexual behaviours **167**
  safe sex interventions 64
sexually transmitted infection (STI) 92, 246, 320
significance testing 145–146
silicosis 7, 168
simple linear regression 153
simple random sampling 96–97, **97**, 98
skinfold thickness 300–301
  measurement **301**
Snow, John 2
snowballing/networking 101
social capital 216
social desirability bias 163
social epidemiology 210–111
  terminology **210**
social networks 214–215, 218–219
social sciences 5
societal perspective 329–330
socioeconomic status 213–214
  schematic representation **212**
source population 82
South African Demographic and Health Survey 10, 86, 190, 212
socioeconomic position **215**
South African Institute for Medical Research 7
South African Medical Journal 8
South African Medical Research Council (MRC) 5, 9, 50, 189
Spearman rank correlation coefficient 152
specificity 16, 158, 314
specific rates 23
split-sample measurements 159
stakeholders 47
standard
  deviation 138
  error 142
standardisation 24, 201–204, 339–342
standardised morbidity/mortality ratio (SMR) 339

standardised mortality rates (SMR) 201–202
standardised questionnaires 109
statistical significance **149**
statistical techniques 72
statistical versus clinical significance 146–147
statistics 142
stem and leaf plot 130–131, **132**
step-down method 332–333
stillbirths **178**
stratification 151
stratified analysis 166
stratified and cluster sampling **99**
stratified random sampling 97–98
STROBE initiative 141
structured interviews 107
study
  2 x 2 table **79**
  design 77, **78**
  eligibility 70
  hypothesis 62
  population and respondent 189–190
  purpose statements 60–62
  synthesising findings 72–73
  target population 94
study protocol 47–48
  contents 48–52
  major headings **49**, 49–52
  purposes 48
subject variation 119
sufficient cause 13–14
summary statistics 138
surveillance systems 182–185, 264
survival analysis 315
susceptibility phase 17
syphilis survey 78
systematic random sampling 100
systematic rveview 68–69, **69**, 75–76

T

targeted sampling 101
technical efficiency 329
technology in workplace 261–262
teenage pregnancy rate **59**
temporality 15
tertiary care 307
tertiary prevention 18, 307
test-retest studies 159
tetanus 183
time
  preference 336
  series analysis 207
  since hire effect **266**
Tolerable Upper Intake Level (UL) 298
total fertility rate 27
training 122, 325
translation 122
transmission of disease 223–224
trends
  interpretation of 181
  over time 206–207
triangulation method 325
t-tests 142, 147

tuberculosis (TB) 7, 9, 13, **14**, 58, 91, 182, 223
  care and control 317
  care and health system **307**
  defaulter rate among patients 58
  drug resistance **308**
  incidence rate **180**
  monitoring 177
  and poverty 212–213, **213**
  register system 175
tuberculous meningitis 179
24-hour recall 296
typhoid 234

U

UNICEF 5, 8
unadjusted association among women **166**
uncertainty 336
understanding (informed consent) 35
unit costs of outpatient clinic 332, **333**
unstructured interviews 107
urbanisation 7, 28–29
utility ratio 334–335

V

vaccination 4
  coverage **179**
  measles 226
  percutaneous BCG 179, **179**
  see also immunisation
validity 155, 313
  criterion-related 121
  of measurement 117, 118, 120
  of studies 72
  of study results 160–168
variables 106, 107, 127
  analysis 147
  scale of measurement 112
  types of **127**
variation, sources of **157**
vector (infection) 222
Verificationists 3
vertical equity 329
vertical integration 308
visiting points 191–192
Voluntary Counselling and Testing (VCT) 175, 330
voluntary nature of informed consent 35
volunteer
  bias 160, 315
  sampling 101

W

Washington Group on Disability Statistics 277
'why' game 56–57, **57**
World Health Organization 5, 8, 9, 34, 176, 307

Y

years lived with a disability (YLD) 205